Assessing and Managing the Acutely Ill Adult Surgical Patient

Edited by

Fiona J McArthur-Rouse *MSc, BSc (Hons), Cert Ed, RGN,*
Principal Lecturer, Department of Adult Nursing Studies,
Canterbury Christ Church University

Sylvia Prosser *PhD, MSc, BEd (Hons), formerly Principal*
Lecturer, Department of Adult Nursing Studies, Canterbury
Christ Church University

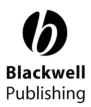

Blackwell
Publishing

Editorial offices:
Blackwell Publishing Ltd, 9600 Garsington Road, Oxford OX4 2DQ, UK
    Tel: +44 (0) 1865 776868
Blackwell Publishing Inc., 350 Main Street, Malden, MA 02148-5020, USA
    Tel: +1 781 388 8250
Blackwell Science Asia Pty Ltd, 550 Swanston Street, Carlton, Victoria 3053, Australia
    Tel: +61 (0)3 8359 1011

First published 2007

ISBN 9781405133050

Library of Congress Cataloging-in-Publication Data

Assessing and managing the acutely ill adult surgical patient / edited by Fiona J. McArthur-Rouse, Sylvia Prosser.
        p. ; cm.
    Includes bibliographical references and index.
    ISBN-13: 978-1-4051-3305-0 (pbk. : alk. paper)
    ISBN-10: 1-4051-3305-8 (pbk. : alk. paper)
    1. Surgical emergencies.   2. Preoperative care.   3. Postoperative care.
  4. Surgical nursing.   I. McArthur-Rouse, Fiona J.   II. Prosser, Sylvia.
    [DNLM: 1. Perioperative Care – Nurses' Instruction.
    2. Acute Disease – therapy – Nurses' Instruction.
  3. Adult.   4. Nursing Assessment – Nurses' Instruction.
  5. Surgical Procedures, Operative – Nurses' Instruction. WO 178 A846 2007]
  RD93.A85 2007
  617′.919—dc22

                                                2006101283

A catalogue record for this title is available from the British Library

Set in 9.5/11.5pt Palatino
by Graphicraft Limited, Hong Kong
Printed and bound in Singapore
by Markono Print Media Pte Ltd

The publisher's policy is to use permanent paper from mills that operate a sustainable forestry policy,
and which has been manufactured from pulp processed using acid-free and elementary chlorine-free practices.
Furthermore, the publisher ensures that the text paper and cover board used have met acceptable
environmental accreditation standards.

For further information on Blackwell Publishing, visit our website:
www.blackwellpublishing.com

Contents

Preface

The aim of this book is to provide a source of information for adult nursing and operating department practitioner (ODP) students and newly qualified nurses working in acute surgical environments. The focus is on major surgical conditions and interventions that are commonly encountered in district general hospitals. Increasingly, patients being nursed in acute wards have complex health care needs and require intensive observation and monitoring. Reasons for this include the fact that technological developments have led to an increase in the number of procedures that are carried out on a day surgical or outpatient basis and a shorter length of stay for patients undergoing inpatient procedures. Thus, patients cared for in acute surgical wards are often older, undergoing major surgical procedures, or are acutely ill (McArthur-Rouse, 2001). Additionally, advancements in anaesthetic and critical care techniques have enabled higher risk patients to undergo major surgical procedures that previously would have been inappropriate. The net effect of these occurrences is an increase in the acuity and dependency of patients being cared for in acute general wards (Coad & Haines, 1999; DoH, 2005).

Traditionally nurses have not been well equipped to assess and manage these patients, missing early warning signs of deterioration, leading to the phenomenon that has become known as 'sub-optimal care'. McQuillan et al. (1998) describe sub-optimal care as avoidable components that contribute to physiological deterioration, with major consequences on morbidity, mortality, requirement for intensive care and cost. Several strategies for reducing the occurrence of sub-optimal care have been implemented including the Critical Care Outreach Initiative (DoH, 2000, 2005) and the use of early warning scoring systems. Additionally, courses have been developed to enable qualified nurses to recognise the early warning signs of critical illness and caring for highly dependent patients in the ward environment and such topics are now addressed in the pre-registration nursing curriculum. This book aims to complement these initiatives with the focus on surgical care. It does not seek to address every surgical intervention; rather it focuses on the common major surgical conditions that could potentially require intensive monitoring and intervention. It seeks to support the use of early warning scoring systems by emphasising the importance of thorough assessment and interpretation of clinical data, thus providing underpinning knowledge to help nurses make sense of their findings and articulate them effectively to the appropriate personnel.

The book is divided into two sections. Part One deals with the principles of surgical care such as pre-operative assessment and preparation, the peri-operative period and post-operative recovery. Additionally the principles of post-operative pain management are considered, as are the psychosocial aspects of surgery. This section deals with the *general* aspects of surgical care as they apply to all patients undergoing surgery and provides underpinning knowledge and rationale for practice.

Part Two considers specific surgical conditions and interventions and the *application* of the principles to particular client groups. The chapters in Part Two are set out according to surgical specialities and each considers the pathophysiology, investigation and diagnosis, assessment, monitoring and management of common acute surgical conditions cross-referenced to Part One.

Nursing and ODP students should find this book useful to consolidate what they learn in lectures and as a guide whilst on surgical placements. Qualified nurses may also benefit from the book to enhance their knowledge and understanding of the rationale for care.

Fiona J McArthur-Rouse and Sylvia Prosser

References

Coad S & Haines S (1999) 'Supporting staff caring for critically ill patients in acute care areas' *Nursing in Critical Care* 4(5): 245–248

Department of Health (2000) *Comprehensive Critical Care – A review of adult critical care services*. London: DoH

Department of Health (2005) *Quality Critical Care – beyond 'Comprehensive Critical Care'*. London: DoH

McArthur-Rouse FJ (2001) 'Critical care outreach services and early warning scoring systems: a review of the literature' *Journal of Advanced Nursing* 36(5): 696–704

McQuillan P, Pilkington S, Allan A, Taylor B, Short A, Morgan G, Nielson M, Barrett D & Smith G (1998) 'Confidential inquiry into quality of care before admission to intensive care' *British Medical Journal* 316: 1853–1858

Contributors

Editors

Fiona J McArthur-Rouse, MSc, BSc (Hons), Cert Ed, RGN, Principal Lecturer, Department of Adult Nursing Studies, Canterbury Christ Church University

Sylvia Prosser, PhD, MSc, BEd (Hons), formerly Principal Lecturer, Department of Adult Nursing Studies, Canterbury Christ Church University

Authors

Tim Collins, BSc (Hons) Acute Care Nursing, PGCLT (HE), Dip HE (Nursing), ENB 100, UK Resuscitation Council Instructor, RN, Senior Lecturer/Practitioner in Critical Care, Department of Adult Nursing Studies, Canterbury Christ Church University

Luke Ewart, BSc (Hons), PGCE, RODP, Senior Lecturer, Department of Adult Nursing Studies, Canterbury Christ Church University

Ian Felstead, BSc (Hons) Nursing, PGCLT (HE), DipHE (Nursing), RN, Senior Lecturer in Acute Care, Department of Adult Nursing Studies, Canterbury Christ Church University

Carma Harnett, Dip Ear Care, RGN, ENT Nurse Practitioner, Medway NHS Trust

Sandra Huntington, MSc, Cert Ed, RODP, Senior Lecturer, Department of Adult Nursing Studies, Canterbury Christ Church University

Jane McLean, BSc (Hons), Dip Nurse Education, RGN, RCNT, Senior Lecturer, Department of Adult Nursing Studies, Canterbury Christ Church University

Ann Newman, BSc (Hons), PGCLT (HE), RGN Senior Lecturer, Department of Adult Nursing Studies, Canterbury Christ Church University

Catherine I Plowright, RN MSc, BSc (Hons) (Nursing), ENB100, DMS, Consultant Nurse Critical Care, Medway NHS Trust

Ann M Price, MSc, PGCE, BSc (Hons), RN, Senior Lecturer, Department of Adult Nursing Studies, Canterbury Christ Church University

Curie Scott, MBBS, BSc, PGCLT (HE), Senior Lecturer, Department of Adult Nursing Studies, Canterbury Christ Church University

Tracey Sharpe, BSc (Hons), RGN, Modern Matron for Head and Neck Services, Medway NHS Trust

Acknowledgements

This book has been the result of collaboration between the authors who would also like to acknowledge with thanks the additional contributions of:

The Operating Theatre Department, William Harvey Hospital, East Kent Hospitals NHS Trust for departmental photographs

Karen E Lumsden, Lecturer Practitioner (Emergency Care), Department of Adult Nursing Studies, Canterbury Christ Church University, for specialist subject advice

Rhonda Barnes, Breast Care Nurse Specialist, William Harvey Hospital, East Kent Hospitals NHS Trust for specialist subject advice

Angela Harman, Ward Manager, Gynaecology, Queen Elizabeth the Queen Mother Hospital, East Kent Hospitals NHS Trust for specialist subject advice

Yvonne Hill, formerly Head of Department, Adult Nursing Studies, Canterbury Christ Church University for her continued support for this project

Part 1

Principles of Caring for Acute Surgical Patients

1 Pre-operative Assessment and Preparation

Curie Scott, Fiona J McArthur-Rouse, Jane McLean

Introduction

This chapter will address the important aspects of assessing and managing a patient before surgery. It will be divided into pre-operative assessment and pre-operative preparation. Box 1.1 identifies the aims of this chapter.

Pre-operative assessment occurs to screen a patient for fitness to undergo anaesthetic and surgery. Formerly, this was conducted by those with medical qualifications. However, with the aim of reducing junior doctors' working hours, other appropriately trained health professionals, mainly nurses, have undertaken some tasks that had been part of the doctors' remit. The screening and assessment process is increasingly carried out prior to

admission by a specifically trained pre-assessment team working to agreed protocols.

A multicentred trial found that appropriately trained nurses performed pre-assessment of surgical patients comparably with medical staff. Three essential components were suggested for preparation of nurses taking on these roles:

- Masters level modules in anatomy, physical examination and test ordering
- The provision of a clinical mentor (senior doctor)
- A requirement to maintain a learning log-book as evidence of developing skills (Kinley *et al.*, 2001)

Although nurses and operating department practitioners (ODPs) are not qualified to decide whether a patient is fit for anaesthetic or surgery, they can identify patients who may be at risk by using agreed questionnaires (Association of Anaesthetists of Great Britain and Ireland (AAGBI), 2001).

Pre-operative assessment

The aim of pre-operative assessment

Pre-operative assessment is a screening process that aims to ensure that patients are in the optimum state before their operation. In addition to evaluating the

---

Box 1.1 Aims of the chapter.

- To discuss the aims and process of pre-operative assessment
- To enable readers to appreciate the pulmonary, cardiac and anaesthetic risks relating to surgery and how these may be assessed
- To discuss the pre-operative preparation undertaken to prevent peri- and post-operative complications
- To identify the limitations of pre-operative assessment for emergency procedures

medical history of the individual and performing an appropriate physical assessment, there is an opportunity to enquire about social circumstances, provide information and allow interventions (such as referral, counselling, ordering and performing investigations) if necessary.

Pre-operative assessment commences when the decision to perform surgery is taken and may take place in a variety of settings and time spans. In addition to the patient's health status, the nature of surgery will dictate whether it could be accomplished in day surgery or whether the patient needs to be admitted as an inpatient. Pre-operative assessment is often conducted at a specified clinic, but screening may begin at the surgical outpatient department by patients completing a questionnaire, or via telephone interview (AAGBI, 2001). These preliminary questionnaires are not a substitute to formal pre-operative assessment, but enable a reduction in the time spent asking the basic questions (Garcia-Miguel *et al.*, 2003).

The ideal situation is to have clinics where pre-operative assessment occurs in a centralised location near departments where investigations take place and with access to anaesthetic opinion (Janke *et al.*, 2002). The timing of a comprehensive pre-operative assessment is influenced by the combination of surgical invasiveness and severity of any existing disease. It needs to be well in advance of the anticipated day of procedure for all elective patients (American Society of Anesthesiologists (ASA), 2002) and the optimum time frame is suggested to be approximately three to four weeks before surgery (Bramhall, 2002). This permits appropriate adjustment and allocation of staffing and resources. Additionally, it avoids surgical delay or cancellation and allows an opportunity for the consolidation of information given to the patient (Ziolkowski & Strzyzewski, 2001).

A pre-operative evaluation includes an interview with the patient (ideally with accessible medical records), a directed examination, investigations when indicated, and other consultations when appropriate (ASA, 2002).

Risk assessment

The risk of surgery to the patient depends on the type of procedure (either minor or major) and the patient's health status, physical fitness and the

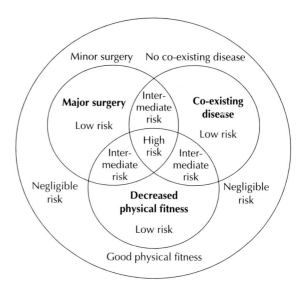

Figure 1.1   Determining risk of surgery by considering type of surgery, co-existing disease and the patient's physical fitness. (Reprinted from *Perioperative Care, Anaesthesia, Pain Management and Intensive Care*, Avidan M *et al.*, p. 7, © 2003 with permission from Elsevier)

presence of any co-existing disease. Avidan *et al.* (2003) suggest that when assessing a patient for surgery and anaesthetic, consideration about the potential benefits of the proposed surgery should be balanced against the risk to the patient. An evaluation of these components will establish whether there is negligible, low, intermediate or high risk to the patient (see Figure 1.1). Those in the low-risk category and those having low-risk surgery may not need further evaluation but for those considered to be of intermediate or higher risk, further testing may be beneficial (Avidan *et al.*, 2003).

Patients' health status can be determined by a simple classification scale produced by the American Society of Anesthesiologists (ASA) describing fitness to undergo an anaesthetic. It is separated into six levels, which are outlined in Table 1.1. They range from a normal healthy patient (ASA grade 1) to a declared brain-dead patient whose organs may be donated (ASA grade 6).

Surgical evaluation

History taking

The initial information collected at pre-operative assessment includes patient demographics, contact

Table 1.1   Patient physical status (ASA classification) (2005).

ASA	Grade Description
P1	A normal healthy patient
P2	A patient with mild systemic disease
P3	A patient with severe systemic disease
P4	A patient with incapacitating systemic disease that is a constant threat to life
P5	A moribund patient who is not expected to survive without the operation
P6	A declared brain-dead patient whose organs are being removed for donor purposes

ASA (2005–06) *Manual for Anesthesia Department Organization and Management* with permission of the ASA, Illinois
www.asahq.org/clinical/physicalstatus.htm

Box 1.2   Specific information collected at pre-operative assessment.

- Current and past medical history
- Surgical history with a focus on anaesthetic risk factors
- Medication and allergies
- Appropriate family history
- Social issues (home transportation and environment, designated caretakers, alcohol intake and smoking habits)

---

details, details of the procedure and relevant medical practitioners involved in the patient's care. Box 1.2 identifies further specific information that is collected.

For pre-operative evaluation, the focus of the history and physical examination is on risk factors for pulmonary, cardiac and anaesthetic complications (Ziolkowski & Strzyzewski, 2001). If the patient has any risks that can be adjusted, then elective surgery can be deferred until his or her health has been optimised. Other areas such as specific endocrine diseases (diabetes and thyroid problems) and neurological conditions (e.g. stroke, muscle disease, epilepsy) are also queried.

Pulmonary risk

Respiratory complications constitute a large proportion of overall morbidity and mortality post-operatively and are more common than cardiac complications. They include:

- Atelectasis (partial or complete collapse of a lung due to obstruction)
- Infection (such as bronchitis and pneumonia)
- Prolonged mechanical ventilation
- Respiratory failure
- Bronchospasm
- Exacerbation of underlying chronic lung disease (Garcia-Miguel *et al.*, 2003)

The most important risk factor for respiratory complications is chronic lung disease, which is more prevalent in smokers. In addition to increased airway irritability and the risk of developing post-operative pneumonia, smoking has a negative effect on cardiac function (Ziolkowski & Strzyzewski, 2001).

Patients with a cold have an increased risk of bronchospasm and laryngospasm following instrumentation of the larynx and pharynx, and this may be life threatening. Additionally, any post-operative coughing may place strain on sutures. Therefore, it is important to ascertain whether a patient has a cold and it is wise to consider delay to surgery until they have recovered (Avidan *et al.*, 2003).

In addition to specific respiratory conditions (such as asthma, emphysema, chronic bronchitis, tuberculosis or obstructive sleep apnoea) it is useful to evaluate the severity of any breathlessness. Table 1.2 outlines the further questions that relate to exercise tolerance, coughs, sputum production and the use of supplemental oxygen therapy.

Cardiac risk

Anaesthesia causes strain on the heart that should not affect a healthy person but if a heart is compromised by ischaemia, it may not be able to withstand the increased demand placed on it by hypoxia, hypotension, hypertension or dysrhythmia (Ziolkowski & Strzyzewski, 2001). Therefore, the patient's current and past cardiac history is confirmed. They are asked several questions to ascertain any history of chest pain, arrhythmias and conditions such as myocardial infarction or hypertension (see Table 1.2).

Anaesthetic risk

Patients are asked if they have previously had an anaesthetic and whether they or any family member has had problems with anaesthetics. Loose teeth, caps, crowns and dentures are noted and

Table 1.2   Pulmonary and cardiovascular risks.
Patients are asked screening questions about the following topics that relate to the relevant system:

Respiratory system	Cardiovascular system
<ul><li>Asthma, chronic obstructive pulmonary disease (emphysema, chronic bronchitis) or tuberculosis (TB)</li><li>Obstructive sleep apnoea</li><li>General breathlessness (dyspnoea), orthopnoea (breathlessness when lying down), paroxysmal nocturnal dyspnoea (wakening in the middle of the night with breathlessness)</li><li>Details of cough and sputum production</li><li>Exercise tolerance</li><li>Use of supplemental oxygen therapy</li><li>Details of any respiratory attacks</li></ul>	<ul><li>Hypertension</li><li>Chest pain, angina, myocardial infarction</li><li>Palpitations, arrhythmias, other cardiac conduction abnormalities</li><li>Heart murmurs, rheumatic fever, valvular dysfunction</li><li>Insertion of a pacemaker</li></ul>

(NHS Modernisation Agency, 2003; Ziolkowski & Strzyzewski, 2001)

patients are informed about the potential risk of chipping to teeth during laryngoscopy (Avidan *et al.*, 2003). Conditions affecting airway management, such as restriction of jaw or neck movements, and states that may impact on the patient's experience, such as depression and anxiety, are also identified.

Medication and allergies

Medication that patients are taking needs to be ascertained and should include prescribed, over the counter and herbal medications as they may adversely affect the outcome of the surgery. For example, warfarin will prolong bleeding time so it needs to be discontinued before surgery commences, especially if blood loss is expected. Patients often regard herbal medications as being safe, but some will have an impact on the surgical procedure or anaesthesia. For example, bleeding time is prolonged by garlic, feverfew, ginger and ginkgo biloba and the sedative effects of anaesthesia are prolonged by valerian and St John's Wort (Flanagan, 2001). It is important to ask specifically about the contraceptive pill, as the patient may not consider this to be medication although it may impact upon treatment. It is often useful if patients attend the clinic with their medications or a list of their drugs with the times they are taken. Allergies to any medications or other substances such as plasters, latex and foods are discussed.

Patients should understand the need to withhold or change some medications before the operation. Often medications can be continued but this should be discussed with the appropriate medical practitioner. Details of some drugs that need to be discontinued or continued are shown in Table 1.3. Patients may benefit from additional medication before surgery. These are termed 'pre-medication' and include anti-emetics, drugs for pain relief or to reduce anxiety.

Physical examination

A general examination of the patient can be conducted during the history taking. This enables the health professional to note the patient's apparent state of health, their posture and gait, their skin colour, any obvious lesions and any signs of distress either from anxiety, breathlessness or pain (Bickley & Szilaygi, 2003). Box 1.3 identifies some minimum evaluations suggested by the ASA (2002).

Box 1.3   Minimum pre-operative evaluations suggested by the ASA (2002).

- Baseline observations:
  - Height
  - Weight
  - Body mass index (BMI)
  - Temperature
  - Blood pressure
  - Pulse rate
  - Respiratory rate
  - Oxygen saturation (SpO_2)
- An airway assessment
- Examination of both the cardiovascular and respiratory systems

---

Table 1.3 Details of some medications that should be continued or discontinued prior to surgery.

	Discontinue	Continue or initiate
Cardiovascular	• ACE inhibitors and potassium-sparing diuretics (morning of surgery)	• Other antihypertensive • Beta blockers and anti-anginals
Respiratory		• Oxygen • Asthma medications (pre-operative nebulisation and steroid cover)
Endocrine	• Long-acting oral hypoglycaemic drugs – convert to insulin sliding scale	• Thyroid replacement • Steroids – additional cover may be required • Insulin – convert to sliding scale
Neurological and psychiatric	• Monoamine oxidase inhibitors (2 weeks)	• Other psychiatric medications • Anti-epileptics – add benzodiazepine
Drugs affecting coagulation	• Warfarin – convert to heparin or low-molecular weight heparin for major surgery • Oral contraceptive pill and hormone replacement therapy – stop for several weeks	• Continue with all anticoagulants where the bleeding risk is low • Provide post-operative thrombosis prophylaxis

(Reprinted from *Perioperative Care, Anaesthesia, Pain Management and Intensive Care*, Avidan *et al.*, p. 9, © 2003 with permission from Elsevier)

Box 1.4 Simple tests are used to evaluate the airway.

• Thyromental distance: the distance between the thyroid notch to the top of the jaw with the head extended should be 6.5 cm or more.
• The patient should be able to insert their middle three fingers vertically into their mouth.
• The Mallampati test: the patient is asked to open their mouth as wide as possible and protrude their tongue out as far as possible. The extent to which the faucial pillars, soft palate and uvula are visualised is then graded from 1 (all visualised) to 4 (not visualised) and is outlined in Figure 1.2. Clinically, grade 1 usually predicts an easy intubation and grade 3 or 4 suggest a difficult intubation.

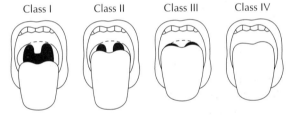

Figure 1.2 Mallampati test to evaluate the airway. The patient is asked to open their mouth as wide as possible and protrude their tongue out as far as possible. The extent to which the faucial pillars, soft palate and uvula are visualised is then classified from 1 (all visualised) to 4 (not visualised). Class I usually predicts an easy intubation and Class III or IV suggest a difficult intubation.
(Reproduced from Mallampati *et al.* (1985) 'A clinical sign to predict difficult tracheal intubation: a prospective study' *Canadian Anaesthesiologists' Journal* 32: pp. 429–434 with permission)

Airway evaluation

Occasionally, there is difficulty in ventilating and intubating patients, particularly obstetric and obese patients. Certain physical characteristics may increase the risk of problems with airway management. These include protruding upper teeth, limited mouth opening, a large tongue, tracheal deviation and immobility of the head, neck and jaw. The patient's teeth are assessed and any caps, crowns, bridges or dentures are noted (Avidan *et al.*, 2003). Box 1.4 identifies some simple tests that are used to evaluate the airway and Figure 1.2 illustrates the various grades of the Mallampati test (Mallampati *et al.*, 1985).

Respiratory examination

The baseline investigations for the respiratory system include the respiratory rate and the peripheral haemoglobin oxygen saturation (SpO_2) while breathing room air. The shape of the spine and chest and any use of accessory muscles are noted and then the chest is more closely evaluated. Movement of the chest with each breath is observed for equality of symmetry and expansion. The patient is asked to cough up sputum that may otherwise be heard on auscultation, then asked to breathe through their mouth moderately deeply. The stethoscope is used to listen at the front and the back of the chest over the lung area. Any added sounds such as wheezes or crackles are recorded. Other techniques include palpation and percussion. The trachea is palpated to check if it is central, and placing hands around the chest wall enables assessment of whether expansion is equal on both sides. Percussion is a technique where the clinician's fingers are used to tap the chest wall in order to produce an audible vibration to assess the density within the lungs (Cross & Rimmer, 2002). Any abnormality is noted and the surgeon or anaesthetist may need to be informed.

Cardiovascular examination
The patient's blood pressure and pulse rate need to be documented. The radial pulse is used to evaluate the rate and rhythm (regular or irregular). If the patient has a history of stroke or transient ischaemic attack (TIA) then they may have narrowed carotid arteries, so a stethoscope is used to listen for a bruit (a swishing sound that indicates increased turbulence) and if one is noted, the surgeon or anaesthetist should be notified (Janke *et al.*, 2002).

A jugular venous pressure (JVP) is measured if the patient has a history of heart failure or if they are breathless. With the patient at 45 degrees, the highest point of the oscillation in the internal jugular vein is noted from the sternal angle. The JVP is useful, as the pressure in the jugular vein reflects right atrial pressure and provides a clinical indicator of cardiac function (Bickley & Szilaygi, 2003).

The chest is then examined for any deformities, surgical scars, visible pulsations or evidence to indicate a pacemaker or cardiac defibrillator (a rectangle under the skin). The heart is auscultated by listening in various regions on the chest wall using the diaphragm (for high-pitched noises) and the bell (for low-pitched noises). The first (S1, 'lub') and the second (S2, 'dub') heart sounds and any additional sounds, such as murmurs, are recorded. Finally, any evidence of peripheral oedema and its extent should be described.

Pre-operative tests and investigations

At pre-operative assessment, patients at high risk are identified for appropriate testing and interventions to reduce their surgical risk. The ASA (2002) states that pre-operative tests are useful only if they affect peri-operative anaesthetic care, and any testing should be informed by the history and examination (Avidan *et al.*, 2003). Investigations in a healthy patient having minor surgery are unnecessary and routine tests are not advised. The argument that they may be useful to discover a disease or disorder in an asymptomatic patient does not make an important contribution to pre-operative assessment (AAGBI, 2001). Specific pre-operative investigations for particular types of surgery are discussed in the relevant chapters in Part Two of this book.

The UK National Institute for Clinical Excellence (NICE) published a comprehensive review of evidence on pre-operative testing for elective surgery (NICE, 2003). The tests relate to the complexity of the operation and to the ASA grades and are highlighted in a visual manner as a series of traffic lights (if red, the test is not recommended; if yellow, the test can be considered; and if green, the test is recommended). Their guidance suggests that, for healthy patients aged 16–80-plus undergoing minor surgery, the only recommended test is an electrocardiogram (ECG) for those over 80 years old. Some tests are to be considered across some of the age-spans (urinalysis, full blood count, renal function) but generally, tests were not considered necessary in this group of people.

Appropriate selection of pre-operative investigations is promoted if departments have policies on which investigations should be performed to reflect the age, co-morbidity and complexity of the surgery (AAGBI, 2001). For example, some tests are useful in certain circumstances and Avidan *et al.* (2003) outline the following:

- Haemoglobin measurement – before surgery where major blood loss is anticipated; may be justified in older people and in menstruating women or if anaemia is suspected
- Platelet count and coagulation (clotting) studies – if the history raises concerns about abnormal clotting
- Urea, creatinine and electrolytes – if the patient is dehydrated, has renal dysfunction or if electrolyte abnormalities are suspected

The AAGBI (2001) suggests that an ECG is not indicated for asymptomatic males under 40 or asymptomatic females under 50 but is valuable in all patients with a cardiac history. Interestingly, Kinley *et al.* (2002) found that house officers ordered almost twice as many unnecessary tests as nurses. This was possibly due to the fact that nurses adhered to protocol more than the house officers.

Blood transfusions
Patients who are likely to require a blood transfusion post-operatively will have blood taken for grouping or cross matching. Although rare, risks of blood transfusions include the possible transmission of hepatitis, HIV/AIDS virus and variant Creutzfeldt–Jakob disease (vCJD), as well as transfusion reactions. Patients should be counselled about the possible need and any objections to receiving blood products should be documented. Autologous transfusion reduces the need for donated blood transfusion and is sometimes used in elective surgery. Box 1.5 identifies the main techniques of autologous blood transfusion.

MRSA screening
Most hospitals have policies for screening patients for methicillin-resistant *Staphylococcus aureus* (MRSA) because whilst colonisation on the individual's skin may be harmless, should the bacteria

be transferred into the patient's wound, severe infection may occur. Also, debilitated patients are more at risk of contracting an infection. This is particularly relevant for patients undergoing orthopaedic surgery (see Chapter 12). Swabs are usually taken from the patient's nose and groin and, if positive, decontamination is recommended according to local policy.

Pressure sore risk assessment

Surgical patients are at increased risk of developing pressure sores because of the increased time that they are immobile during and immediately after their operation. The Waterlow Risk Assessment Scale (Waterlow, 1988) is frequently used to assess the patient's level of risk and enables staff to implement appropriate plans of care and allocate the necessary pressure-relieving devices. In older patients and those at increased risk of developing pressure sores it is important to inspect, assess and document the status of the pressure areas on admission.

Nutritional screening and assessment

In an important study undertaken in the early 1990s, McWhirter and Pennington (1994) highlighted that many patients are admitted to acute hospitals in a nutritionally compromised state. Additionally, during hospitalisation, further deterioration in their nutritional status can occur. Surgical patients are at particular risk of developing malnutrition, due in part to the nature of the surgery and any pre-existing disease, and also to factors such as prolonged fasting pre-operatively and restriction of oral intake post-operatively.

Older people in particular may have pre-existing poor general physical and mental health causing a loss of appetite. Chronic ill health and acute episodes of illness are often associated with an impaired appetite, as are depression and drug treatments such as chemotherapy. Patients who have difficulty swallowing or who are fasting for surgery or other tests may miss meals. If an operation is cancelled, the fasting period may be prolonged if pre-operative nutritional support is not instigated.

During nutritional *screening*, patients at risk of malnutrition who may require a more comprehensive nutritional *assessment* are identified.

Box 1.5 Types of autologous blood transfusion.

Pre-operative donation – patients who are otherwise fit for surgery may donate their own blood, which can be stored for up to 35–42 days. Contraindications to autologous transfusion include sepsis and severe myocardial infarction.

Isovolaemic haemodilution – up to 1.5 litres of blood may be withdrawn before the induction of anaesthesia and replaced by intravenous saline infusion. This results in haemodilution and a reduction in the red blood cells lost during surgery. The withdrawn blood can be reinfused either intra- or post-operatively.

Cell salvage – blood is collected from the patient either by suction directly from the operation site or via collection devices attached to surgical drains (see Chapter 12). The blood is reinfused either intra- or post-operatively, with or without washing.

(Green & McClelland, 2004)

Box 1.6   Nutritional screening – observations and questions that may be asked when taking a dietary history.

- Age – older patients are at increased risk of malnutrition
- History of recent unintentional weight loss – how much weight has been lost? How quickly? Do the patient's clothes appear to be loose? Body mass index.
- Appetite – does the patient finish meals or leave all or part of each meal? Are meals skipped?
- Physical ability to prepare meals and eat – does the patient require assistance with the preparation of meals and/or with eating? Is a particular diet required? What is the condition of the patient's mouth and teeth?
- Gastrointestinal function – does the patient suffer from constipation or diarrhoea, indigestion, heartburn, or nausea and vomiting?
- Social factors – does the patient eat alone or with family? Who shops and which products are bought? How much exercise does the patient have?
- Medical factors – does the patient have any pre-existing diseases that may influence nutritional intake and demand (e.g. diabetes, thyroid disease, malignancy,

food allergies)? Is the patient taking any medication that may influence appetite?
- Psychological factors – does the patient appear depressed? Has he or she suffered a recent bereavement?
- General appearance – the following should be observed:
  - Skin – tone, texture, colour, signs of bruising
  - Nails – white patches, dry, brittle
  - Eyes – colour and condition, sunken
  - Mouth – moist, pink mucosa or discoloured
  - Lips – are they dry and cracked?
  - Tongue – is it dry or moist, clean or furred? Does the breath smell?
  - Gums – do they bleed for no reason? Do they recede?
  - Dentures – do they fit?
  - Cheek bones – are they overly prominent?
  - Clothes and rings – are they loose?

Nutritional screening involves taking a dietary and clinical history from the patient (see Box 1.6). If nutritional screening highlights a deficit, further assessment may be undertaken, usually by a dietician. This will include more intense measurements, such as anthropometric indices and biochemical indicators (see Edwards (2000) for further discussion of these). If a nutritional deficit is identified, it is important to instigate pre-operative nutritional support in order to optimise the patient's condition pre-operatively. This may take the form of dietary supplements, enteral or parenteral feeds. (See Chapter 3 for a further discussion of the nutritional demands of surgery.)

Assessment of home circumstances

In order to prevent delays in discharging the patient post-operatively, an assessment of the individual's home circumstances and support mechanisms should take place pre-operatively, preferably as part of the pre-admission assessment. This includes providing the patient with an anticipated date of discharge and, if long-term convalescence is likely to be required, commencing the necessary arrangements, including any specialist referrals

(e.g. social work, occupational therapist). Any changes that need to be made to existing care packages should also be noted.

Pre-operative preparation

Preparing patients for surgery involves both psychosocial and physical dimensions. Psychosocial preparation includes assessing and managing anxiety and stress, patient education and informed consent, whilst physical preparation is concerned with the prevention of peri- and post-operative complications.

Psychosocial preparation

This aspect of pre-operative preparation often commences when the patient visits the pre-assessment clinic. Sometimes they have the opportunity to visit the ward or intensive care unit and meet the staff who will be caring for them. Alternatively, theatre staff may come to the ward once the patient has been admitted, to introduce themselves and answer any questions the patient may have. Chapter 5 provides further discussion of the management of anxiety and stress in surgical patients.

Informed consent

Before undergoing any surgical procedure, the patient must give consent that is based on a realistic understanding of the procedure and potential complications. The surgeon explains the operation to the patient, who is given the opportunity to ask questions prior to signing the consent form. It is important that language is used that the patient understands and that the use of medical terminology is avoided. The patient must receive sufficient information to make an informed choice. Cable *et al.* (2003) identify three areas of consideration when obtaining consent: legal, professional and ethical. These include issues such as age/adulthood, mental capacity and professional duty of care. Some patients, however, lack the capacity to consent and Plant (2004) identifies these as:

- Minors
- Those with transient or irreversible cognitive impairment
- Those with mental illness
- Those who are receiving undue coercion to consent

In the acutely ill adult surgical patient, transient cognitive impairment may arise due to the effects of illness or its treatment and in such situations it may be necessary to administer treatment in the patient's best interests (Plant, 2004). In situations such as these it may be necessary to seek legal advice. (See Plant (2004) for further discussion of this issue.)

Accuracy of the documentation is vital in order to avoid a catastrophe and numerous checks are carried out to ensure that patient safety is maintained. Often the patient's skin will be marked with an indelible pen at the site of operation to ensure that the correct procedure is carried out.

Physical pre-operative preparation

The main aims of pre-operative preparation are to prevent peri- and post-operative complications such as wound infection, deep vein thrombosis and chest infection. This section considers measures to help prevent such complications from occurring.

Pre-operative fasting

Patients are often fasted for elective procedures and they may be referred to as being 'nil-by-mouth' (NBM). This is to reduce the potentially fatal complication of aspiration of the gastric contents into the lungs (causing aspiration pneumonia). Webb (2003) states that a patient is at higher risk of reflux during surgery for two main reasons:

- Increased pressure in the abdominal cavity, especially during bowel or stomach surgery
- Muscle relaxation caused by drugs used in anaesthesia

Patients were often fasted from midnight for a procedure the following day. However, a comprehensive report produced by the ASA (1999) made recommendations that are supported by the AAGBI (2001). They state that the minimum fasting periods are:

- Six hours for solid food or milk
- Two hours for clear non-particulate and non-carbonated fluids

Avidan *et al.* (2003) state that, despite precautions, some patients remain at high risk of aspiration due to impaired gastric emptying. These include trauma patients; those who have underlying gastrointestinal pathology or autonomic dysfunction; patients who are on opioid medications and patients who are pregnant or obese.

If the above fasting times are adhered to, fluid and nutritional supplementation is usually not required. However, it is valuable to note that there are some patients who may need intravenous fluid support due to their vulnerability to dehydration. These include older people, those who have had bowel preparation, sick patients, children and breast-feeding mothers (AAGBI, 2001).

Benefits of implementing the above evidence-based pre-operative fasting times include reduced anxiety, thirst and post-operative nausea and vomiting (Oshodi, 2004, Figure 1.3).

Skin preparation

The aim of pre-operative skin cleansing is to reduce the bacterial skin flora, particularly *Staphylococcus aureus* (Simmons, 1998), which is a common cause of wound infection. Patients admitted on the day of surgery may undertake their own skin preparation

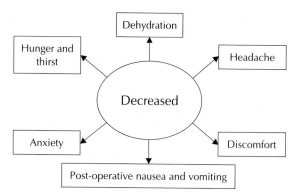

Figure 1.3   Benefits of implementing evidence-based pre-operative fasting times. (Adapted from Oshodi, 2004)

prior to admission. They are usually advised to have a bath or shower to remove dirt and microbes from the skin and to wash their hair because this can act as a reservoir for bacteria (Simmons, 1998). Patients admitted a day or more before surgery will need to have their bath or shower using the ward facilities and will be provided with clean linen. Following the bath or shower, the patient will be given a clean theatre gown to wear and will be asked to remove his or her own clothing (depending on the type of operation). Controversy exists regarding the effectiveness of soap versus whole-body disinfection in patients showering pre-operatively, with few recent studies effectively examining this issue. In a review of the literature Simmons (1998) argues that:

> '. . . although chlorhexidine 4% appears to reduce the incidence of skin flora, its impact on the incidence of wound infection is not conclusive . . .'
>
> (Simmons, 1998, p. 447)

Another controversial aspect of skin preparation is the removal of body hair from the surgical site. Numerous studies have been undertaken to evaluate the effectiveness of this in reducing the incidence of wound infection with little by way of definitive conclusions (Dawson, 2000). Box 1.7 identifies the arguments for and against this practice.

Anticoagulant therapy and antiembolic stockings

To prevent the complication of deep vein thrombosis (DVT), patients are encouraged to mobilise pre-

---

Box 1.7   Arguments for and against the removal of body hair in pre-operative skin preparation.

- The argument **for** hair removal suggests that leaving body hair in place encourages the bacteria around the hair follicles to be introduced to the wound because of their proximity to the operation site.
- The argument **against** suggests that removing body hair increases the potential for infection because:
  ○ The process of removing body hair (shaving and use of depilatory creams) destroys the body's natural defence mechanism by destroying the natural flora that occur on the skin.
  ○ Depilatory creams, being chemical agents, destroy the natural barrier of the skin.
  ○ Shaving causes nicks in the skin that offer bacteria an ideal environment to reproduce.
- If hair is to be removed, clipping or trimming may be preferred.

(adapted from Dawson, 2000)

---

operatively and may be taught limb exercises by the physiotherapist to promote venous return. Antiembolic stockings are frequently used, and the patient must be given the correct size as badly fitting stockings can cause excessive pressure and heel necrosis. Anticoagulant therapy is sometimes prescribed pre-operatively or commences in the immediate post-operative period. See Chapter 3 for further discussion of the prevention of DVT.

Prophylactic antibiotics

Because surgery involves a breach in the body's natural defence mechanisms, there is potential for infection of various types, for example wound infection, chest infection and infection of prostheses. For this reason, prophylactic antibiotics are often prescribed to be administered immediately before the operation (often on induction of anaesthesia) and during the post-operative period. The type of antibiotic varies according to the type of surgery.

Pre-operative checks

Before transferring the patient to the operating department, a number of pre-operative checks are undertaken (see Box 1.8). Patients who use a hearing aid or dentures should be able to keep these in

> **Box 1.8** Checks undertaken and recorded pre-operatively.
>
> - Baseline observations
> - Time of last food and drink
> - Pre-medication and prophylactic antibiotics administered (if applicable)
> - Skin preparation/hair removal (if applicable)
> - Removal of make-up, nail varnish, jewellery, personal clothing, prosthesis (if applicable)
> - Presence of dentures, loose or capped teeth is documented
> - Identification bracelet with correct details is checked
> - Allergies are identified and documented
> - Notes, X-rays, blood results, ECG results, etc., are collated
> - The consent form is signed with the correct procedure and the patient can explain in his/her own words the procedure to be carried out

place until they arrive in the operating department. The patient's notes, including the results of any pre-operative investigations and X-rays are collated in readiness to accompany the patient to theatre. The patient is then transferred, usually on his or her bed, to the operating department, escorted by a member of the ward or theatre staff. Throughout the transfer, it is necessary to maintain close observation of the patient and attempt to put him or her at ease.

Emergency procedures

In pre-operative assessment and preparation the primary objective is to enable the patient to undergo surgery in the best physiological and psychological condition. This remains true for those undergoing emergency surgery, where time is often limited and adequate assessment and pre-operative resuscitation of the patient are key. However, Avidan *et al.* (2003) note that cardiac complications are between two and five times more likely following emergency procedures. Patients in this category are those who present with trauma or a condition that requires fairly immediate surgery.

Chapter 13 discusses the assessment of acutely unwell patients using the ABCDE system and this is normally undertaken in emergency situations. It is important to optimise the patient's condition as

much as possible before surgery in order to achieve the best possible outcome.

Trauma patients are not often fasted and will have delayed gastric emptying due to a variety of mechanisms (Sarmah *et al.*, 2004) so they often have a gastric tube inserted to empty the stomach (Dowds, 2000). Nasogastric insertion is the most common route except where there is a possibility of a basal skull fracture or facial fractures.

As part of the assessment process, various investigations may be conducted on the patient. When inserting wide bore cannulae, blood specimens should be extracted for cross matching, electrolytes, full blood count, clotting studies and glucose. Arterial blood gases are often measured and if there is a urine specimen, this can also be tested for abnormalities and the presence of pregnancy in women of childbearing age. Further investigations such as an ECG, X-rays or those specific to the patient can be completed as appropriate (Dowds, 2000).

When there is adequate time before an operation, the blood bank can complete a 90–95% cross-match referred to as 'type specific' blood but if not, the ordering of six units of O-positive blood (and for women of childbearing age an equal number of O-negative blood) is valuable (Sarmah *et al.*, 2004).

The consent form for surgical intervention should be completed, and all necessary information related to the procedure and the possible complications should be explained to the patient if his or her condition allows. Obviously, factors such as being under the influence of alcohol and drugs may impair the patient's comprehension or ability to comply with this. Children undergoing surgery also need consent from a legal guardian unless their condition is critical (Dowds, 2000). Relatives must be kept well informed both pre-operatively and post-operatively.

Self-test questions

1. Match each statement with the correct ASA grade.
   a. A patient with severe incapacitating disease
   b. A fit, healthy patient
   c. A patient who is not expected to survive more than 24 hours
   d. A patient with mild systemic disease

2. State if the following are **true** or **false**.
   a. All medication can be continued until midnight before the operation day
   b. Surgical patients are at particular risk of developing malnutrition
   c. Once evidence about a surgical intervention has been presented, a competent adult has the right to refuse it
   d. Patients should always have hair removed from the surgical site
3. Which of the following tests should be carried out on all surgical patients? (answer **yes** or **no**)?
   a. Blood pressure
   b. ECG
   c. Liver blood tests
   d. Waterlow risk assessment
4. How much more likely are cardiac complications in those following an emergency procedure?
   a. 1–2 times
   b. 4–8 times
   c. 2–5 times
   d. 2–4 times
5. What is the minimum recommended fasting period before surgery? (choose one answer)?
   a. 10 hours for solid food/milk and 2 hours for clear fluid
   b. 6 hours for solid food/milk and 2 hours for clear fluid
   c. 6 hours for solid food/milk and 4 hours for clear fluid
   d. 2 hours for solid food/milk and 6 hours for clear fluid
6. The Waterlow Risk Assessment Scale is used to assess the patient's:
   a. Nutritional risk
   b. Pressure sore risk
   c. Anaesthetic risk
   d. Cardiac risk
7. Identify three types of autologous blood transfusion.
8. Briefly explain the difference between nutritional screening and nutritional assessment.
9. Briefly explain the purpose of pre-operative skin preparation.
10. List the checks that are carried out before the patient is transferred to the operating department.

References and further reading

American Society of Anesthesiologists (1999) Task Force on Preoperative Fasting 'Practice guidelines for preoperative fasting and the use of pharmacologic agents to reduce the risk of pulmonary aspiration – application to healthy patients undergoing elective procedures: report from the American Society of Anesthesiologists Task Force on Preoperative Fasting' *Anesthesiology* 90(3): 896–905

American Society of Anesthesiologists (2002) 'Practice Advisory for Preanesthesia Evaluation: report from American Society of Anesthesiologists Task Force on Preanesthesia Evaluation' *Anesthesiology* 96(2): 485–496

American Society of Anesthesiologists (2005) *Manual for Anesthesia Department Organization and Management* (online) www.asahq.org/clinical/physicalstatus.htm (Accessed 08.01.07)

Association of Anaesthetists of Great Britain and Ireland (2001) *Role of the anaesthetist.* (online). www.aagbi.org/publications/guidelines/docs/preoperativeass01.pdf (Accessed 07.01.07)

Avidan M, Harvey A, Ponte J, Wendon J & Ginsburg R (2003) *Perioperative Care, Anaesthesia, Pain Management and Intensive Care.* Edinburgh: Churchill Livingstone

Bickley LS & Szilaygi PG (2002) *Bates' Guide to Physical Examination and History Taking* (8th edn). Philadelphia: Lippincott Williams and Wilkins.

Bramhall J (2002) 'The role of nurses in preoperative assessment' *Nursing Times* 98(40): 34–35

Cable S, Lumsdaine J & Semple M (2003) 'Informed Consent' *Nursing Standard* 18(12): 47–55

Clevenger FW & Tepas J (1997) 'Preoperative management of patients with major trauma injuries' *Association of Peri-Operative Registered Nurses* 65(3): 583–594

Cross S & Rimmer M (2002) *Nurse Practitioner: Manual of Clinical Skills.* London: Baillière Tindall

Dawson S (2000) 'Principles of preoperative preparation' *in:* Manley K & Bellman L (2000) *Surgical Nursing – Advancing Practice.* Edinburgh: Churchill Livingstone

Dowds P (2000) 'Surgical Emergencies' *in:* Dolan B & Holt L (eds) *Accident and Emergency: Theory into Practice.* London: Baillière Tindall

Edwards SL (2000) 'Chapter 27 – Maintaining Optimum Nutrition' *in:* Manley K & Bellman L (2000) *Surgical Nursing – Advancing Practice.* Edinburgh: Churchill Livingstone

Flanagan K (2001) 'Preoperative assessment: safety considerations for patients taking herbal products' *Journal of Perianesthesia Nursing* 16(1): 19–26

Garcia-Miguel FJ, Serrano-Aguilar PG & Lopez-Bastida J (2003) 'Preoperative assessment' *The Lancet* 362(9397): 1749–1757

Green R & McClelland DBL (2004) 'Chapter 4 – Transfusion of blood and blood products' *in:* Garden

OJ, Bradbury AW & Forsythe J (eds) (2004) *Principles and Practice of Surgery* (4th edition). Edinburgh: Elsevier Churchill Livingstone

Janke E, Chalk V & Kinley H (2002) *Pre-operative assessment – setting a standard through learning, NHS Modernisation Agency.* Southampton: University of Southampton

Kinley H, Czoski-Murray C, George S, McCabe C, Primrose J, Reilly C, Wood R, Nicolson P, Healy C, Read S, Norman J, Janke E, Alhameed H, Fernandez N & Thomas E (2001) 'Extended scope of nursing practice: a multi-centred randomised controlled trial of appropriately trained nurses and pre-registration house officers in pre-operative assessment in elective general surgery' *Health Technology Assessment* 5(20): 1–87

Kinley H, Czoski-Murray C, George S, McCabe C, Primrose J, Reilly C, Wood R, Nicolson P, Healy C, Read S, Norman J, Janke E, Alhameed H, Fernandes N & Thomas E (2002) 'Effectiveness of appropriately trained nurses in preoperative assessment: randomised controlled equivalence/non-inferiority trial' *British Medical Journal* 325(7376): 1323–1328

Mallampati SR, Gatt SP, Desai SP, Waraksa B, Freiberger D & Liu PL (1985) 'A clinical sign to predict difficult tracheal intubation: a prospective study' *Canadian Anaesthesiologists' Journal* 32: 429–434

McWhirter JP & Pennington CR (1994) 'Incidence and recognition of malnutrition in hospital' *British Medical Journal* 308: 495–498

National Institute for Clinical Excellence (NICE) (2003) *Guidance on the use of peri-operative test for elective surgery* (NICE Clinical Guideline, number 3). London: NICE

Ormrod G & Casey D (2004) 'The educational preparation of nursing staff undertaking pre-assessment of surgical patients – a discussion of the issues' *Nurse Education Today* 24(4): 256–262

Oshodi TO (2004) 'Clinical skills: an evidence-based approach to preoperative fasting' *British Journal of Nursing* 13(16): 958–962

Plant WD (2004) 'Chapter 7 – Ethical and legal principles in surgical practice' *in*: Garden OJ, Bradbury AW & Forsythe J (eds) (2004) *Principles and Practice of Surgery* (4th edn). Edinburgh: Elsevier Churchill Livingstone

Sarmah A, Lam-McCulloch J & Yee D (2004) 'Anaesthesia concerns in the management of the trauma patient' *Current Orthopaedics* 18(6): 441–450

Simmons M (1998) 'Pre-operative skin preparation' *Professional Nurse* 13(7): 446–447

Thomson PJ, Fletcher IR & Downey C (2004) 'Nurses versus clinicians – who's best at pre-operative assessment?' *Journal of Ambulatory Surgery* 11: 33–36

Waterlow JA (1988) 'The Waterlow card for the prevention and management of pressure sores; towards a pocket policy' *Care – Science and Practice* 6(1): 8–12

Webb K (2003) 'What are the benefits and the pitfalls of preoperative fasting?' *Nursing Times* 99(50): 32–33

Ziolkowski L & Strzyzewski N (2001) 'Perianesthesia assessment: foundation of care' *Journal of Perianesthesia Nursing* 16(6): 359–370

2 The Peri-operative Phase

Luke Ewart and Sandra Huntington

Introduction

The peri-operative experience of the surgical patient may involve various processes. However, all patients will undergo the same three phases of anaesthesia, surgery and immediate post-anaesthetic care as part of the peri-operative journey. Each of these processes impacts on the care required and will be affected by factors such as the surgical procedure and type of anaesthesia administered. This chapter will explore the principles of peri-operative care, taking into account the need to view the patient as an individual. Box 2.1 identifies the aims of this chapter.

Box 2.1   Aims of the chapter.

- To discuss the different types of anaesthesia that may be used on the surgical patient
- To identify the physiological changes that occur as a result of the anaesthetic and surgical experience (pharmacology)
- To examine evidence-based care of the peri-operative patient
- To discuss the management of care for the surgical patient
- To provide the reader with a general overview of the peri-operative setting

---

The peri-operative environment

Access into the operating department is restricted. The number and type of personnel permitted entry is controlled to limit potential contamination and to provide a safe, therapeutic environment for the patient. The layout of the operating department can broadly be explained as three distinct 'zones'. The 'dirty zone' is an unrestricted area that generally includes the entrance and exit to the operating department, as well as holding bays, offices and changing rooms. Access to these areas is permitted to personnel in outside clothing. The 'clean zone' is a semi-restricted area that allows access to support areas within the operating department. This zone includes the anaesthetic and post-anaesthetic recovery rooms (see Figures 2.1 and 2.2), areas of storage for clean and sterile supplies and areas for the processing of instruments and equipment. Access is restricted in this zone to the patient and authorised personnel wearing appropriate theatre footwear and clothing, with covered hair. The 'sterile zone' is a restricted area that includes the operating theatre itself (Figure 2.3), the scrub areas and 'laying up' or preparation rooms. In this zone, hair must be covered and theatre footwear and clothing worn at all times.

Operating theatres are designed to minimise the risk of infection. The walls and ceiling are covered with a non-porous material that is impervious to

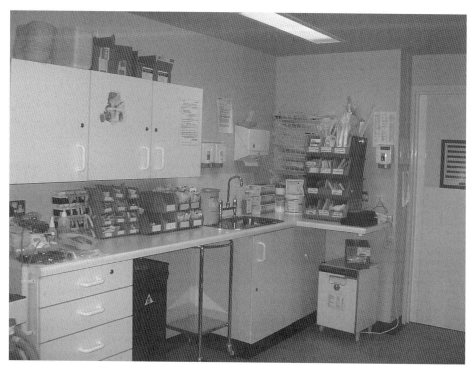

Figure 2.1   The anaesthetic room.

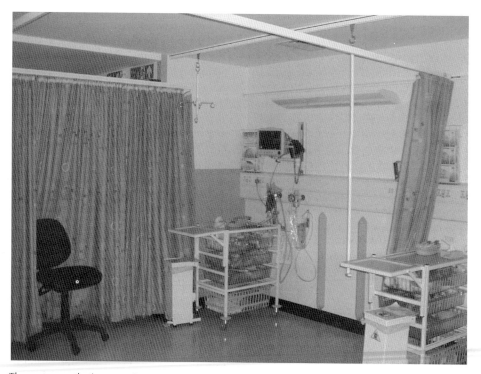

Figure 2.2   The post-anaesthetic care unit.

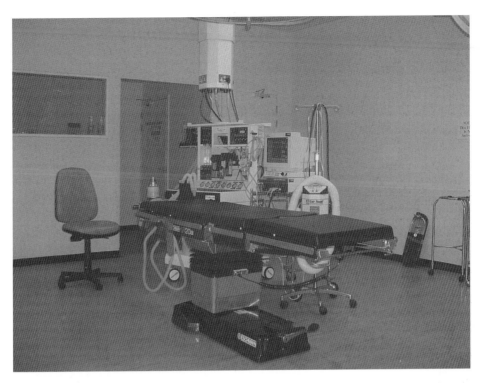

Figure 2.3   The operating theatre.

bacteria and easily cleaned with disinfectant. Joints between the walls and ceiling or floor are curved to limit microbial deposits and promote effective cleaning and drying. As modern anaesthetic gases do not present a risk of explosion, floors are no longer required to be antistatic. Therefore, the most common form of flooring in the operating theatre is now seamless vinyl, which may be cushioned to prevent personnel fatigue (Fortunato, 2000).

In order to minimise the amount of micro-organisms within the operating department, all theatre staff must maintain a high level of personal hygiene, remove jewellery and change into theatre trouser suits before entry into theatre. Hair should be covered with an appropriate theatre hat to prevent the spread of bacteria, in particular *Staphylococcus aureus*, which is commonly found in hair. Theatre footwear is no longer required to be antistatic, although it must cover the toes to prevent injury and should be specific to theatre to prevent contamination. The wearing of facemasks either with or without an attached visor is generally regarded as being for the benefit and safety of the surgical team rather than to prevent the spread of micro-organisms to the patient. However, it is considered prudent to wear a facemask for surgery involving prosthetic implants due to an increased potential for surgical site infection. Although this is still a slightly contentious issue, the wearing of a facemask may lead to an increase in the shedding of *Staphylococcus aureus* from the skin of the face and neck, and it may become saturated with oral and nasal bacteria (Lipp & Edwards, 2002). If facemasks are worn, it is advisable that these are handled by the tapes only and are discarded between cases.

Patients undergoing any form of surgery become vulnerable to infection when barriers such as the skin or mucous membranes are breached by surgical incision during the operative procedure. To minimise the risk of cross-infection and contamination, the theatre environment is controlled to help prevent the accumulation of potentially harmful bacteria and pollutants. Conventional operating theatres are equipped with a humidifying positive air pressure filtering ventilation system, as well as a gas scavenging system, which removes waste anaesthetic gases. The ventilation system regularly changes the air within the operating theatre at a rate of 20–30 changes per hour, and ancillary areas at a slightly reduced rate of 10–15 changes per hour in the 'clean zone' and 5–7 changes per hour in the 'dirty zone'.

This system normally maintains the temperature in theatre between 20°C and 24°C to provide a comfortable working environment for staff. However, this may be adjusted according to the requirements of the patient and the risk of hypothermia. Additionally, the level of humidity in the theatre is controlled. Low levels of humidity promote a dry, statically charged atmosphere that is uncomfortable to work in and potentially dangerous if flammable anaesthetics are used. High levels of humidity result in a 'sticky' atmosphere, which is also uncomfortable and may lead to sterile packs becoming damp, and potential contamination by bacteria. Levels of humidified air are therefore maintained within these two extremes at 50–55% which provides a safe and comfortable environment to work in and suppresses bacterial growth.

The risk of infection increases in the operating theatre according to the amount and movement of micro-organisms present. To minimise this risk, the amount of personnel in theatre should be kept to a minimum, any equipment brought into the theatre should be decontaminated before use and all equipment should be prepared in advance to prevent unnecessary movement. The efficiency of the air conditioning system is compromised each time the theatre doors are opened. Contamination should be minimised by reducing the number of times the doors are opened to the outside. This may be assisted by personnel entering and leaving the operating theatre through the anaesthetic room, which is attached to the theatre and acts as a buffer zone for the air conditioning.

Patient admission to the operating department

During the peri-operative phase the patient is highly dependent upon healthcare professionals functioning as a team. Upon admission to the operating department, all relevant documentation and required information must be present (see Box 2.2). The patient's medical records will be

---

> **Box 2.2**   Checklist of information required for admission to the operating department.
>
> - Patient wristband confirming identity, date of birth, hospital number and any allergies
> - Appropriate consent form
> - Drug/fluid charts
> - Medical/nursing notes
> - X-rays (if applicable)
> - Operative site marked (if applicable)
> - Time of last food/drink
> - Known allergies
> - Relevant medical history, e.g. diabetes
> - Presence of prosthesis/implants
> - Dentures/caps/crowns
> - Jewellery including body piercings should be taped or removed

checked for specific information and where appropriate a verbal confirmation will be encouraged (see Chapter 1 for discussion of pre-operative assessment and preparation).

Once the details have been checked, the patient will be transferred to the anaesthetic room either in their own bed or on a theatre trolley. It is becoming increasingly common practice for acutely ill patients arriving for operative procedures to bypass the anaesthetic room and be transferred straight into the operating theatre.

Physiological monitoring of the surgical patient

Monitoring equipment is attached to the patient in the anaesthetic room. This is considered essential for the safe conduct of anaesthesia irrespective of duration and type of anaesthetic used (Association of Anaesthetists of Great Britain and Ireland (AAGBI), 2002). Routine monitoring devices are described in Table 2.1.

It may be necessary to attach additional invasive monitoring owing to the physiological condition of the patient or the extent and complex nature of the surgical procedure. Regardless of the type of anaesthetic, venous access is required for all patients. This provides a safe and effective route for the administration of drugs and fluid therapy peri-operatively.

Table 2.1   Routine monitoring devices.

Type of monitoring	Purpose
Electrocardiogram (ECG)	To monitor the electrical activity of the heart. This is obtained by placing electrodes in a specific configuration, during anaesthesia the most common is the three-lead called the CM5.
Non-invasive blood pressure	To monitor systolic, diastolic, mean arterial pressures and pulse rate. The correct size cuff must be placed on a limb, for example a standard adult cuff is 12 cm.
Pulse oximetry	To detect changes in the oxygen saturation of haemoglobin. This is obtained by positioning a probe on a finger, toe, ear lobe or nose.
Capnography	To measure carbon dioxide levels in the exhaled end tidal gases. It is very useful for monitoring the adequacy of ventilation in the unconscious patient and confirming correct positioning of an endotracheal tube. It is attached to the patient's breathing system usually via the heat and moisture exchanger humidifier (HME).
Additional monitoring: invasive arterial pressure	This will provide continuous measurement and a greater accuracy of information about the state of the heart and circulation. It is obtained via an arterial cannula inserted into the radial artery (most common), which is attached to a transducer and a continuous infusion of pressurised heparinised saline.
Central venous pressure (CVP)	This indicates the state of circulating volume during anaesthesia, thus allowing assessment and management of fluid therapy. It involves catheter insertion of a large vein such as the internal jugular or subclavian, which is attached to a transducer and an infusion of heparinised saline.
Bi spectral index (BIS)	Depth of anaesthesia has proved difficult to assess for all anaesthetic agents. BIS monitors use a mathematical technique combined with information on EEG power and frequency to record the state of the brain as opposed to the effect of the drug. BIS monitors are used to guide titration of sedatives, analgesics and anaesthetic agents.

The triad of anaesthesia

The triad of anaesthesia is a concept that was developed to describe the three basic requirements of a general anaesthetic – narcosis, analgesia and relaxation (Whelan & Davies, 2000). The aim is to achieve a balanced anaesthetic appropriate for the surgical procedure. This may involve narcosis alone, analgesia alone, a combination of narcosis and analgesia, or a combination of narcosis, analgesia and relaxation (see Figure 2.4).

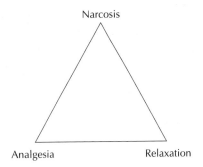

Figure 2.4   The triad of anaesthesia.

Narcosis

Narcosis is the sleep-inducing part of a general anaesthetic. This is usually divided into two parts – induction and maintenance.

Induction

Anaesthesia is induced to produce a state of unconsciousness in which the patient does not perceive or recall stimuli. Usually, but not exclusively, induction of anaesthesia is achieved by intravenous injection, as this route is more predictable, rapid and smooth than other methods (see Table 2.2 for a description of the more commonly used intravenous induction agents). Narcosis is achieved as the drug diffuses from arterial blood across the blood-brain barrier into the brain. Exactly how intravenous anaesthetic agents induce narcosis is not fully understood, since the different agents

Table 2.2 Commonly used intravenous induction agents.

Agent	Properties	Physiological effects
Thiopentone	<ul><li>Barbiturate</li><li>No analgesic properties</li><li>Rapid onset – usually within 1 minute depending upon arm–brain circulation time</li><li>Alkaline solution, therefore irritant especially if injected into tissues</li><li>Usually diluted to 2.5% solution (25 mg/mL)</li><li>Diluted solution is unstable and must be discarded within 24 hours of dilution</li><li>Redistributed into the tissues rapidly – therefore awakening time fairly quick 5–15 minutes</li><li>Slow metabolism up to 24 hours – hangover effect</li><li>Repeated doses have cumulative effect</li><li>Thiopentone overdose is potentially lethal</li></ul>	**Central nervous system** – Anticonvulsant properties make thiopentone suitable for epileptic patients. Decreases in cerebral blood flow, intraocular and intracranial pressure makes thiopentone a useful induction agent for neuro-anaesthesia and head injury patients. **Cardiovascular system** – Cardiac output is often decreased with an accompanying fall in blood pressure and an increase in heart rate. Therefore thiopentone is not the induction agent of choice for patients who are cardiovascularly compromised **Respiratory system** – Following induction, a transient decrease in respiratory rate is common with accompanying apnoea.
Etomidate	<ul><li>Rapid recovery time</li><li>No hangover effect</li><li>High incidence of post-operative nausea and vomiting</li><li>Painful on injection</li><li>Usually 2% (20 mg/mL)</li><li>Repeated dose may impair adrenocortical function</li></ul>	**Central nervous system** – Involuntary muscle movements or tremor are often associated with etomidate during induction. Decreases in cerebral blood flow, intraocular and intracranial pressure are also observed, although to a lesser extent than thiopentone. **Cardiovascular system** – Etomidate causes less hypotension than thiopentone and may therefore be used in patients with a compromised cardiovascular system. **Respiratory system** – A decrease in tidal volume and respiratory rate may be seen to a lesser extent than thiopentone.
Ketamine	<ul><li>Can be given IV or IM</li><li>Good analgesic properties</li><li>Long onset time – longer than arm–brain circulation time</li><li>Muscle tone is increased and upper airway is usually maintained</li><li>Causes hallucinations – although less so in children</li></ul>	**Central nervous system** – Produces a state of dissociative anaesthesia, which is a combination of profound analgesia and superficial sleep (Sasada & Smith, 2003). Cerebral blood flow, intraocular and intracranial pressure all increase. Hallucinogenic effects are the main disadvantage associated with this drug particularly in adults and are more marked if patients are disturbed during the recovery period. **Cardiovascular system** – A stimulatory effect, with increases in heart rate, cardiac output and blood pressure, makes ketamine unsuitable for patients with pre-existing hypertension. **Respiratory system** – Minimal effects, airway reflexes are usually preserved which, combined with the good analgesic properties, makes this a useful anaesthetic agent for off-site 'field' anaesthesia. Ketamine may also be used as a treatment for severe unresponsive asthma.
Propofol	<ul><li>Currently most popular IV induction agent</li><li>May be used for both maintenance of anaesthesia and sedation</li><li>Rapid recovery without hangover</li><li>May cause pain on injection</li><li>Less incidence of post-operative nausea and vomiting (PONV)</li><li>Non-cumulative effect makes this an ideal agent for an infusion technique</li><li>Emulsion contains soya bean oil and egg phosphatide, therefore is contraindicated in patients with egg or soya allergy</li></ul>	**Central nervous system** – Produces a smooth rapid induction with minimal side effects. **Cardiovascular system** – Although heart rate remains largely unchanged, the vasodilatory effect can produce a profound hypotension. **Respiratory system** – Respiratory depression following induction is common and is often preceded by a decrease in tidal volume and increase in respiratory rate.

have no common chemical structure and there is no known reversal agent. However, these agents commonly bind to the cell membranes of excitable cells such as nerve and muscle cells and so may work through an effect on the bi-phospholipid layer of the cell membrane; in particular the cell membrane proteins that regulate action potential within the neurons (Fryer, 2001).

Once asleep, the patient is given a mixture of gases. Oxygen (O_2) is given to the patient for obvious reasons. However, during anaesthetic oxygen is usually delivered as a higher percentage (25–33%) than is present in room air (21%), to ensure that the partial pressure (PaO_2) is more than

adequate for metabolic demands during surgery. In addition to oxygen, nitrous oxide (N_2O), also known as 'laughing gas', is commonly administered. Nitrous oxide acts as an analgesic and may also be used in other departments, commonly as a mixture of 50% oxygen and 50% nitrous oxide, known as Entonox.

Maintenance

This is often achieved by use of an inhalational agent (see Table 2.3 for a description of the more commonly used inhalational anaesthetic agents). Because these inhalational anaesthetic agents are in

Table 2.3 Commonly used inhalational anaesthetic agents.

Physiological effects	**Central nervous system** – All inhalational anaesthetic agents cause some degree of cerebral vasodilation and therefore an increase in both cerebral blood flow and intracranial pressure. **Cardiovascular system** – All inhalational anaesthetic agents affect the cardiovascular system adversely, although the exact mechanism varies from agent to agent. Halothane has the most profound effect and Sevoflurane the least. **Respiratory system** – All inhalational anaesthetic agents cause a dose-related depressed response to hypercarbia and hypoxia. Although tidal volume is often reduced, the respiratory depressant effects of halothane are the least of all the volatile anaesthetic agents.
Halothane	● Fairly smooth induction, non-irritant ● Low incidence of coughing or breath holding ● Low incidence of PONV ● Hepatotoxicity especially in repeated doses – rarely leading to 'halothane hepatitis' ● Cardiovascular depression – may cause bradycardia and hypotension ● Respiratory depression ● Myocardial depression ● May cause cardiac sensitivity to adrenaline resulting in ventricular dysrhythmias ● Some bronchial dilation
Isoflurane	● Slightly less potent than halothane ● Less is metabolised than halothane ● Noxious to inhale – may cause coughing or breath holding unless dose is increased gradually ● Heart rhythm generally stable but rate may rise in younger patients ● Respiratory depression ● Vasodilation causing hypotension ● Muscle relaxant drugs potentiated
Desflurane	● Low potency (about 20% that of isoflurane) ● Not recommended for induction of children because of: ○ Increased incidence of coughing ○ Increased incidence of breath holding ○ Increased incidence of laryngospasm ○ Increased secretions ○ Increased risk of apnoea ● Vaporiser must be pre-warmed by electrical supply
Sevoflurane	● Rapid acting ● Rapid awakening means patients may require post-operative pain relief earlier ● Some agitation observed in children – stage 2 depth of anaesthesia ● Relatively new and therefore expensive

a liquid state, they need to be 'carried' in the form of a vapour by another gas. To achieve this, the oxygen and nitrous oxide are passed over the agent in a specialised device called a vaporiser. This enables the oxygen and nitrous oxide to 'pick up' an adjustable amount of the vapour of the inhalational anaesthetic agent as it evaporates. The amount of vapour required is worked out by a minimum alveolar concentration (MAC) value. This is the percentage of inhalational anaesthetic agent in oxygen that is needed to prevent movement in response to a surgical incision in 50% of the population. The oxygen, nitrous oxide and chosen inhalational anaesthetic agent are 'maintained' throughout the operative procedure in order to keep the patient asleep.

Total intravenous anaesthesia (TIVA) through target-controlled infusions (TCI)

This is an alternative technique for the induction and maintenance of anaesthesia. Using a specialised programmable syringe pump, a continuous infusion of intravenous agent is delivered to provide a target plasma concentration. The microprocessor in the syringe pump incorporates a pharmacokinetic model and a set of parameters for the drug to be infused. Data specific to the patient, such as age and body weight, are fed into the syringe pump before anaesthesia is started. The microprocessor uses this information to select the best set of available pharmacokinetic parameters to calculate the variable infusion rates required to give a predicted blood concentration

in that particular patient. This concentration is maintained until a new target is set. Propofol is particularly well suited to this technique as this agent undergoes a rapid distribution and metabolic clearance.

Analgesia

Analgesics used during general anaesthesia can broadly be divided into three groups:

- Local anaesthetics (LA)
- Opioids
- Non-steroidal anti-inflammatory drugs (NSAIDs)

Local anaesthetics

These drugs are not usually given systemically through an intravenous route, but may be administered in other ways to reversibly prevent or abolish peripheral nerve impulses. The benefit of using this group of drugs as part of a balanced general anaesthetic is that they provide excellent analgesia both during surgery and post-operatively. (See Table 2.4 for a description of the more commonly used local anaesthetic agents.)

Local anaesthetics produce analgesia while consciousness is maintained. By reducing the inward flow of positively charged sodium ions into neurons, the depolarisation of nerve cells needed to generate an electrical nerve impulse is inhibited. The first sensation lost is that of pain, followed by temperature, touch, proprioception and, finally, musculoskeletal tone. The duration of action of

Table 2.4   Commonly used local anaesthetic agents.

Lidocaine (Lignocaine)	• Rapid onset – within 2–20 minutes, duration is dependent on dosage, concentration and degree of vasoconstriction • Has few haemodynamic effects when used in low doses • Can be administered topically, by infiltration or epidurally
Bupivicaine	• Slow onset – up to 30 minutes, duration of action is 5–16 hours • Often used in lumbar epidural blockade • 'Heavy' preparation contains glucose and is the most commonly used local anaesthetic for spinal anaesthesia
Levobupivacaine hydrochloride (Chirocaine)	• Similar to bupivacaine with less cardiovascular toxicity • Increasingly used for local infiltration and peripheral nerve blockade
Cocaine (paste or solution)	• Administered topically to mucous membranes • Use restricted to otolaryngology
Tetracaine/Amethocaine	• Used in ophthalmology in the form of eye drops and skin preparations prior to venepuncture

these drugs depends upon the rate of removal from the site of administration rather than the rate of metabolism. Increasing the dose of the local anaesthetic shortens the onset time and increases the duration of the block. The duration of local anaesthetic action is also affected by the extent of vasodilation at the site of administration. Vasoconstrictors such as adrenaline can be added to local anaesthetics to adjust the amount of vasodilation at the site, quicken the onset time and prolong the extent of the block.

Local anaesthetics may be administered topically, for example, application of cocaine to nasal mucosa can provide vasoconstriction and local anaesthesia prior to nasal surgery. Local anaesthetic eye drops can be used to provide anaesthesia during ophthalmic surgery. A eutectic (easily melted and absorbed) mixture of local anaesthetics (EMLA) preparation can also be used to provide a localised area of anaesthesia on skin, prior to cannulation or skin grafting. Another commonly used method of administering these drugs is a subcuticular injection along the site of the surgical incision. This technique is effective as it prevents pain signals being generated from the numerous nerve endings in the dermis and provides good post-operative pain relief.

Regional block techniques are also used to provide anaesthesia. The extent of the anaesthetised area depends largely on where the nerve supply to the surgical area is blocked. Generally, the nearer to the main nerve trunk the local anaesthetic is injected, the larger the area of anaesthesia will be. For example, if the brachial plexus in the axilla is blocked, the field of anaesthesia will extend throughout the hand and forearm. If the digital nerves supplying one finger are blocked, the field of anaesthesia will only extend to that finger. Other techniques, such as a spinal or epidural anaesthesia, block the nerve signals at the level of the spinal cord and can provide a still wider field of anaesthesia (see Chapter 4). Unfortunately, local anaesthetic agents have drawbacks. Regional techniques in particular can be difficult to administer and vasodilatory effects can cause a marked drop in blood pressure.

Opioids

Opioids modulate the pain signals that are generated by acting on specific receptors in the brain and spinal column concerned with the sensation of pain. This group of drugs raise the pain threshold and reduce the psychological and emotional components of pain. These effects are associated with a dose-related euphoria, which may lead to drowsiness and eventually sleep.

Despite the ability to induce sleep, intravenous opioids are given as a part of a balanced general anaesthetic to provide peri-operative analgesia, not as induction agents. However, these drugs do reduce the minimum alveolar concentration (MAC) requirement of inhalational anaesthetic agents and can also help stabilise the cardiovascular system following the stimulation of endotracheal intubation. Opioids are used for moderate to severe peri- and post-operative pain management, with morphine being considered the 'gold standard'. Morphine provides good analgesia for all types of pain, but is particularly effective at treating dull, throbbing pain such as post-operative pain or pain associated with major trauma (see Table 2.5 for a description of opioids commonly used peri-operatively). The advantage of using these drugs to provide peri-operative analgesia is that they are easily administered and provide adequate pain relief for a relatively long period of time (up to four hours).

Undesired complications of opioid administration include varying degrees of respiratory depression, although this may be reversed with an opioid antagonist such as naloxone. Post-operative nausea and vomiting (PONV) is a potential side-effect and can lead to further complications, such as wound breakdown, increased pain and a delayed recovery time. The neurological effects of opioids can lead to a delayed post-operative recovery time and, in the long term, these drugs can cause dependence.

Non-steroidal anti-inflammatory drugs (NSAIDs)

NSAIDs suppress inflammatory pain by preventing the formation of prostaglandins that are released as a result of cell damage. Prostaglandins are naturally occurring chemicals associated with the inflammation, redness and swelling of tissues at the site of injury. The release of prostaglandins increases the sensitivity of pain receptors to other stimuli and decreases the threshold needed to generate an action potential to send pain signals. NSAIDs have become an increasingly useful

Table 2.5   Opioids commonly used peri-operatively.

Morphine	• The gold standard opioid
	• May be administered via intravenous, intramuscular, oral, rectal, subcutaneous or intrathecal routes
	• Analgesia lasts up to 4 hours
	• Can cause histamine release
	• May cause hypotension, particularly in cardiovascularly compromised patients
	• Can cause delayed respiratory depression, particularly if used intrathecally
	• Continued use can lead to dependence
Pethidine	• More rapid onset than morphine
	• May be administered via intravenous, intramuscular or oral routes
	• Duration 2–3 hours
	• Less potent than morphine
	• Respiratory depressant, although less so than morphine
	• When used as an analgesic during labour, pethidine causes less respiratory depression in the newborn than morphine
Fentanyl	• More rapid onset than morphine
	• May be administered via intravenous, transdermal or epidural routes
	• Potent but short duration of analgesia via intravenous route of 30–60 minutes, limits usefulness of fentanyl to peri-operative setting
	• Cumulative effect of repeated intravenous doses
	• Transdermal fentanyl 'patches' are becoming more common in the treatment of chronic pain
	• Cardiovascular depressant, particularly causing bradycardia
	• Potent respiratory depressant
Alfentanil	• Very rapid onset of action, within 90 seconds
	• Administered via intravenous route
	• Very potent action but short duration of 5–10 minutes makes alfentanil suited for use in a continuous infusion in the peri-operative setting
	• Some cardiovascular depression, due to bradycardia
	• Potent respiratory depression
	• Limited hypnotic or sedative effect

Both fentanyl and alfentanyl are used primarily in the operating theatre because they are of short duration and high potency. This means that they provide a good analgesia during surgery but have worn off by the post-operative period.

alternative to opiates for both peri-operative and post-operative analgesia. They do not depress respiration or circulation, cause post-operative nausea and vomiting or lead to dependence. However, on their own, NSAIDs may not be adequate for the relief of severe pain. For this reason, they are often given in conjunction with opioids (see Chapter 4 for a further discussion of the use of NSAIDs post-operatively).

Relaxation

The passage of an impulse down a nerve fibre is an electrical one, as is the spread of an impulse across a muscle fibre. However, the transmission of an impulse from the nerve fibre across a synapse to the muscle fibre is chemical. This occurs at the neuromuscular junction, an area between the nerve fibres. As the electrical impulse reaches the pre-synaptic area it triggers the release of synaptic vesicles, containing acetylcholine. This chemical travels across the synapse and arrives at special receptor sites. The arrival of enough acetylcholine on these receptors triggers a rapid electrical depolarisation in the muscle, which results in contraction. This effect is rapidly reversed by the enzyme cholinesterase, which is present at the motor end plate.

Muscle relaxants are a group of chemicals that block the transmission of signals at the neuromuscular junction, thereby preventing the contraction of muscle fibres, and should not be confused with neurological relaxants. Muscle relaxant drugs may be used to enable surgical access, endotracheal intubation or mechanical ventilation. They are only administered to an unconscious patient and can

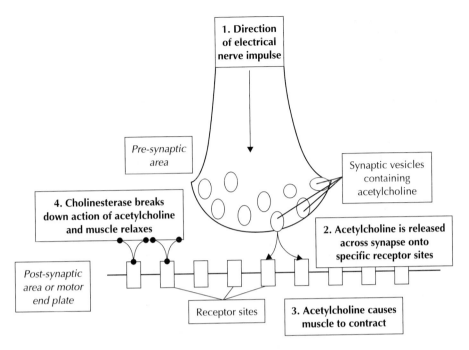

Figure 2.5   The neuromuscular junction.

be divided into two groups, depolarising and non-depolarising muscle relaxants:

Depolarising muscle relaxants

There is only one drug of note in this group: suxamethonium chloride. Agents of this group produce relaxation at the post-synaptic membrane in a similar way to acetylcholine (see Figure 2.5). However, once relaxation is produced, it is maintained, thus negating the effect of further acetylcholine release.

Non-depolarising muscle relaxants

Drugs of this type include all of the other muscle relaxants. Non-depolarising muscle relaxants attach themselves to the receptor sites on the post-synaptic membrane to which acetylcholine normally attaches. Acetylcholine is thus prevented from reaching the end plate in sufficient quantity to produce depolarisation. Although these muscle relaxants will be eventually broken down by metabolism or degradation, they may also be reversed by administering intravenous neostigmine. However, neostigmine has unwanted side-effects, including bradycardia and stimulation of bronchial and salivary secretory glands. These effects may be overcome by concurrently administering atropine or glycopyrronium.

Airway management of the anaesthetised patient

Respiratory depression, often with an accompanying period of transient apnoea, is a common side-effect of general anaesthesia. In order to treat this complication, the patient's airway is managed to ensure patency and to allow administration of anaesthetic gases required to maintain anaesthesia. Airway management devices used to assist in this vary in their degree of invasiveness (see Figure 2.6). The simplest method is simply to support the patient's airway in the 'sniffing the morning air' position by tilting the head back and lifting the lower jaw forward. A facemask is then placed over the patient's mouth and nose to deliver the anaesthetic gases. This method may be further aided by the use of either an oropharyngeal or nasopharyngeal airway to prevent the tongue from causing an obstruction.

A laryngeal mask is an anatomically shaped airway that consists of a silicone mask with inflatable

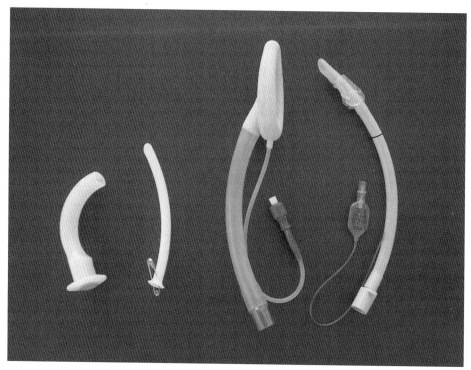

Figure 2.6   Airway management devices.
Left to right: oropharyngeal airway (Guedel type), nasopharyngeal airway, laryngeal mask, endotracheal tube.

cuff and connecting tube. It is inserted blindly through the patient's mouth into the pharynx where the cuff is inflated to form a low-pressure seal around the laryngeal opening. Laryngeal masks sit on the larynx and hold the airway open, but do not protect against aspiration of gastric contents.

Pre-operative fasting is considered essential prior to a general anaesthetic to reduce the risk of vomiting and regurgitation leading to a possible aspiration of gastric contents (Beesley & Pirie, 2004). Aspiration of gastric contents is a rare but potentially disastrous complication for patients, occurring in 3–5 per 10 000 anaesthetics (Thorne *et al.*, 2005). However, despite this potential complication, there are instances when it is inappropriate to follow a pre-operative fasting regime, such as the non-elective trauma or emergency situation. There is the additional complication of delayed gastric emptying in these patients, which increases the risk of vomiting and regurgitation.

Endotracheal tubes (ETTs) provide a more invasive method of airway management that also secures against the risk of aspiration of gastric contents.

ETTs come in a variety of shapes and designs, with or without a cuff, and may be inserted either orally or nasally. Adult ETTs are usually cuffed, whereas paediatric ETTs are usually uncuffed. This difference reflects the anatomical differences between the adult larynx, which is narrowest at the glottis, and the paediatric larynx, which is narrowest at the level of the cricoid cartilage.

ETTs are inserted through the larynx into the trachea under direct vision during laryngoscopy. The tip of the endotracheal tube is passed through the vocal cords to a predetermined point marked on the tube and once in position, the cuff is inflated to the point where no gas leak is audible on positive pressure ventilation. This provides an airtight seal between the cuff and the tracheal wall to protect against aspiration of gastric contents. Once in situ, the ETT is securely tied or taped in place.

A rapid sequence induction is required for those patients who, despite a fasting period, are considered to be at risk of regurgitation. This may be due to a non-elective trauma or emergency situation, or as a result of pregnancy, obesity, hiatus hernia or gastric reflux. The term 'rapid sequence' relates to the amount of time between the onset of the induction agent, muscle relaxation and intubation. This technique begins with pre-oxygenation of the awake patient in order to achieve the maximum possible oxygen saturation prior to anaesthetic induction. The induction agent is rapidly followed by administration of a muscle relaxant, normally suxamethonium chloride, due to its fast onset and short duration of action. As the patient loses consciousness, pressure is applied by pressing either two or three fingers against the cricoid cartilage. This manoeuvre is thought to compress the oesophagus between the ring of cricoid cartilage and the cervical vertebrae to prevent regurgitation of gastric contents. Pressure is maintained until the endotracheal tube has been passed and the cuff inflated to secure the airway.

Transfer and positioning of the patient

Transfer to the operating table usually follows the anaesthetic procedure in an anaesthetic room. However, in emergency situations or patients arriving from the Intensive Care Unit (ICU), transfer will be immediate and it is important that all members of the peri-operative team have the necessary training to transfer all patients safely.

Those patients who are acutely ill will have invasive central venous and arterial pressure monitoring as well as other intravenous infusions. If the patient has been transferred from the ICU, there may also a portable ventilator, infusion pumps and the standard monitoring devices such as electrocardiogram (ECG) and oxygen saturation. These patients often have a urinary catheter in situ and chest or abdominal drains may possibly be present. In order to ensure the comfort, dignity and safety of the patient transfer from a bed or trolley requires careful co-ordination by the peri-operative team (Beesley & Pirie, 2004).

Patient positioning

Positioning should ensure optimal surgical access without compromising homeostasis or causing injury to soft tissues and the musculoskeletal system. The surgical procedure will dictate the position required and as there are several variations of patient position, only a selection of the most commonly used will be discussed in this chapter. Although the anaesthetist will usually be in charge of the co-ordinated transfer, the surgeon is ultimately responsible for the safety of the patient and will often take an active role in patient positioning. It is important that practitioners have a thorough understanding of the physiological implications of patient positioning (Beesley & Pirie, 2004).

The anaesthetised patient is also at risk from soft tissue and musculoskeletal injury because they cannot adjust their position in response to discomfort or pain. The majority of nerve injuries seen in the immediate post-operative period are caused by short-term compression and/or traction. Fortunately, these are quite rare. However, any pain, numbness, lack of motor control or other unexpected sensations should be investigated. Different positions require specific considerations and some of these are now described further.

Supine position

This position is the standard for most surgical procedures such as appendicectomy, mastectomy or laparotomy. The patient will be flat on their back with arms usually to the side; however, sometimes an arm board is used to allow IV access. It is important to maintain alignment of the hips and spinal column. Extra padding and support is usually required for specific pressure areas such as elbows, knees, sacrum, heels, greater trochanter of the femur and occiput. Potential effects are:

- *Cardiovascular* – This is already affected by the anaesthetic and hypotension is common. This is particularly important in pregnant patients who are prone to aorto-caval compression by the gravid uterus. For this reason a 20-degree lateral tilt is applied to the supine position. Compression of a blood vessel against a bony structure will compromise blood flow in any position, thus care must be taken not to hyperextend limbs or apply excessive restraints. Venous stasis or ischaemia could result.
- *Respiratory* – Dependent lung regions are better perfused and ventilated. However, functional residual capacity (FRC), which is the air remaining in the lungs after normal expiration, is reduced by about 20% in the supine patient and

this is reduced by a further 20% with anaesthesia and ventilation (Malan & McIndoe, 2003).

- *Nerve injury* – This is due to direct trauma, compression and overstretching. Several types of nerves are at risk through inappropriate patient positioning. The most common injury is to the ulnar nerve and is a result of proximation of the nerve to the elbow joint. The radial nerve can also be affected and the usual cause is compression against the edge of the operating table, which

can occur in all positions. The preventive measure is to supinate the arm, lifting the ulnar nerve away from the table edge. Brachial plexus nerve injury is the result of stretching when the arm is abducted greater than 90 degrees, this may occur when using an arm board attachment for surgical or venous access. Ensuring that the shoulder is not hyperextended further than 90 degrees and supinating the arm on the arm board will prevent injury (see Figure 2.7 for nerve location.)

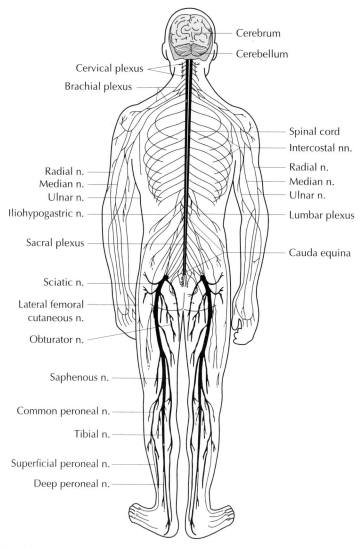

Figure 2.7   Nerve location diagram.
The central and peripheral divisions of the nervous system. The central nervous system consists of the brain and spinal cord. The peripheral nervous system is composed of the cranial and spinal nerves.
(reprinted from *Medical Surgical Nursing* (7th edn) Phipps *et al.*, p. 1300, ©2003, with permission from Elsevier)

Prone position

This position is used for surgery involving the posterior surface of the body such as spinal surgery, lower extremities such as buttocks, heels and also neurosurgery. Initially, the patient is anaesthetised in the supine position and once the airway is secured the patient will be rolled on to his or her abdomen from the bed or trolley to the operating table. This requires a well co-ordinated and safe team manoeuvre to ensure that the endotracheal tube and any intravenous lines are not dislodged. Preparation of the operating table includes a cushioned horseshoe support for the face to maintain alignment of the cervical spine; pillows or a preformed support will be used for the thorax and pelvis; and protection for the feet is also necessary. The arms are usually rotated and with elbows bent, positioned next to the patient's head on a large padded arm board. It is important to move the arms simultaneously and symmetrically with no more than a 90-degree flexion or abduction. Specific areas to be protected are the face and eyes, shoulders, breasts, genitalia, patella and toes. Prolonged prone positioning may lead to oedema and swelling of the face and upper airway (Malan & McIndoe, 2003). Potential effects are:

- *Cardiovascular* – Effects are few but pressure on the inferior vena cava and femoral veins can reduce venous return which in turn will affect the blood pressure. This is usually due to incorrect positioning.
- *Respiratory* – Although dependent lung regions are better perfused and ventilated and FRC is usually maintained, there is the risk of increased abdominal pressure owing to body weight against the abdominal wall. This will impair diaphragmatic movement and may increase airway pressure, making ventilation difficult. There is also the risk of passive regurgitation.
- *Nerve injury* – Examples include the lateral cutaneous nerve of the thigh due to pressure against the anterior-superior iliac spine and the cervical spinal cord as a result of overextension of the neck. The brachial plexus and ulnar nerve can also be affected for the same reasons as in the supine position. Gel pads, extra padded and preformed supports should be used to prevent the possibility of these nerve injuries.

Lithotomy position

This position is used in urological procedures, gynaecological procedures involving the perineum and surgery of the lower gastrointestinal system involving the rectum and anal region. Initially the patient is placed in the supine position; the patient's buttocks will be aligned with the break in the operating table at the level of the lithotomy poles and the hips and knees flexed to allow the thighs and legs to be placed into stirrups. Simultaneous movement when flexing the knees is important to avoid straining the patient's lower back. Flexion of more than 90 degrees of the knees and hips may cause injury to the sciatic, femoral and obturator nerves. Buttocks must not overhang the edge of the table and legs are usually placed on the outside of the lithotomy poles to protect the common perineal nerve. The ankles and feet are supported by straps on the lithotomy poles. Alternatively, gas-assisted lithotomy stirrups allow for the same positioning but the legs and feet are enclosed within a boot. Arms are usually placed either on the abdomen or on an arm board. If this is not possible, measures must be taken to ensure protection of the hands. Potential effects are:

- *Cardiovascular* – There can be circulatory pooling in the lumbar region from this position. There is the potential for compression of abdominal contents on the inferior vena cava and abdominal aorta, which will compromise circulation. Both of these effects can lead to a reduced venous return, affecting cardiac output. As with all positions there is the consequence of postural hypotension and the redistribution of blood volume. Rapid changes in position may cause sudden hypotension, for example, if the legs are lowered quickly from the lithotomy poles. A head-down tilt may be required for certain procedures. If this is for a prolonged time it can cause oedema of the head and neck and increased venous return and preload, which may precipitate acute heart failure in patients with poor cardiac reserve (Malan & McIndoe, 2003).
- *Respiratory* – There may be reduced respiratory efficiency due to pressure from the raised thigh area onto the abdomen and pressure from the diaphragm on abdominal viscera causing a restriction on breathing.

- *Nerve injury* – Several nerves may be affected in this position and they are femoral, due to hips being flexed against the abdomen; obturator, due to compression at the obturator foramen when there is full flexion of the hips; sciatic, from stretching between neck of fibula and sciatic notch when hips are flexed and thighs abducted; common peroneal, from pressure against the head of the fibula; saphenous, resulting from compression against the medial tibial condyle and tibial nerve due to pressure against the stirrups. The cervical spine can also be affected and must be protected in all surgical positions.

Peri-operative fluid management

Irrespective of the surgery, there is usually a disruption to the normal fluid balance of the patient owing to the required restriction on oral fluids prior to anaesthesia. The impact on individual patients depends upon medical status, surgical procedure and type of anaesthetic. Pre-operative assessment should identify the fluid status of each patient with specific information being documented, such as fasting time, intravenous infusions, vomiting or diarrhoea, bleeding, and medication such as diuretics. Knowledge of the operative procedure and the potential effect on fluid and electrolyte balance and ability of the patient to cope with any deficits must also be considered when deciding on a fluid therapy regimen. Clinical condition and pre-existing diseases such as renal or hepatic failure will increase the potential for fluid and electrolyte imbalances; as will gastrointestinal surgical procedures where an excessive loss of intestinal fluid may result in low sodium and potassium levels. Where possible, patients with a deficit should have had fluid and electrolyte resuscitation pre-operatively, as this will improve their condition and enhance their ability to cope with the surgical procedure. The aim of fluid replacement is to adjust imbalances approximately and thus allow the body to respond homeostatically.

It is not always necessary to administer intravenous fluid to the peri-operative patient, but factors contributing to an inevitable loss of fluid are usually in excess of normal physiological losses. Local policy for pre-operative fasting will usually allow patients to have clear fluids until two hours before surgery. However, the timing of this is both variable and ritualistic in practice (Oshodi, 2004). This means that some patients may have endured far more than the required two hours without fluids. This practice, combined with the additional fluid losses incurred as a result of surgery and anaesthesia, means that the majority of surgical patients will require replacement fluids. If the patient is critically ill, then overall losses will be greater and replacement of fluids will be larger, so a central venous line and central venous pressure monitoring will be used.

Fluid losses

Third space losses

These are a common reason for replacement fluids in major surgery, where there may be tissue trauma, inflammation or infection. Sequestration of fluids into a potential space is called 'third spacing' and is associated with a loss of sodium-rich fluid and water from the interstitial space affecting plasma volumes (Knighton & Smith, 2003). This fluid is not lost from the body but is unavailable for use and will expand the extracellular fluid (ECF) volume; ultimately this leakage may lead to circulatory hypovolaemia. These losses are not preventable but can be treated by maintaining the circulating volume with isotonic fluids or colloids. Major bowel surgery is a procedure for which large fluid loss is expected and may be as much as 8–10 mL/kg/hour, therefore requiring adequate fluid replacement both during and after surgery (Knighton & Smith, 2003). Third space fluid loss will usually return to the circulation around the second to third day post-operatively.

Additional fluid losses

Though predictable, these will vary according to the procedure, degree of evaporation and redistribution of fluid. This may be due to nasogastric tubes, surgical site drainage, diarrhoea, vomiting, excessive sweating and urine output. Measurement of fluid loss via tubes, drains, swabs and catheter bags is usually accurate but losses from a pyrexial patient who is sweating excessively or the patient who has ascites is based on estimation. The principle for replacement of fluids is to return that which has been lost. However, understanding volume, electrolyte concentration and which compartment is affected is important for effective peri-operative care of surgical patients.

Effect of anaesthesia on fluid balance

General and regional anaesthesia decrease blood pressure. Vasodilation or myocardial depression and a reduced sympathetic tone are contributing factors and thus vasopressors and intravenous fluids are used to minimise their effects (Thornberry, 2002). Surgical stimulus can sometimes correct a reduced blood pressure, but mechanical ventilation can increase evaporative loss if gases are not adequately humidified.

Blood loss

Reduced blood volume results in reduced venous return and cardiac output. Blood loss can be measured by recording the contents of suction bottles and weighing swabs. However, accuracy is not possible for estimated blood losses such as spillage onto surgical drapes and the floor. Massive unaccountable blood loss may necessitate assessment of the patient's condition by monitoring the physiological signs and symptoms. For example, in a 70 kg male patient with a 30% blood volume deficit, the signs and symptoms are tachycardia of more than 120 beats/minute; moderate hypotension; tachypnoea; cool, clammy and pale appearance and oliguria. In the conscious patient, aggression and anxiety

might also be present (Thornberry, 2002). These patients will require continuous direct blood pressure monitoring and will have an arterial line inserted; this will also facilitate blood gas sampling. Central venous pressure (CVP) measurement is useful for indicating falling blood volumes and a CVP line will also facilitate administration of fluids including blood. Haemoglobin and haematocrit levels will also be closely monitored. Table 2.6 discusses commonly used peri-operative fluids.

Blood transfusion

In procedures such as tonsillectomy, where blood is not routinely required but there is the potential for loss, a specimen of blood will have been collected to establish the blood group and an aliquot saved in case subsequent cross-matching is required. Anticipated blood loss is usually based on factors such as surgical procedure and pre-operative condition of the patient; thus cross-matching blood would be a standard procedure for an aortic aneurysm repair. Emergency requests for blood may occur when there is unexpected acute or severe loss and it is also important to note that, for a transfusion to be of any benefit to the patient, surgical control of bleeding is imperative, especially where there is massive blood loss.

It is preferred that transfusion is limited to unavoidable situations as there are inherent risks; where possible, alternative methods such as pre-operative autologous donation (PAD) are becoming normal practice. Indications for transfusing the surgical patient are usually because it has become

Table 2.6   Commonly used peri-operative fluids.

Normal saline or 0.9% saline (crystalloid)	Initially distributed into the intravascular compartment then disperses throughout the ECF. It is used to replace third space loss, blood loss and any additional losses and is considered isotonic with plasma.
Hartmann's solution (crystalloid)	Initially distributed into plasma but will disperse into ECF. It has an electrolyte content very similar to ECF so is considered suitable for general fluid replacement.
Dextrose solution (crystalloid)	Initially distributed into the intravascular compartment and then it rapidly disperses through all body compartments. It is used to replace intracellular and extracellular water depletion and in the treatment of hypoglycaemia.
Dextran solution (colloid)	Dextran 70 is used for immediate short-term plasma volume replacement in haemorrhage and burns. A 500 mL infusion will increase the plasma volume by approximately 750 mL.
Gelatins (colloid)	Plasma volume expanders replacing intravascular losses, Haemaccel® and Gelofusine® are considered better than a crystalloid but not as effective as albumin.

necessary to increase the oxygen-carrying capacity of red cells and thus haemoglobin (Hb) concentration. It is generally accepted that an Hb of less than 7 g/dL is a good indicator for transfusion. Red cells, platelets and fresh frozen plasma are some of the products derived from whole blood that are used for transfusion purposes. Transfusion checking procedures must be undertaken when blood administration is required to ensure correct patient identification and compatibility of blood to be infused. All fluids administered must be recorded.

Peri-operative temperature management

Normal thermoregulation is inhibited during anaesthesia and surgery, affecting the ability of the hypothalamus to regulate the body's temperature. All peri-operative patients are potentially at risk of inadvertent hypothermia. The definition of peri-operative hypothermia is a core temperature of less than 36°C. There are three categories of hypothermia: mild (32–35°C), moderate (30–32°C) and severe (below 30°C). The main causes are general or regional anaesthesia, low ambient temperature, the nature of the surgical procedure and cold fluid administration. Patients most likely to develop hypothermia include those patients who are debilitated, have a small body mass or have an impaired metabolic rate or circulatory system. Although there is debate about age, this has also been identified as a contributing factor. Older and particularly frail patients undergoing surgery are more at risk due to a lack of insulation from adipose tissue and a reduced basal metabolic rate affecting their ability to generate heat (Parker, 2004). Box 2.3 explains the ways in which heat is transferred from the patient's body.

The consequences of peri-operative hypothermia are considerable and there are several adverse effects for the surgical patient. Anaesthesia can affect body temperature through inhibition of the autonomic system by anaesthetic agents. Although the hypothalamus regulates body temperature, the ability to maintain and respond to temperature change is depressed under anaesthesia. Vasoconstriction and shivering are natural responses to cold, but inhalational anaesthetic agents will cause vasodilation and muscle relaxants will prevent shivering. Eventually the patient will

---

Box 2.3   Ways in which heat is transferred from the patient's body.

Radiation – from the patient's body to the colder environment, i.e. walls, ceiling, floor in the form of radiant energy and contributes to the greatest proportion of heat loss
Convection – loss of heat as cold air moves over the patient's body, absorbing heat, and out through the ventilation system
Conduction – transfer of heat from the patient to an inanimate object such as the operating table or via unwarmed fluids
Evaporation – heat loss from body surfaces and open body cavities

---

lose heat through redistribution as blood flows freely to the periphery and this is followed by further heat loss in any one of the four previously mentioned transfer methods. Thermoregulatory responses may not activate until approximately 3–4 hours after anaesthesia (Deacock & Holdcroft, 1997). Patients who have undergone a local anaesthetic regional block procedure will often feel warm due to incorrect perceptions of the thermoreceptors in the nerve block area. However, there is also impairment of shivering and vasoconstriction, so that hypothermia may go undetected. Patients recovering from anaesthesia may shiver excessively either due to the anaesthetic agents or from heat loss. Irrespective of the cause, apart from the discomfort to the patient it increases oxygen consumption by 400–500% above basal requirements (Bernthal, 1999). Increased oxygen demand will impact on the cardiovascular system and could be detrimental to patients with impaired cardiac reserves as the extra effort required may induce cardiac arrhythmias.

Hypothermia alters drug metabolism and results in prolonged duration of action, which delays recovery from the anaesthetic. This is due to poor perfusion of the liver, brain and kidneys. Coagulopathy is another adverse effect of hypothermia. In particular, decreased clotting and reduced platelet functions will cause increased blood loss. There can be an increase in wound breakdown and infection due to reduced tissue perfusion. A core temperature of 2°C below normal can triple the incidence of infection and this will prolong a hospital stay by 20% (Sessler, 2001).

Unnecessary exposure of the patient is avoided until surgical access is required and then the blanket can be folded to expose only the surgical site. Current modalities commonly used for warming include forced warm air systems; fluid heating systems for intravenous fluids and blood; heat moisture exchangers (HMEs), which humidify anaesthetic gases; warming cabinets for irrigation fluids and blankets; and thermal drapes. While heat loss is inevitable, using one or more of these measures will contribute to both prevention and a reduction in the amount of heat lost (McNeil, 1998).

Immediate post-operative care

Following surgery, patients are transferred to the post-anaesthetic care unit (PACU) or 'recovery'. Supplementary oxygen is administered to all transfer patients and it is the anaesthetist's responsibility to hand over care of the patient to a qualified recovery practitioner (AAGBI, 2002), although it is standard practice for the scrub practitioner or a member of the surgical team to accompany the patient and contribute to the handover of care. Regardless of the anaesthetic technique, once admitted to recovery, the patient's clinical condition and vital signs will be closely monitored until sufficient physiological stability has occurred to allow transfer to a lower dependency setting. Immediate post-operative care will be on an individual basis until the patient can be safely transferred. The critically ill patient may have to remain in the recovery area until they can be transferred to either a high dependency or intensive care unit. Box 2.4 lists the clinical observations that should be recorded.

Airway management is extremely important during the immediate post-anaesthetic phase of recovery and the recovery practitioner must assess the airway for possible obstruction to determine whether the patient can protect his or her own airway. Inadequate oxygenation of the tissues may lead to hypoxia and maintenance of the cardiorespiratory system is vital. Upper airway obstruction is one of the most common complications in the post-anaesthetic patient (Yates, 2000). This is largely due to a loss of muscle tone, resulting in the tongue falling back and obstructing the pharynx. There may also be excessive secretions such as

> **Box 2.4**   Recommended clinical observations to be recorded.
>
> - Level of consciousness
> - Haemoglobin oxygen saturation and oxygen administration
> - Blood pressure
> - Respiratory rate and depth
> - Heart rate and rhythm
> - Pain intensity
> - Intravenous infusions
> - Drugs administered
> - Temperature, urinary output, CVP, end-tidal carbon dioxide, surgical drainage – these are dependent on circumstances

blood or saliva and an increased risk of vomiting. Laryngospasm is one example of a common cause of airway obstruction in patients such as children, smokers and asthmatics, and occurs when the vocal cords are irritated by insertion of an airway in a semi-conscious patient, excessive secretions, or during extubation (Tuckey, 2000). Other potential complications include hypoventilation due to an opiate-induced respiratory depression; inadequate reversal of a muscle relaxant; or restricted respiration caused by pain. It has become common practice for patients to be handed over to the recovery practitioner with a laryngeal mask airway in situ, which will require removal once the patient is conscious. Assessment for appropriate removal will be the task of the recovery practitioner and as this type of airway does not protect the patient from aspiration, careful observation is necessary while it remains in situ.

The patient's cardiovascular status may be affected by any number of factors, including hypoxia and hypothermia. Hypertension is common and causes include pain, pre-existing hypertension, hypervolaemia and even a full bladder! Alternatively, hypotension may be caused by epidural or spinal anaesthesia, reduced preload due to blood loss or third space loss, residual effects of anaesthetic drugs or cardiac arrhythmias. Prompt and accurate recognition of the causes will facilitate appropriate treatment.

It is normal practice for the anaesthetist to prescribe pain relief, anti-emetics, oxygen and fluid therapy. Effective management of pain and post-operative nausea and vomiting (PONV) is an important aspect of post-anaesthetic care. Patients should not be returned to the ward until both pain and emesis have been controlled as much as is possible (AAGBI, 2002; Beesley & Pirie, 2004) (see Chapters 3 and 4). Anaesthesia and surgery may compromise the cardiovascular and respiratory systems, so it is necessary to use higher inspired oxygen percentages to maintain adequate oxygenation (Maguire, 2000). Every patient will receive oxygen in the recovery area and this is usually via a Hudson multivent mask, nasal cannulae or a T-piece, depending on the method of airway management. As discussed earlier, fluid loss is expected and post-operative fluid management is guided by pre- and peri-operative loss. Further losses may occur from surgical drains or continuous irrigation as required in some urological surgery. See Chapter 3 for more information on surgical drains.

Specific criteria for discharge from recovery must be fulfilled; if the patient does not fulfil the criteria or there have been difficulties with the recovery, the anaesthetist will usually assess the situation and make the decision as to whether discharge is appropriate. A scoring system is used by many recovery units for assessing and monitoring patients and used as the basis for a safe discharge. Handover of the patient to ward staff will include all peri-operative care documentation relating to the anaesthetic, surgical and recovery phases. Further instructions for post-operative care will include oxygen therapy, pain relief and fluid therapy requirements.

Self-test questions

Circle the correct answer(s).

1. The ventilation system in an operating theatre regularly changes the air at a rate of:
   a. 10–20 changes per hour
   b. 20–30 changes per hour
   c. 40–50 changes per hour
   d. 50–60 changes per hour
2. High levels of humidity in an operating theatre will result in:
   a. A dry statically charged atmosphere
   b. Potential contamination of sterile packs
   c. Increased risk of hypothermia
   d. Suppressed bacterial growth
3. The triad of anaesthesia is comprised of:
   a. Narcosis, analgesia and relaxation
   b. Induction, maintenance and relaxation
   c. Anaesthesia, analgesia and anti-emetic
   d. Oxygen, nitrous oxide and isoflurane
4. Which of the following analgesics works by preventing formation of prostaglandins?
   a. Opiates
   b. Local anaesthetics
   c. NSAIDs
   d. Nitrous oxide
5. Which of the following airway management devices protects against aspiration of gastric contents?
   a. Guedel airway
   b. Nasopharyngeal airway
   c. Laryngeal mask airway
   d. Endotracheal tube
6. In a supine position, which nerve may become injured by abducting the arm greater than 90 degrees on an arm board?
   a. Ulnar nerve
   b. Radial nerve
   c. Brachial plexus nerve
   d. Sciatic nerve
7. Peri-operative hypothermia is defined as a core temperature below which level?
   a. 34°C
   b. 35°C
   c. 36°C
   d. 37°C
8. Thermoregulatory responses may not activate until how long after anaesthesia?
   a. 1–2 hours
   b. 2–3 hours
   c. 3–4 hours
   d. 4–5 hours
9. Whose responsibility is it to hand over care of the patient to the recovery practitioner?
   a. Scrub practitioner
   b. Surgeon
   c. Circulating practitioner
   d. Anaesthetist
10. The most common complication following a general anaesthetic is:
    a. Hypothermia
    b. Hallucinations
    c. Vomiting
    d. Upper airway obstruction

References and further reading

Association of Anaesthetists of Great Britain and Ireland (2002) *Immediate Post Anaesthetic Recovery*. London: AAGBI

Beesley J & Pirie S (eds) (2004) *NATN Standards and Recommendations for Safe Peri-operative Practice*. Harrogate: NATN

Bernthal EMM (1999) 'Inadvertent hypothermia prevention; the anaesthetic nurse's role' *British Journal of Nursing* 8(1): 17–25

Deacock S & Holdcroft A (1997) 'Heat retention using passive systems during anaesthesia: comparison of two plastic wraps; one with reflective properties' *British Journal of Anaesthesia* 79(6): 766–769

Fryer M (2001) 'Intravenous induction agents' *Anaesthesia and Intensive Care Medicine* 2(7): 277–281

Fortunato N (2000) *Berry and Kohn's Operating Room Technique*. London: Mosby

Green D, Ervine M & White S (2003) *Fundamentals of Peri-operative Management*. London: Greenwich Medical Media

Knighton J & Smith GB (2003) 'Peri-operative fluid therapy' *Anaesthesia and Intensive Care Medicine* 4(10): 324–326

Lipp A & Edwards P (2002) 'Disposable surgical face masks: a systematic review' *Journal of Advanced Peri-operative Care* 1(2): 41–46

Malan T & McIndoe AK (2003) 'Positioning the surgical patient' *Anaesthesia and Intensive Care Medicine* 4(11): 360–363

Maguire M (2000) 'The recovery of patients from anaesthesia and surgery' *in*: Davey A & Ince CS (eds) *Fundamentals of Operating Department Practice*. London: Greenwich Medical Media

McNeil B (1998) 'Addressing the problems of inadvertent hypothermia in surgical patients' *British Journal of Theatre Nursing* 8(5): 25–33

Oshodi TO (2004) 'Clinical skills: an evidence-based approach to pre-operative fasting' *British Journal of Nursing* 13(16): 958–962

Parker A (2004) 'Principles of surgical practice' *in*: Radford M, County B & Oakley M (eds) *Advancing Peri-operative Practice*. London: Nelson Thornes

Phipps WJ, Monahan F, Donovan Sands JK, Marek JF & Neighbours M (2003) *Medical-Surgical Nursing: Health and Illness Perspectives*. London: Elsevier

Sasada M & Smith S (2003) *Drugs in Anaesthesia and Intensive care* (3rd edn). Oxford: Oxford Medical Publications

Sessler DI (2001) 'Complications and treatment of mild hypothermia' *Anaesthesiology* 95(2): 531–543

Thorn K, Thorn SE & Wattwil M (2005) 'The effects of cricoid pressure, remifentanil and propofol on oesophageal motility and the lower oesophageal sphincter' *Anaesthesia and Analgesia* 100: 1200–1203

Thornberry EA (2002) 'Peri-operative fluids' *Anaesthesia and Intensive Care* 3(11): 414–417

Tuckey J (2000) 'Care of the post-operative unconscious patient' *Anaesthesia and Intensive Care* 1(1): 3–6

Whelan E & Davies H (2000) 'The pharmacology of drugs used in general anaesthesia' *in*: Davey A & Ince CS (eds) *Fundamentals of Operating Department Practice*. London: Greenwich Medical Media

Yates A (2000) 'The recovery room' *Anaesthesia and Intensive Care* 1(1): 1–3

3 Post-operative Recovery

Sylvia Prosser and Fiona J McArthur-Rouse

Introduction

The post-operative recovery phase is a period when patients depend upon healthcare professionals to maintain their safety through close monitoring and early intervention to prevent complications. The immediate recovery phase typically takes place in the post-anaesthetic recovery unit and is discussed in Chapter 2. However, patients undergoing major surgical procedures or those at increased risk of complications may require overnight intensive recovery or a longer period in the intensive care unit (ICU). Post-operative care will be largely determined by the nature of the surgery undergone and the type of anaesthetic administered. It is therefore important to receive a comprehensive handover from the staff of the recovery unit. This chapter considers the principles of caring for patients during the immediate and longer-term post-operative period in the surgical ward and should be read in conjunction with the chapter on the specific surgical procedure that the patient has undergone. Box 3.1 summarises the aims of this chapter.

When the patient is ready to be discharged from the recovery unit, all relevant documentation must be completed and any specific post-operative instructions recorded and prescribed. Patients are ready for transfer to the surgical ward when they meet the following criteria:

> **Box 3.1** Aims of the chapter.
>
> - To discuss the observation and monitoring of patients post-operatively in the light of the underlying physiological rationale
> - To discuss issues relating to the collection and transfer of patients from the recovery unit to the surgical ward
> - To discuss the care required to reduce the potential for post-operative complications

- They are able to maintain their own airway
- They are conscious and responding to verbal stimuli
- There is no evidence of haemorrhage
- Vital signs including temperature, pulse, respiratory rate, oxygen saturation, blood pressure and level of consciousness are within the patient's normal range and stable
- Pain and nausea are controlled
- Oxygen and fluid treatments are prescribed

Throughout the transfer observation of the patient is maintained. On return to the ward the nurse reassesses the patient and continues regular observations and monitoring as required. Some wards have specific guidelines for the frequency and duration of post-operative observations; however some patients will require more intensive monitoring than others and these should be undertaken as required.

As patients recover from the initial effects of anaesthesia they will need additional nursing interventions to help them return to their normal level of
independence. However, appropriate observation
and monitoring must be maintained. Goldhill (1997)
undertook a review of national confidential enquiries
into peri-operative deaths and noted that approximately two thirds of these patients died three
or more days after surgery and most deaths took
place on wards. Further studies (Goldhill *et al.*,
1999a, b) attempted to identify the early warning
signs of deterioration and found that despite severity of illness, the results of routine observations
were often not found in the notes and data were
often recorded improperly or imprecisely. Hence
there is a need to ensure accurate recording and
documentation of the patient's condition.

During surgery, a number of physiological processes may have been affected: breathing; circulation;
fluid balance; nutrition; elimination; thermoregulation; nervous function; and tissue integrity. Each of
these will be considered in this chapter.

The respiratory system

Applied physiology

Surgery may put the patient at risk for a number of
reasons. Even if the patient has not received a general anaesthetic, he or she will have been required
to lie still in a position which best allows surgical
access, for the length of time needed for the procedure. This position is unlikely to be one enabling
maximal respiratory function. We have evolved
to use an upright posture. When sitting upright
with the thoracic wall unrestricted the muscles of
ventilation are best able to increase the anterior–
posterior thoracic dimensions and draw air into the
respiratory passages by creating a negative pressure. Similarly, when sitting upright, the abdominal contents respond to the force of gravity and
fall away from the diaphragm, thus enabling the
diaphragm to flatten, increasing the superior–
inferior dimensions to enable intermittent large
breaths to be taken. This helps to expand basal alveoli
and small airways. When normally active, regular
changes in position promote these processes.

The respiratory system serves a range of physiological purposes, firstly to bring oxygen in the

inspired air into contact with red blood cells (RBCs)
at the interface between the alveoli and the pulmonary capillaries. Oxygen is needed for the cellular mitochondria to make adenosine triphospate
(ATP), the energy compound. ATP is then used to
power inflammation, protein synthesis and cell
division, all of which are needed for wound healing
to occur. So, at the most basic level, if sufficient
oxygen is not taken into the body, then the process
of wound healing is compromised at the outset.
The respiratory system also removes excess carbon
dioxide, one of the waste products of cell metabolism, and contributes to the control of acid–base
balance of the blood. The erythrocytes act as fac-
tories converting water and carbon dioxide to car-
bonic acid, which then splits to liberate hydrogen
ions – which reduce pH, or hydroxyl ions – which
increase pH. The respiratory system provides a
medium-speed control of acid–base balance. If the
blood pH is inappropriate, then the extracellular
fluid pH is similarly affected, impairing cellular
function and therefore, amongst other processes,
wound healing. Normal blood gas values are
shown in Table 3.1. The relationship between respiratory function and wound healing is shown
in Figure 3.1.

Table 3.1   Normal arterial blood gases.

Measurement	Normal range
pH	7.35–7.45
PaO_2	10–13.3 kPa
$PaCO_2$	4.6–6 kPa
HCO_3	22–26 kPa
Base excess/deficit	−2 to +2
Oxygen saturation	above 95%

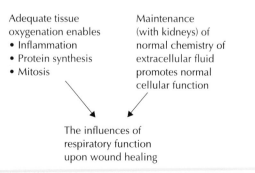

Figure 3.1   Diagram to show the influences of respiratory
function on wound healing.

If the patient has undergone a general anaesthetic for a procedure that required muscular relaxation, the muscle relaxant agent may have suppressed spontaneous ventilation. This should not be a problem during the operation, as the anaesthetist will use a mechanical ventilator, and the patient's blood chemistry should remain normal during this time. When the operation nears completion, the muscle relaxant must be reversed to enable the patient to resume normal ventilation, and for a while, depending on the speed and consistency of removal of the anaesthetic agents, breathing may be compromised. This is carefully monitored in the recovery unit and suitable positioning and oxygen therapy are used to promote optimal respiratory function.

The effect of a general anaesthetic for a straightforward surgical procedure appears in healthy people to be minimal. A study in Germany by Loick *et al.* (1997) compared the respiratory function of elderly patients who had had light anaesthesia and found that there was little difference in terms of blood oxygen saturation and alteration to breathing from those encountered during a normal night's sleep. So, in summary, a light anaesthetic given to a healthy person should not produce untoward respiratory effects. However, post-operative alterations in respiratory vital signs may herald important changes in the patient's condition.

Clinical observations and monitoring

Throughout the post-operative period it is important to monitor and document respiratory rate and depth. Several studies have identified changes in respiratory rate as an early warning sign of deterioration (Goldhill *et al.*, 1999a) and this parameter is frequently not observed or documented by nursing staff. From the discussion of the factors that may impair normal ventilation during surgery, the rationale for observing the rate, depth and symmetry of the respiratory effort becomes clear. Not only might respiratory control be impaired due to the residual effect of anaesthetic agents: prolonged abnormal posture during surgery may result in areas of atelectasis – collapse of areas of pulmonary tissue which have been compressed for a period of time. In addition, observation of the patient's skin colour and mucous membranes for cyanosis will help determine whether the haemoglobin is adequately saturated with oxygen – well-saturated haemoglobin produces the bright red colouration of the erythrocytes, which provides the normal pinkness of lips, oral mucosa, conjunctiva and the nails.

Oxygen saturation

Oxygen saturation monitoring may be a useful adjunct to observing respiratory rate and depth but few wards have enough monitors to carry out this observation continuously on all post-operative patients. Intermittent measurements are of limited benefit and trends are more important than absolute figures (Woodrow, 1999). As stated above, saturated haemoglobin produces the characteristic bright red colouration of arterial blood, reduced haemoglobin the dark red of venous blood. Pulse oximetry (see Figure 3.2) uses these principles to provide a measurement of the percentage of saturation of the haemoglobin.

The tissue under the probe is transilluminated by a light-emitting diode. The amount of bright red light from saturated haemoglobin is compared

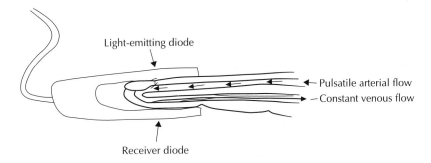

Light-emitting diode

Pulsatile arterial flow

Constant venous flow

Receiver diode

Figure 3.2   Pulse oximetry.

with the darker red produced by the venous blood, and the result is expressed as a percentage. Because saturated blood flows through arteriolar capillaries, the pulse oximeter needs a pulsatile flow through the tissue under the probe in order to be able to function properly. The probe will work with the skin colours of all races. A finger is commonly used for the positioning of the oximeter probe: if the patient wears green or blue polish this may reduce the accuracy of the measurement.

Oxygen saturation measures the concentration of oxygen being carried in combination with haemoglobin. However, what really matters is the amount of oxygen dissociating from the haemoglobin to diffuse through the extracellular fluid to the cells and into the mitochondria. Usually, it can be predicted that the oxygen attached to the haemoglobin will dissociate at a certain rate and therefore will be made available to the cells. Carbon monoxide causes the haemoglobin to retain the oxygen molecules, making them less available to cells. The most extreme example of this is carbon monoxide poisoning, which is beyond the scope of this book. Cigarette smoking produces carbon monoxide in the plasma. This will slightly hinder the release of oxygen to the cells. Checking the patient's smoking history may yield some information about the possible state of the respiratory mucosa and efficiency of the cilia. For example, cigarette smoke inflames the respiratory epithelium, increasing mucus production and additionally paralyses cilia, reducing the ability of the airways to move the increased volumes of mucus up the respiratory tract to be coughed out. It also reduces the predictability of oxygen saturation as a means of assessing supply of oxygen to the tissues.

Management

Supplemental oxygen

Normal room air contains 20.9% of oxygen as part of its an appropriate make-up. In health and with normal respiratory function, this provides adequate oxygen to the cells. When respiratory function is compromised following surgical intervention, oxygen therapy may be used for varying lengths of time post-operatively. The concentration of oxygen used will depend upon the extent of the patient's oxygen lack, so may vary from 100% in the immediate post-operative period to 24% – whatever concentration provides sufficient oxygen to allow normal functioning. Surgery imposes increased physiological demands (a stress) upon the body, and this increases the metabolic needs of the cells. The extent of the surgery will therefore influence the concentration of additional oxygen that is used.

The amount of extra oxygen required by the patient must be balanced against the adverse effects of inhaling an enhanced oxygen/air mix. Oxygen molecules are usually bonded together in stable pairs (O_2). However, in the turbulence of the gas escaping from the storage container, some molecules become split into single oxygen atoms (oxygen free radicals), which seek to combine with other substances to regain atomic stability. Within the respiratory tract, the substance most easily encountered is the epithelium of the airways, so the free radicals may form bonds with the protein of the respiratory tissue. This process alters the chemical composition of the tissue and stimulates the immune system, which mounts an inflammatory reaction against the now 'abnormal' tissue. So more oxygen is not necessarily better – excessive concentrations can inflame and damage the respiratory system. Table 3.2 considers the advantages and disadvantages of post-operative oxygen therapy.

Some patients need continuous oxygen therapy post-operatively. Those who are receiving high flow oxygen or therapy for a prolonged time require some form of humidification as the piped oxygen dries the upper airway and destroys the ciliated epithelium. This stops secretions from being cleared from the lungs and increases the risk of infection (Shelly & Nightingale, 1999). Maintaining adequate hydration levels will also help to prevent drying of the airways.

Prevention of respiratory infection

Patients who have undergone major surgical intervention, particularly chest and abdominal procedures, are at increased risk of post-operative chest infection. In addition to factors discussed above, pain, or the fear of pain, may prevent full expansion of the lungs, reducing tidal volume and increasing the anatomical dead space. This leads to stasis and the accumulation of secretions that the patient finds difficult to expectorate. The dehydrating effects of

Table 3.2 Advantages and disadvantages of oxygen use in the post-operative patient.

Advantages	Disadvantages
• Improves oxygenation of tissues with increased metabolic demands due to stress associated with surgery • Increases patient's feeling of energy/well-being • Promotes wound healing	• Risk of tissue damage from O_2 free radicals • May be perceived by patient or relatives as a sign of critical illness • Oxygen equipment may restrict patient's mobility or increase the risk of complications of immobility • Risk of dehydration of mucous membranes: humidification needed

continuous oxygen therapy may thicken secretions and reduced mobility post-operatively contributes to stasis in the lungs.

Prevention of chest infection begins pre-operatively with assessment of those at risk (see Chapter 1). During the post-operative period adequate pain relief to enable lung expansion and encouragement to practise regular deep breathing exercises will help to reduce the risk and prevent alveolar collapse. Breathing exercises may be taught by the physiotherapist and should be further encouraged by nursing staff. Mobilising patients post-operatively is an important way of preventing chest infection. This enables the adoption of an upright posture to maximise lung expansion and encourages gas exchange by improving circulation. The movement and change of position also promote expectoration of secretions.

Prevention of thromboembolism

If overall mobility and the depth of respiration are reduced, this diminishes the venous return, which may predispose to the formation of thrombi. Should a large venous thrombosis become detached and travel within the circulation, a pulmonary embolism may result. The outcome of a blood clot travelling into the pulmonary circulation depends upon the size of the pulmonary embolism. Figure 3.3 demonstrates how pulmonary emboli form.

A small pulmonary embolism may produce pleuritic pain as an infarction develops in the peripheral lung tissue adjacent to the pleura. The resulting inflammation then causes pain from the pleural nerve endings. A large pulmonary embolism may obstruct either the pulmonary trunk, in which case collapse and sudden death will occur, or the right or left pulmonary arteries, in which case acute hypoxia and dyspnoea will result from the sudden

failure of perfusion of an entire lung. Prevention is clearly much better than cure in relation to pulmonary embolism. Diagnosis is by ventilation–perfusion lung scanning. Treatment involves the administration of oxygen and anticoagulant or thrombolytic therapy to reduce the size of the clot. A further discussion of venous thrombosis is provided in the section in this chapter discussing the cardiovascular system. Management of the hypoxic patient is discussed in Chapter 13.

The cardiovascular system

Applied physiology

Surgery presents a physiological challenge to the cells of the body. If the cells' metabolic needs increase, the cardiovascular system must increase its output in order to meet these enhanced demands.

Risk of haemorrhage

Surgery involves deliberate intervention upon the tissues, and this may result in the opening of small or large blood vessels and subsequent blood loss. The use of cutting implements such as scalpels will increase this risk: use of lasers and heat coagulation, while causing inflammation, should reduce the risk of haemorrhagic blood loss. An appreciation of the techniques used during surgery will help in predicting the extent of possible blood loss. The vascularity of the area being treated will also influence the risk of blood loss. Dissection of the vascular supply to an area carries an enhanced risk of haemorrhage, as will trauma, in which highly vascular tissue may have been damaged by shearing forces, producing dramatic blood loss. The prediction of blood loss will help determine

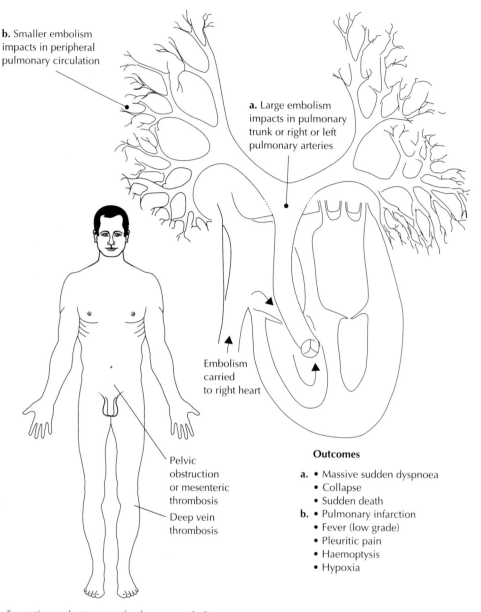

b. Smaller embolism impacts in peripheral pulmonary circulation

a. Large embolism impacts in pulmonary trunk or right or left pulmonary arteries

Embolism carried to right heart

Pelvic obstruction or mesenteric thrombosis

Deep vein thrombosis

Outcomes

a. • Massive sudden dyspnoea
   • Collapse
   • Sudden death
b. • Pulmonary infarction
   • Fever (low grade)
   • Pleuritic pain
   • Haemoptysis
   • Hypoxia

Figure 3.3 Formation and outcomes of pulmonary embolism.

whether the surgeon inserts a drain at the wound site. Knowledge of the surgery undertaken and an awareness of the trend of loss via the drain or wound will help to determine the frequency of observation of fluid balance.

Normal haemostasis requires vessel closure, either surgically in the case of large vessels, or through vasospasm and the formation of a platelet plug if small vessels are involved. Failure of these initial haemostatic mechanisms will produce a primary haemorrhage, possibly requiring a return to the operating theatre to find and seal the bleeding point. A surgical ligature might have slipped, or a blood vessel spasm ceased to control flow through a damaged vessel.

Reactionary haemorrhage

During anaesthesia and surgery, blood pressure may have been reduced, either pharmacologically

Table 3.3   Normal blood values for haemoglobin and red blood cells.

Haemoglobin		Erythrocytes	
Male	13–18 g/dL	Male	$4.5–6.0 \times 10^{12}$/litre
Female	11.5–15.5 g/dL	Female	$3.9–5.1 \times 10^{12}$/litre

to control the likelihood of haemorrhage, or as a result of opening of a large wound, for example in the abdomen, or due to loss of blood or other tissue fluids. As the hypotensive effects created during surgery decrease and the patient's blood pressure returns towards normal, small bleeding points may reopen, causing a reactionary haemorrhage some hours after completion of the surgical procedure. So for the first 12–24 hours post-operatively, observations for excessive loss of blood are maintained, at levels of frequency appropriate to the trends of blood loss. Before surgery, baseline measurements of the haemoglobin and red cell count may be made. In addition, if blood transfusion will be needed, grouping and cross-matching will be undertaken. Table 3.3 shows normal blood values of haemoglobin and the red cell count.

Shock

Shock is a syndrome produced by the failure of the circulatory system to meet the metabolic needs of the tissues. It may be mild and self-limiting, but severe forms can result in permanent tissue damage, or the death of the patient. Early detection and correction of the circulatory function are extremely important in minimising the morbidity and mortality of shock. There are many causes of shock: myocardial dysfunction, severe pain and fear, anaphylaxis, dehydration and hypovolaemia. A comprehensive discussion of shock will be found in Chapter 13.

Clinical observations and monitoring

Haemodynamic monitoring

On a busy operating day, the convenience offered by mechanised sphygmomanometers that also record pulse rate is appealing, but there are some important considerations to remember. Mechanised

sphygmomanometers are reliable when the patient's state is stable, with a regular pulse rate and normal blood pressure. These machines 'expect' one pulse to follow another in a recognisable rhythm, and will record the onset of the pulse in relation to the cuff pressure accordingly. If either the pulse rate or blood pressure becomes erratic, their recordings may become less reliable, abnormal fluctuations being missed.

When observing and monitoring cardiovascular status, it is necessary to pay attention not only to pulse rate and blood pressure, but also to pulse volume and regularity, limb temperature (systemic vascular resistance), capillary refill time and urine output. These cannot be assessed using a mechanised sphygmomanometer; however the machine may be useful in providing a mean arterial pressure (MAP). MAP is the arterial pressure averaged during one cardiac cycle and is useful in determining perfusion pressure (Bassett & Makin, 2000). It gives particular weighting to the diastolic pressure, which is significant in relation to perfusion; a MAP of less that 70 mmHg indicates inadequate perfusion particularly to the kidneys. MAP is calculated using the following equation:

$$MAP = \frac{(2 \times \text{diastolic pressure}) + \text{systolic pressure}}{3}$$

Again there is a need to monitor trends and to consider the patient's baseline observations for comparison. Another trend that is useful to observe post-operatively is the pulse pressure. This is the difference between the systolic and the diastolic pressure and a narrowing pulse pressure is often a sign of falling cardiac output (Ahern, 2002). Other factors that may affect blood pressure include the administration of opioid analgesia and the use of spinal or epidural anaesthetic or analgesia.

Wound drains

Towards the end of a surgical procedure a drain may be inserted to drain potential collections of blood or inflammatory exudate. The use of drains is, however, controversial and Box 3.2 identifies their advantages and disadvantages. There are a number of different types of drain and Henry & Thompson (2005) classify them as 'active' and 'passive' and 'open' and 'closed'. Active drainage involves the use of vacuumed containers, which provide suction to draw out the fluid; whereas

> **Box 3.2**   Advantages and disadvantages of surgical drains.
>
> **Advantages**
> - The drainage of fluid removes a potential source of infection
> - The drain prevents further fluid collection
> - Excessive drainage may warn of haemorrhage or anastomotic leak
> - Following removal there is a route for residual fluid to discharge
>
> **Disadvantages**
> - The drain is a potential focus and entry route for infection
> - The use of suction and mechanical pressure may cause tissue damage
> - The drain may cause healing to be delayed
> - In certain situations the drains are sealed off within six hours and may therefore be ineffective
>
> (adapted from Henry & Thompson, 2005)

passive drains rely on gravity and differential pressures between the body and the exterior (Henry & Thompson, 2005). Closed drains have a tube that drains directly into a container; whereas open drains (for example, a corrugated drain) drain into a dressing or bag. A Redivac™ drain is an example of an active, closed drain. Drains are sometimes sutured into place and care needs to be taken, when moving and handling the patient, not to pull on the drains. Passive drains should not be raised above the level of the body, as there is a risk of reversal of

the fluid movement back into the patient's body with subsequent increased risk of infection.

During the post-operative period it is necessary to observe the wound site and any drainage systems for excessive bleeding. The amount of bleeding that occurs will depend partly on the surgical procedure performed, and it is important to be aware of what can be considered normal in each case. All drainage should be recorded on the fluid balance chart.

Management

Most patients returning to the ward following major surgical intervention will have an intravenous infusion (IVI) and/or central venous catheter (CVC) in situ. This will enable fluid replacement therapy to maintain intravascular volume and ensure that the patient remains adequately hydrated. (Fluid replacement therapy is discussed later in this chapter.)

Some patients may require a blood transfusion, either in the immediate post-operative period or several days later. A low haemoglobin level may be identified either through observation of particular symptoms, for example dizziness, nausea, fatigue, breathlessness and tachycardia, or a routine blood count. During the transfusion, regular observations and monitoring will need to be undertaken according to local policy. Table 3.4 lists blood transfusion observations that may be used.

Table 3.4   Observations undertaken during a blood transfusion.

Observations	Rationale
Pulse	Detect signs of improvement or worsening of cardiac output
Arterial blood pressure	Detect signs of improvement or worsening of cardiac output
Estimation of core temperature (usually tympanic)	To detect signs of pyrexia if an immune reaction to the transfusion occurs. If a rapid transfusion is required before a blood warmer is available, to detect the onset of hypothermia
Respirations	Older patients may develop cardiac failure if over-transfused, in which case tachypnoea or bubbling respirations may be observed – diuretics and/or reduction of transfusion rate may be needed
Observation of skin for urticarial rashes or itching	May indicate hypersensitivity reaction to proteins within the transfused blood – may need to discontinue transfusion and give prescribed antihistamines
Fluid balance	Ensure that urine output appropriate for input; monitor for signs of acute renal failure which may occur either due to shock or transfusion reaction
Note any reports from patient of loin pain	May indicate transfusion reaction/renal involvement

Box 3.3 Signs and symptoms of DVT.

- Abnormal swelling of affected limb
- Warmth of the affected limb
- Localised pain
- Dilation of veins
- Colour changes of the leg
- Pyrexia
- Asymptomatic

(adapted from Wallis & Autar, 2001)

Venous thrombosis

Another complication that patients may develop following surgery is deep vein thrombosis (DVT). This can occur due to one or a combination of three factors, known as Virchow's triad: trauma to veins, blood coagulation factors and stasis of venous circulation. Patients who have undergone surgery, particularly orthopaedic, major pelvic or abdominal procedures, are at increased risk, as are older patients and those with malignant disease (Wallis & Autar, 2001). The main contributing factors are reduced mobility leading to stasis of blood and hypercoagulation due to dehydration or malignancy. Prevention of DVT commences pre-operatively by identifying those at risk, providing compression hosiery and administering prophylactic anticoagulant therapy such as low molecular weight heparin. Post-operatively it is necessary to remove antiembolism stockings in order to undertake regular observation of the legs and to encourage active leg exercises and early mobilisation. Box 3.3 lists the signs and symptoms of DVT.

Fluid and electrolyte balance

Applied physiology

Body water is needed as a medium for chemical reactions, for transport of dissolved cell substrates and metabolites and for the dissipation of heat generated by cellular metabolism. The average 70 kg male's body composition includes around 45 litres of water, which is disposed within the cell cytoplasm (around 30 litres); within the extracellular space (around 12 litres) and in the circulation (around 3 litres). The proportion of body water varies according to age and gender. Older people have a lower proportion of body water than do the very young. Males have more water in their body composition than do females. This is because there is usually more muscle mass in males and more fat in females. Muscle has a comparatively high water content, and fat less water.

The proportion of body water and electrolytes is monitored by osmoreceptor cells in the hypothalamus and kidneys. These cells monitor the concentration of solutes in the tissues. If the tissue fluid becomes too concentrated, antidiuretic hormone is secreted by the posterior pituitary to reduce urinary water loss. In addition, the hypothalamic thirst centre is stimulated and the individual seeks fluid to drink, and also increases the salt intake. So patients who are denied food and fluids prior to a lengthy operation are likely to suffer thirst post-operatively. The effect of tracheal intubation combined with the anaesthetic agents may produce a dry mouth and marked thirst; so clear fluids will probably be appreciated if there are no contra-indications (see specific chapters for guidance related to resuming normal patterns of eating and drinking after particular types of surgery). Fluids and electrolytes are important for the maintenance of volume in the body fluid compartments. Tissue cells and the extracellular space need to be adequately hydrated for wound healing to be effective and the intravascular compartment needs to be maintained within normal limits to ensure effective circulation of blood to the tissues. Table 3.5 shows normal values and functions of commonly encountered electrolytes.

A number of factors may cause a reduction in urine output post-operatively. These include the release of antidiuretic hormone (ADH) as part of the stress response. The hormone may continue to be released for a few days after surgery so reduced urine volume (oliguria) should be anticipated.

Other causes of oliguria include hypovolaemia due to bleeding, excessive pre-operative fasting and inadequate fluid replacement. If significant hypotension occurred during surgery, renal function may be impaired, and there is a possibility that the patient could develop acute renal failure. In older patients, this risk may be increased if non-steroidal anti-inflammatory drugs have been

Table 3.5   Normal values and functions of common electrolytes.

Electrolyte	Function	Homeostasis
Sodium (135–145 mEq/L)	Controls water distribution and ECF volume	ICF/ECF levels maintained by the Na$^+$K$^+$ pump. Intake via diet, excretion via kidneys, GI tract and sweating
Potassium (3.5–5.0 mEq/L)	Neuromuscular function	ICF/ECF levels maintained by the Na$^+$K$^+$ pump. Intake via diet. Excreted via kidneys, bowel and sweat
Calcium (total = 8.9–10.3 mg/dL or 2.23–2.57 mmol/L)	Sedative action on nerve cells and major role in transmission of nerve impulses; regulates muscle contraction and relaxation	Parathyroid hormone promotes transfer of calcium from bones to plasma and augments intestinal absorption of Ca^{++}. Calcitonin inhibits bone resorption (reducing serum levels)
Magnesium (1.3–2.1 mEq/L or 0.65–1.1 mmol/L)	Enzymatic reactions particularly those involving production and utilisation of ATP. Neuronal control, neuromuscular transmission and CV tone	Intake via diet and excretion via kidneys
Phosphorous (0.81–1.45 mmol/L or 2.5–4.5 mg/dL)	Source of high-energy bonds of ATP. Muscle function, RBCs and nervous system	Intake via diet and excretion via kidneys

used for analgesia (Worsley, 1993) as these can exacerbate pre-renal failure by interfering with renal internal regulation. NSAIDs and some antibiotics may also contribute to intrarenal failure as they are nephrotoxic, so renal function should be monitored. The onset of cardiac failure may cause oliguria due to inadequate perfusion of the kidneys from a low mean arterial pressure of less than 70 mmHg. It is important, therefore, to ascertain the cause of oliguria and ensure that the correct treatment is given, as inappropriate fluid or diuretic administration can have disastrous results. A further discussion of oliguria can be found in Chapter 13.

Clinical observations and monitoring

Fluid balance is another area of nursing practice that is often poorly documented (National Confidential Enquiry into Perioperative Deaths (NCEPOD), 1999, 2001), resulting in difficulty in ascertaining the patient's hydration status. Hypotension and oliguria are common post-operative problems and the causes include fluid loss, cardiac failure, renal failure and the effects of epidural or spinal analgesia (NCEPOD, 2001). Therefore, full assessment and accurate interpretation of vital signs are essential in ensuring appropriate treatment. The NCEPOD (2001) enquiry lists numerous cases where this was not evident and patients died as a result.

For these reasons it is common practice for the first voiding to be noted and, also, for a fluid balance chart to be used for the first 24 hours following surgery. If a patient is catheterised, the normal urinary output for an adult is usually more than 1 millilitre per kilogram (mL/kg) body weight per hour. The threshold below which advice should be sought for an adult is 30 mL per hour or, more accurately, 0.5 mL/kg/hour. In cases when this is in question, use of a metered system for collecting urine is helpful to keep watch on the hourly output. This is obviously not possible without a urinary catheter, and explains why catheterisation is sometimes undertaken in a patient who has resumed normal patterns of micturition, but whose kidneys are at risk of failing. See Chapter 13 for a further discussion of the assessment of fluid balance.

Renal function is assessed by plasma levels of urea and electrolytes. Urea is produced by the liver as a waste product of amino acid metabolism. The

Table 3.6 Intravenous fluids commonly used post-operatively.

Type of solution	Use
Whole blood or blood products (for example, whole blood; packed cells; plasma protein fraction)	Augment circulatory blood volume Increase oxygen-carrying capacity of circulation. Replace clotting factors if large haemorrhage has previously occurred (in this case fresh, rather than stored blood is needed).
Colloids (solutions of large molecular weight)	Will remain in the circulation rather than passing into the extracellular space via the capillary walls. Augment blood volume and draw water from tissues by osmosis.
Crystalloids (small molecular weight glucose and electrolyte solutions)	Will provide electrolytes and a small amount of calories to the extracellular space and thus to the cells.

normal range of blood urea for an adult or child is 2.5–6.7 mmol/litre. These levels will be raised above normal if the patient is dehydrated. Creatinine is a waste product of skeletal muscle breakdown. Amongst other causes, creatinine levels may become elevated in renal disease or in association with obstructive conditions of the urinary tract. For an adult, normal values range between 60 and 100 micromoles (µmol) per litre.

It is important that fluid balance is monitored accurately and if a central venous catheter is in situ, central venous pressure (CVP) measurements should be obtained if there is any doubt regarding the patient's hydration status. The benefit of CVP monitoring is that it demonstrates conditions within the right atrium. In contrast to the left side of the heart and the arterial system, the large veins and right atrium are relatively unaffected by changes due to sympathetic compensation, so there is no masking of any developing state of shock.

Management

Dehydration

According to the extent of the surgery undertaken, the patient returning to the ward may have one or more intravenous lines delivering blood, colloid or crystalloid solutions. The type of fluid administered will depend upon the nature of the fluid loss. Post-operative fluid replacement needs to take into account normal maintenance, fasting, blood losses, gastrointestinal, third space and insensible losses. The nurse will need to ensure that intravenous fluids are administered safely, using an infusion pump if necessary, and ensure that the cannula is patent and not inflamed. The infusion should continue until the patient is able to tolerate adequate amounts of oral fluids. Table 3.6 shows some intravenous fluids that are commonly used post-operatively.

Patients who are severely dehydrated and oliguric may be subjected to a 'fluid challenge' in order to determine the cause of the oliguria. A bolus of intravenous fluid, approximately 500 mL, is given over a short period of time with careful cardiopulmonary monitoring (Metheny, 2000). A positive response is indicated by a rise in CVP measurement and increased urine output (see Chapter 13 for further discussion of the management of hypovolaemia and oliguria).

Overhydration

As discussed above, some patients may retain fluid post-operatively due to excessive ADH secretion, renal failure or cardiac failure. Overhydration may also be due to excessive administration of sodium-containing fluids. Initially the cause should be ascertained and, if possible, reversed. Otherwise, symptomatic treatment is required and will usually involve the administration of a diuretic such as frusemide, which acts on the loop of Henle causing loss of sodium, chloride, potassium and water (Metheny, 2000). Care should be taken when using diuretics post-operatively as it is possible to cause the patient to become dehydrated.

Nutrition

Applied physiology

On transfer to the ward from the recovery unit, the resumption of normal nutrition will depend upon what surgical procedure the patient has undergone, and this should be checked before giving food and drink.

For optimal wound healing, it is important that the patient resumes a balanced diet as soon as possible. Surgery imposes a metabolic demand because it constitutes a physiological challenge, so an increased energy intake would be helpful. However, the effects of the anaesthesia may mean that the patient does not immediately feel like resuming a normal eating pattern. They may suffer from post-operative nausea and vomiting which will need to be treated first. It is important to be aware of the nutritional limitations of intravenous glucose and electrolyte solutions. These preparations are designed to help restore normal chemical composition to the circulation and the tissues, but a 24-hour regimen of solutions such as normal saline, dextrose saline and 5% dextrose does not provide sufficient energy for normal metabolism, let alone allow for recovery from anaesthesia and surgery. As soon as is possible, the patient needs to resume a palatable diet of normal or enhanced nutritional value.

Nutritional demands of surgery

Following surgery, the effects of starvation and increased catabolism promote the loss of body proteins and fat (Holmes, 1998). However, these losses may be masked by sodium and water retention in the first few post-operative days. In uncomplicated surgery, energy requirements may be increased by 10%; and if surgery is preceded by multiple fractures or trauma, this may be up to 25% (Holmes, 1998). A detailed discussion of wound healing and the prerequisites will be found later in this chapter. The surgical patient needs a diet that supplies proteins for tissue building, fats and carbohydrates for energy production, vitamins and zinc for the formation of collagen and epithelium. During a normal sleep–wake cycle, there are times when food is ingested, absorbed and metabolised to provide raw materials for cellular function. This is the absorptive phase of metabolism, and leads to building up of tissue (anabolism). During the absorptive phase, there is an increase in available glucose in the blood and insulin is secreted by the pancreatic islets of Langerhans. Insulin makes glucose available to all body cells, by enabling uptake via active cellular transport mechanisms.

During sleep, food is not ingested, and energy must be found from stores of glycogen within the liver. The person enters a fasting phase of metabolism. The supply of glucose is now limited and priority for its use is given to the brain. Insulin secretion diminishes, which means that glucose can only be taken into the brain cells, which have the ability to use it in the absence of insulin. So the secretion of insulin acts as a rationing system – in times of plenty, glucose is made available for general use, in times of scarcity, the brain becomes the main user. The two opposite metabolic states contribute to an 'ebb and flow' pattern of function. During sleep, growth hormone is released which is needed in adults for tissue growth and repair. If the fasting period becomes prolonged, fuel for making cellular ATP must come from other sources, namely fatty acids and glycerol. When there is a lack of available carbohydrates, the conversion of fats is incomplete, and ketone bodies are formed, which can be used for energy creation by tissue cells.

When physiological insult is great, such as when extensive surgery is undertaken or major trauma has occurred, particularly when the original nutritional state of the patient is poor, a state of nutritional crisis develops in the tissues. Muscle protein must be used to provide amino acids in addition to the liberation of fatty acids and glycerol from adipose tissue stores for the creation of cellular energy. The patient now enters a catabolic stage, in which there is a significant decrease in body mass (muscle and fat) in order to maintain normal cellular activity. If the catabolic state continues unchecked, wound healing, muscular strength and immune activity are all compromised, which will have a detrimental effect upon the surgical patient's recovery. In such situations, nutritional support is needed, either enterally using formulae designed for use via the gastrointestinal tract, or directly into the bloodstream, using specific products that are administered into a large vein as total parenteral nutrition (TPN).

Clinical observations and monitoring

Identification of patients at risk of post-operative malnutrition is carried out pre-operatively with nutritional screening and assessment (see Chapter 1). Post-operatively, close observation of dietary intake is required to ensure adequate intake of required nutrients. This may take the form of a food chart or monitoring of enteral or parenteral feeds.

Management

The main principle is the need to commence oral or enteral nutrition as soon as possible after surgery (Scottish Intercollegiate Guidelines Network (SIGN), 2004). If the patient can tolerate diet, then this should be encouraged unless contraindicated. A number of studies have suggested that post-operative infections can be reduced and hospital stay shortened by starting early post-operative enteral nutrition (Silk & Gow, 2001).

Post-operative nausea and vomiting (PONV) is a common complication, which is often underestimated. It is important to control PONV as it can cause discomfort, embarrassment, exhaustion,

Table 3.7 Risk factors for PONV.

Patient factors	Surgical factors
• Age	• GI surgery
• Gender	• Gynaecological
• Obesity	surgery
• Anxiety	• Laparoscopy
• Past medical history	• ENT surgery
• Gastroparesis	• Eye surgery
• Pre-operative fasting	• Orthopaedic
• Duration of operation	surgery
• Operative procedure	• Emergency surgery

Anaesthetic factors	Post-operative factors
• Pre-medication	• Pain
• Anaesthetic agent	• Opioid analgesia
• Dose of anaesthesia	• Movement
• Gastric distension and	• Hypotension/
suctioning	dizziness
• Oropharyngeal stimulation	• Hypoxaemia
• Reversal of neuromuscular	• Oral intake
blocking agent	• Psychological
• Opioid administration	factors

Box 3.4 Types of anti-emetic commonly used.

- Phenothiazines, e.g. prochlorperazine
- Serotonin antagonists, e.g. ondansetron; dolasetron; granisetron (particularly effective against vomiting)
- Dopamine antagonists, e.g. droperidol; promethazine; prochlorperazine (droperidol is particularly effective against nausea)
- Combined dopamine and serotonin-3 receptor antagonist – metoclopramide
- Antihistamines, e.g. cyclizine

Combination therapy is usually more effective than a single medication. Serotonin antagonist with dopamine antagonists or corticosteroid, e.g. dexamethasone, may be used for persistent cases.

The use of propofol as an intravenous anaesthetic during surgery has been found to reduce PONV (Gan, 2002).

---

wound disruption, electrolyte imbalance, dehydration and malnutrition. There may be delays in mobilisation, increased morbidity and delayed discharge. A number of factors increase the risk of suffering from PONV and these are listed in Table 3.7.

Management of PONV is typically pharmacological and should be used prophylactically, particularly if the patient is receiving opioid analgesia. A variety of anti-emetics can be used and work in different ways. Classifications vary according to sources, but they are generally categorised according to the site and mode of action (see Box 3.4). The nurse must be aware of the different types of anti-emetic, their side-effects and which can be used together.

Various non-pharmacological methods of managing PONV have been investigated and appear to have some effect. These include acupressure, ginger root capsules taken by mouth and the inhalation of peppermint oil (Tate, 1997; Mann, 1999; Thompson, 1999).

Elimination

Applied physiology

On return from the operating department, the nurse should note the patient's urinary output, whether that be as a result of normal micturition or via a urinary catheter. This is for two main reasons. Firstly, and most commonly, the neurological effects of anaesthesia may produce a temporary inhibition of the normal feedback mechanisms that allow micturition to take place. This may occur following general or epidural anaesthesia, and also if the surgery has involved tissues in the vicinity of the sacral nerves, for example within the pelvis. In cases where the mechanism of micturition is temporarily inhibited, the lower abdomen may be distended and the patient may be aware of the need to empty the bladder but unable to do so at first. If the patient has a urinary catheter in situ, it is wise to check that this is draining freely and is not obstructed, for example by the patient sitting on it.

Following surgery, gut motility may be reduced and constipation may be a problem. This is due to a number of factors including reduced mobility, reduced oral intake and the effects of opioid analgesia. In some cases, particularly in abdominal surgery, a paralytic ileus may occur. This is a form of non-mechanical gastrointestinal obstruction and is discussed in Chapter 9. If this does occur, the patient may become extremely ill. The nurse needs to be alert to the signs and symptoms of a paralytic ileus and to act upon them if a patient does not appear to be recovering as expected.

Clinical observations and monitoring

It is important to establish that the post-operative patient has voided. The significance of monitoring urine output is discussed above in relation to fluid balance and in Chapter 13. In some cases, patients may pass a small amount of urine but not empty the bladder completely. This can give a false impression about fluid status or may cause urinary retention to go undiagnosed.

The nurse needs to ascertain whether bowel function is returning to normal post-operatively. Listening for bowel sounds can be misleading as the presence or absence of sounds does not necessarily relate to function. If possible, it is more reliable to ask patients if they have passed flatus, have sensations of intestinal movement or feel hungry. It is also possible to examine the patient for signs of abdominal distension.

Management

Some patients may have difficulty voiding urine in unnatural surroundings. It is often easier to resume normal micturition if the patient is taken to a toilet. The use of a mobile commode with a bedpan for a woman will enable the nurse to check that an adequate volume of urine has been passed and note it on the fluid balance chart. Men often find it easier to resume micturition if they are able to stand up to use a urinal. In such cases it is important to check that the blood pressure is relatively normal for that person and that they can tolerate the change of position without becoming faint and dizzy and risking falls and injuries. If there is any doubt, the patient should not be left alone, although this may cause further inhibition. It would be sensible for the nurse to be able to observe the patient whilst being as unobtrusive as possible.

Patients who have difficulty opening their bowels post-operatively may require an aperient. However, encouraging mobilisation and a high-fibre diet with plenty of oral fluids can replace this medication in those who are able to tolerate an oral diet.

Thermoregulation

Applied physiology

As can be seen in Chapter 2, there are well-known risks to thermoregulatory control associated with the intra-operative period. Recovery staff are vigilant for the signs of inadvertent hypothermia and the patient ready for transfer to the ward should have a core temperature that is within the normal range. Operating department staff are aware that a core temperature of less than 36°C can be linked with an increase in wound infection rate; tendency to bleed post-operatively and raised incidence of cardiac dysfunction (Hudson et al., 1999). A few patients react to the anaesthetic and develop malignant hyperpyrexia or malignant hyperthermia, which is a potentially fatal complication of an inherited muscular disorder. It is precipitated by the administration of some volatile anaesthetics and neuromuscular blocking agents and is characterised by skeletal muscle rigidity and a hypermetabolic state (McCarthy, 2004). Such patients are likely to have been stabilised in intensive care before they return to the ward. However, they would need to be made aware of their reaction and their notes should give details of the problem so that appropriate precautions can be taken by the anaesthetist should any future anaesthesia be needed. For further reading on this subject see McCarthy (2004).

The tissue damage caused by an incision will provoke the inflammatory response, which may be sufficient to cause low-grade pyrexia. This, coupled with the normal redness of inflammation, which is the first stage of the healing process, needs to be understood and differentiated from a developing infection. Because much post-operative pain is related to inflammatory processes, non-steroidal anti-inflammatory (NSAID) analgesics may provide effective pain relief. As the patient stabilises after surgery, these signs should abate, but if an infection is present, the inflammatory signs will persist and frank signs of infection become apparent (see below). If infection is present, a blood specimen may reveal a raised white cell count. A normal white cell count for an adult is between 4 and 11×10^9/litre.

Clinical observations and monitoring

In the days following surgery, the patient will be observed for a rise in temperature that may indicate the presence of infection. Whilst a slight rise during the first and second post-operative days is part of the body's normal inflammatory response to the invasive surgical procedure, persistent low-grade pyrexia, or a temperature that spikes intermittently over a period of several days, is often a sign that infection is present. It is then necessary to ascertain the cause by taking wound swabs, blood cultures, sputum and urine specimens. Some patients will have been given prophylactic antibiotics post-operatively and these should be noted when sending specimens to the laboratory.

Management

Management of pyrexia is a controversial subject, with some authors recommending that it should be allowed to run its natural course as long as no

detrimental effects are present. This is because the high temperature has a beneficial protective effect in infective states and lowering it may deprive the patient of an important host defence mechanism (Edwards, 1998). Detrimental effects of high temperature include an increased basal metabolic rate; increased heart and respiratory rates; vasodilation – making the patient appear hypovolaemic; discomfort; weakness and loss of appetite. If these symptoms are present, the use of antipyretics may help to relieve them and make the patient more comfortable; however, the temperature should not be reduced too rapidly. The use of tepid sponging and fanning should be avoided, as they will ultimately increase temperature by causing heat-generating mechanisms such as shivering (Edwards, 1998).

Nervous system function

Applied physiology

When fully recovered from the anaesthetic and analgesia, the patient should have the same level of neurological function that was present prior to the surgery. During the immediate post-operative period, the return of basal protective reflexes such as coughing and swallowing will have been monitored, and the patient should be able to respond to simple requests by the time he or she returns to the ward. The type of analgesia given may cause drowsiness, and morphine-based analgesia may cause respiratory depression in susceptible people such as those with pre-existing respiratory disease. For a more detailed consideration of post-operative pain, see Chapter 4. The homeostatic control mechanisms may be less efficient in older people who may also have less efficient renal function; this may impair their ability to excrete medication. For this reason, renal function should have been assessed as part of the pre-operative screening process, when a blood sample is likely to have been sent for biochemical analysis of urea, electrolyte and creatinine levels. If during their operation a patient has been immobile, with the limbs maintained in an unusual position for any significant length of time, there may be impaired mobility or sensation of the affected limb. Although this will have been observed for during the immediate recovery period (Chapter 2), the effect of anaesthesia and analgesia may mask the signs, so it is important for the ward staff to continue to notice and report any signs or complaints from the patient related to loss of motor or sensory function.

Acute confusional state

Older people may respond adversely to biochemical alteration within their central nervous system. Hypoxia, pH shifts, pain, or the effects of analgesia may cause them to become disoriented. This acute confusional state should subside as the underlying cause is detected and treated. This may be particularly important when the patient comes to the ward directly from the operating department as an emergency admission. In such cases, the ward staff will not have had the chance to know the patient beforehand and as such may not appreciate the change from the patient's normal self. It is important to heed the comments of relatives and friends who may be the only ones to appreciate how unlike their normal self the patient currently is. (See Chapter 12 for further discussion of this condition.)

Clinical observations and monitoring

Because the neurological state may give warning of a number of post-operative complications, it is important to observe the patient's level of consciousness and investigate any change. One simple method of assessing level of consciousness is the alert-voice-pain-unresponsive (AVPU) scale (see Chapter 13); however, limitations of this include the fact that it does not differentiate between subtle changes in mental state that only prior knowledge of the patient can determine.

Consciousness may also be affected by medications such as opioid analgesia, and patients receiving this regularly should undergo assessment and scoring of sedation level. Whilst being cared for in the ward the post-operative patient should always be responsive to verbal stimulus or touch. If the patient's level of consciousness deteriorates, assistance should be sought immediately and the patient should not be left unaccompanied. (See Chapter 4 for treatment of opioid-related respiratory depression and the assessment and management of pain.)

Tissue integrity

Applied physiology

Wounds occur due to trauma, surgical intervention, or due to cellular damage resulting from a lack of oxygen or nutritional substrates. Different body tissues have different abilities to repair themselves. This depends upon the type of cell that makes up the tissue. Some tissues, such as those of the epidermis, heal rapidly because their component cells are capable of undergoing mitotic division throughout their lifespan. Other tissues can regenerate as long as the appropriate growth factors are secreted and there is a supportive tissue framework for the new cells to grow along. Embryonic tissue cells, which are freely able to replicate, can repair themselves with no scar tissue being formed, so babies who required intrauterine surgery tend to have little scarring. Most tissues use connective tissue for repair. In this case, cells which have not been able to regenerate are replaced with scar tissue, which restores tissue integrity, but which lacks the specific properties of the original structure.

Before a wound can heal, blood loss must be halted and then tissue inflammation must occur. The inflammatory process brings an increased blood supply to the area, following which capillary permeability increases and phagocytic white cells migrate to the tissues, ingesting debris from damaged and dead cells and any bacteria which are present. During this time, the wound appears red and slightly swollen, but this is due to inflammation, rather than to the presence of infection. There is pain and increased heat. The pain serves as a protection to diminish further tissue damage that might result from constant movement of the damaged area. As the inflammatory process concludes, the healing process commences.

Wounds heal via one of two main processes, depending upon the extent of the wound surface. A small clean cut will heal by primary intention; as long as the wound edges are held in apposition (see Figure 3.4).

Healing by primary intention

The cut surfaces of surgical wounds, which are expected to heal by primary intention, are held together either by adhesive strips, tissue adhesive,

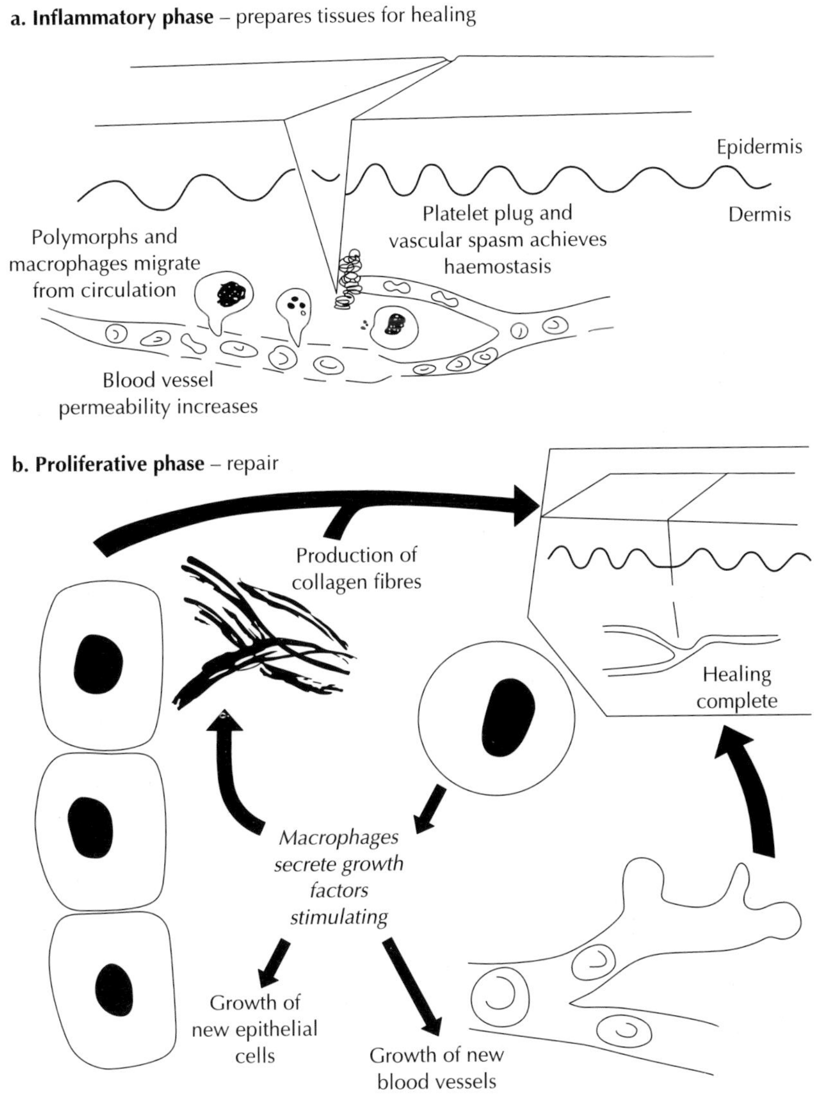

a. Inflammatory phase – prepares tissues for healing

Epidermis

Dermis

Platelet plug and
vascular spasm achieves
haemostasis

Polymorphs and
macrophages migrate
from circulation

Blood vessel
permeability increases

b. Proliferative phase – repair

Production of
collagen fibres

Healing
complete

*Macrophages
secrete growth
factors
stimulating*

Growth of
new epithelial
cells

Growth of new
blood vessels

Figure 3.4   Wound healing by primary intention.

sutures or clips. In healing by primary intention, the cut surface of the wound has a preliminary seal within 24–48 hours. A well-sutured wound has regained around 70% of the strength of the original tissue as long as the sutures are present, but after removal of sutures, the wound may only have around 10% of its original strength, so it is instinctive (and sensible) for a patient to support the wound with the hands during moving or coughing. Between two and three months post-surgery, the wound will probably have regained 70–80% of the original strength. Unless the wound closure is biologically absorbable, it must be removed once healing is well in progress, as the presence of a foreign substance will become a focus for infection and will otherwise cause the healing process to break down.

Healing by secondary intention

This occurs when larger surfaces have to be repaired. The wound comprises a cavity, which may become filled with exudate or necrotic tissue.

a. Large wound with exudate and necrotic tissue

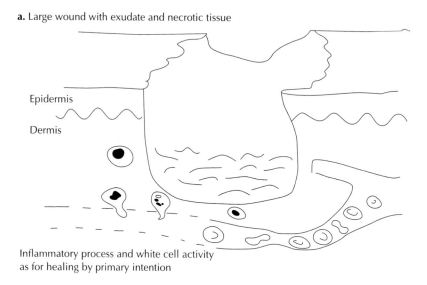

Epidermis

Dermis

Inflammatory process and white cell activity
as for healing by primary intention

b. Necrotic tissue ingested by macrophages – growth factors produced

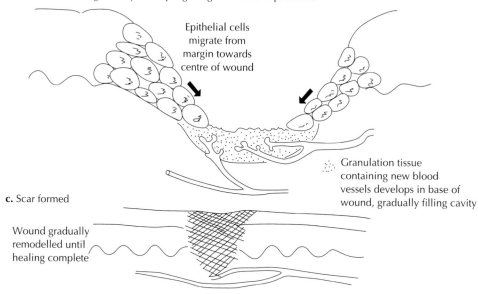

Epithelial cells
migrate from
margin towards
centre of wound

Granulation tissue
containing new blood
vessels develops in base of
wound, gradually filling cavity

c. Scar formed

Wound gradually
remodelled until
healing complete

Figure 3.5   Wound healing by secondary intention.

Necrotic tissue must be removed before healing can take place. A range of wound preparations exist which are designed to encourage healing from the base of the wound, rather than allowing surface closure with a sinus underneath, in which case, trapped exudate may become a focus for infection and prevent healing (see Figure 3.5).

During this process, the floor of the wound cavity becomes covered by granulation tissue, which is fragile and contains budding capillaries. Epithelial cells proliferate from the wound edges and migrate towards the centre of the wound, providing a protective surface layer. Collagen tissue is laid down within the wound and a scar is modelled to restore the wound integrity. Scar tissue is often considerably less strong than the tissue of origin. If a scar lies over a joint, then as it contracts during the later stages of healing, it may significantly diminish joint mobility.

Prerequisites for wound healing

For a wound to heal, a diet containing adequate protein is needed. This enables an effective immune response to occur, and also enables appropriate fibroblast activity. Protein is needed for creation of the necessary protein and collagen structures within the tissues, also for wound remodelling and development of new blood vessels. Carbohydrates are needed for energy to power cell mitosis, so as to leave amino acids available for tissue rebuilding. Carbohydrates also provide energy to fuel white blood cell activity. Fats are required to enable the synthesis of new cell membranes and vitamins A and C for collagen formation. Zinc is thought to be needed for the formation of new epithelium.

All of these nutrients, plus oxygen, must be delivered to the tissues by the bloodstream, which must also remove tissue metabolites. A good blood supply to the area is therefore necessary. In addition to its role in ATP formation, oxygen is needed for the formation of stable collagen, and is also used by white cells during the process of phagocytosis of infective micro-organisms. The presence of shock, tissue oedema or blood vessel pathology,

which reduces the vessel lumen, will impair wound healing.

Wounds need to be clean, and to have a warm, moist undisturbed environment. The young have more effective wound healing mechanisms than do older people. The inflammatory process brings white blood cells and immune products to the area so as to remove foci of infection. Cells that will create collagen and fibrous scar tissue are also drawn to the area. If infection occurs, the inflammatory process is prolonged, the formation of granulation tissue is delayed and fibroblast activity and collagen deposition are delayed. If a wound is heavily infected, the white cell defences may become overwhelmed. The use of corticosteroids impairs the inflammatory process, delaying healing, as does the pre-existence of diabetes mellitus. The use of corticosteroid medication reduces capillary permeability, diminishes protein synthesis by cells and inhibits the activity of fibroblasts and phagocytic white cells. Diabetes mellitus causes delayed wound healing due to small blood vessel abnormalities. It also results in poor collagen formation, the production of weak scar tissue and impaired phagocyte activity. Figure 3.6 shows factors necessary for wound healing to occur.

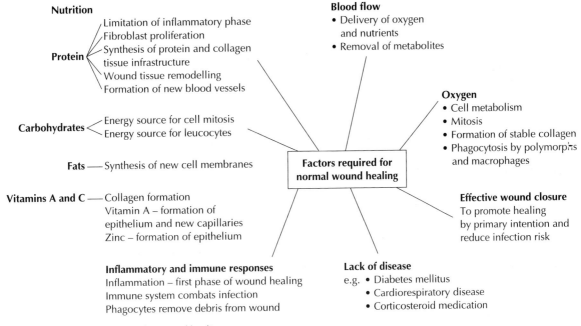

Figure 3.6   Factors necessary for wound healing.

Clinical observations and monitoring

Surgical wound infection is a key outcome indicator of surgery (Reilly, 2002), having serious implications for mortality and morbidity rates as well as increased financial cost to the NHS. A number of risk factors are associated with the development of a surgical wound infection including age, smoking, body mass index, pre-operative skin preparation and post-operative dressings (pre-operative skin preparation is discussed in Chapter 1). Post-operatively, it is necessary to observe the wound regularly and to ensure that it is healing appropriately, although the dressing should not be removed less than 24 hours post-operatively (see below). Some local inflammation is not unusual but excessive redness, warmth and swelling may indicate infection. The presence of exudate may or may not indicate infection as bacteria may colonise some wounds without active infection being present. The patient's temperature may also indicate the presence of infection. If infection is suspected a wound swab should be obtained.

Management

Cleansing

There has been controversy about whether wounds should be cleaned, and if so, with what. Betts (2003) suggests that the use of water for wound cleansing produces comparable results to the use of more sophisticated solutions. Fernandez et al. (2005) undertook a systematic review to assess the use of water as an effective means of cleansing a wound, and made the following points: in terms of infection rate, acute wounds appear to heal just as well if cleaned with tap water of high quality (i.e. safely drinkable) as when they are cleaned with normal saline or not cleaned at all. However, the temperature of the fluid used may be important: if the solution is too warm, it is readily contaminated by micro-organisms; if it is too cold, the rate of mitotic division may be reduced. There is evidence that the use of antiseptic substances is detrimental to the healing process. Some suggestions have been made that the use of any sort of cleaning solutions to remove wound exudate may be detrimental because they remove growth factors and other active chemicals that promote wound healing. Overall, the evidence to support cleansing of a healthy patient's surgical wound remains uncertain. Fernandez et al. (2005) suggest that further research would be useful, but point out the need for a reliable set of criteria to standardise the assessment of the presence of wound infection.

Dressing

The aim of the surgical wound dressing is to absorb secretions and to protect the wound from injury and bacterial contamination (Reilly, 2002). Because adherent dressings can damage the wound when removed, non-adherent dressings should be used on surgical wounds. As discussed above, wounds healing by primary intention are usually sealed by fibrin within 24–48 hours. Therefore, the theatre dressing should normally be removed on the second day post-operatively. It is acceptable for the wound to remain exposed after this period if there is not excessive exudate. However, some patients may prefer to have it covered for aesthetic reasons or for personal comfort. Skin closures are usually left in situ for several days post-operatively (this varies according to the type of surgery), but should normally be removed within 10 days to reduce the risk of wound infection (Reilly, 2002). The appearance of the surgical wound can have a psychological impact on the patient and this is discussed further in Chapter 5.

Self-test questions

1. List three advantages and three disadvantages of oxygen therapy for the post-operative patient.
2. What is a narrowing pulse pressure often indicative of?
3. List four signs or symptoms of deep vein thrombosis.
4. Complete the following sentence:
   The proportion of body water and electrolytes are monitored by _____ cells present in the _____ and _____.
5. Identify three causes of reduced urine output in the post-operative patient.
6. Identify three advantages and three disadvantages of surgical drains.

7. Which hormone, needed by adults for tissue growth and repair, is released during sleep?
8. Identify three factors that increase the risk of suffering from post-operative nausea and vomiting.
9. In what ways is the management of pyrexia controversial?
10. Identify three prerequisites for wound healing.

References and further reading

Ahern J (2002) 'Assessing acutely ill patients on general wards' *Nursing Standard* 16(47): 47–56

Amdipharm (2004) *Post-operative nausea and vomiting* (online). www.nauseaandvomiting.co.uk (Accessed 20.01.07)

Basset CC & Makin L (eds) (2000) *Caring for the Seriously Ill Patient.* London: Arnold

Betts J (2003) 'Review: wound cleansing with water does not differ from no cleansing or cleansing with other solutions for rates of wound infection or healing' *Evidence-based Nursing* 6(3): 81

Edwards S (1998) 'High Temperature' *Professional Nurse* 13(8): 521–526

Fernandez R, Griffiths R & Ussia C (2005) 'Water for wound cleansing' *Cochrane Database of Systematic Reviews (4)* 2005

Gan TJ (2002) 'Post-operative nausea and vomiting – can it be eliminated?' *Journal of the American Medical Association* 287(10): 1233–1236

Goldhill DR (1997) 'Introducing the postoperative care team: Additional support, expertise, and equipment for general postoperative patients' *British Medical Journal* 314: 389

Goldhill DR, White SA & Sumner A (1999a) 'Physiological values and procedures in the 24h before ICU admission from the ward' *Anaesthesia* 54: 529–534

Goldhill DR, Worthington L, Mulcahy A, Tarling M & Sumner A (1999b) 'The patient-at-risk team: identifying and managing seriously ill ward patients' *Anaesthesia* 54: 853–860

Henry MM & Thompson JN (eds) (2005) *Clinical Surgery* (2nd edn). Edinburgh: Elsevier Saunders

Holmes S (1998) 'The aetiology of malnutrition in hospital' *Professional Nurse Study Supplement* 13(6): S5–S8

Hudson G, Beaver M, Scott J & Heichemer D (1999) 'Warming up to better surgical outcomes' *AORN Online* 69(1): 247–248; 251; 253

Loick HM, Schwann G, Radwig-Thomas H & Theissen JL (1997) 'The effect of general anaesthesia on breathing patterns in elderly patients during the early post-operative period' *European Journal of Anaesthesiology* 14(3): 258–265

Mann E (1999) 'Using acupuncture and acupressure to treat post-operative emesis' *Professional Nurse* 14(10): 691–694

McCarthy EJ (2004) 'Malignant hyperthermia – pathophysiology, clinical presentation and treatment' *AACN Clinical Issues: Advanced Practice in Acute and Critical Care* 15(2): 231–237

Metheny NM (2000) *Fluid and Electrolyte Balance* (4th edn). Maryland: Lippincott

National Confidential Enquiry into Perioperative Deaths (1999) *Extremes of Age.* London: NCEPOD

National Confidential Enquiry into Perioperative Deaths (2002) *Functioning as a Team?* London: NCEPOD

Place B & Graham S (2000) 'Non-invasive vital organ assessment' *NT Plus* 96(20): 6–9

Reilly J (2002) 'Evidence-based surgical wound care on surgical wound infection' *British Journal of Nursing (Tissue Viability Supplement)* 11(16): S4–S12

Shelly MP & Nightingale P (1999) 'ABC of intensive care – respiratory support' *British Medical Journal* 318: 1674–1677

Scottish Intercollegiate Guidelines Network (SIGN) (2004) *Postoperative management in adults – a practical guide to postoperative care for clinical staff.* Edinburgh: SIGN

Silk DBA & Gow NM (2001) 'Post-operative starvation after gastrointestinal surgery: early feeding is beneficial' *British Medical Journal* 323(7316): 761–762

Tate S (1997) 'Peppermint oil: a treatment for post-operative nausea' *Journal of Advanced Nursing* 26: 543–549

Thompson HJ (1999) 'The management of post-operative nausea and vomiting' *Journal of Advanced Nursing* 29(5): 1130–1136

Wallis M & Autar R (2001) 'Deep vein thrombosis: clinical nursing management' *Nursing Standard* 15(18): 47–54

Woodrow P (1999) 'Pulse oximetry' *Nursing Standard* 13(42): 42–46

Worsley M (1993) 'NSAIDs in the post-operative period' *British Medical Journal* 307(6898): 257

4 Post-operative Pain Management

Jane McLean, Sandra Huntington, Fiona J McArthur-Rouse

Introduction

Pain is virtually inevitably linked with surgical treatment, so it is important that staff caring for such patients have an understanding of the relevant mechanisms and a readiness to institute effective pain control. Within this chapter, the physiology and assessment and management of pain will be considered. Box 4.1 identifies the aims of this chapter.

The International Association for the Study of Pain endorsed the definition proposed by Merskey *et al.* (1979) that pain is

'. . . a sensory and emotional experience associated with actual or potential tissue damage or described in terms of such damage . . .'
(cited in Cambitzi *et al.*, 2000, p. 467)

Meanwhile, McCaffery's (1979, p. 11) oft-quoted definition of pain as

'. . . whatever the experiencing person says it is, existing whenever the person says it does . . .'

highlights the subjectivity of the experience (Carr & Thomas, 1997).

This definition implies that the patient's experience of pain is always believed – a fundamental concept for effective pain management. However, numerous studies have indicated that healthcare staff consistently underestimate the amount of pain that patients experience post-operatively and that although patients themselves expect to experience pain, this is often greater than anticipated (Carr & Thomas, 1997; Cambitzi *et al.*, 2000).

Types of pain

Pain may be classified as acute, chronic non-malignant, or chronic malignant. It must be remembered that patients with chronic malignant pain may also experience acute pain. Acute pain, such as that experienced post-operatively, is characteristically of recent onset with a relatively short duration, lasting no more than days or weeks. Its intensity is variable and anxiety may be prominent when the pain is severe or the cause unknown.

Pain occurs when tissues are either damaged or at threat of being damaged. In the context of this book, pain may be an effect of the underlying pathology for which surgery could be required, or

---

Box 4.1 Aims of the chapter.

- To discuss the physiology of pain
- To consider the effects of unrelieved pain in the post-operative patient
- To discuss the process of assessing post-operative pain
- To discuss the principles of post-operative pain management

it may be an outcome of the surgical intervention itself. The pain response evolved as a warning of potential tissue damage, and specialist nerve receptors and fibres called nociceptors developed to respond to the situation.

Nociceptive pain is the normal reaction to a painful stimulus transmitted through intact neural pathways and is the process that transmits pain from the injury to the brain. Acute pain is short-lived, and disappears once the injury has healed or the disease is treated. The physiological responses are involuntary; the sympathetic part of the autonomic nervous system (ANS) predominates, leading to an increase in cardiac and respiratory rate as well as blood pressure, diaphoresis (sweating), and dilated pupils and increased muscle tension. (Behavioural responses to pain are discussed later in this chapter.)

Nociceptive pain can be subdivided into somatic and visceral pain. Somatic pain is experienced in superficial structures, muscle and fascia, and is usually described as dull or achy, well localised and consonant with the underlying lesions; for example, post-operative pain. Visceral pain arises in hollow organs and is usually poorly localised, deep squeezing and cramp-like. Examples include intestinal obstruction and tissue infarction. It is frequently associated with autonomic sensations such as nausea and often has referral sites, for example, the pain of ureteric colic (see Chapter 10) may radiate from the loin to the groin.

Pain may occur due to nerve pathology, in which case it serves no protective function, but causes distress to the patient. Causalgia is a painful condition which is due to oversensitivity of the nerve tract. It may be a cause of back pain, or neuralgic pain elsewhere in the body. Although this type of pain does not have a cause that can be treated surgically, such patients may undergo investigations to exclude conditions that require surgical treatment.

Pain threshold and pain tolerance

Nociceptive pain has a threshold defined as an intensity of stimulation below which it is not perceived. The pain perception threshold is relatively constant and does not vary widely between individuals and cultures. The maximum amount of pain an individual will stand is the pain tolerance threshold (Melzack & Wall, 1965). This may vary both between and within individuals at different times and will be influenced by emotional, psychological and cultural factors. It is often thought that pain results from physical damage and that its intensity relates to the severity of the injury. However, the relationship between pain and injury does not always equate and the same operation may produce dissimilar pain experiences in differing people.

The physiology of pain

Receptors are modified nerve endings that convert the stimulus into electrical potentials, which are propagated along the nerve fibres. Trauma, surgery and inflammatory disease cause a reaction at the site of the tissue damage followed by a physiological response through the body. Tissue damage results in the release of local chemicals, such as histamine, prostaglandins, bradykinin, substance P and 5-hydroxytryptamine (5-HT), which react with each other and on nerve endings. These chemicals activate receptors, whereupon signals travel to the dorsal horn of the spinal cord and then up to the cortex of the brain, where the perception of pain occurs. Algesic (pain-producing) chemicals are released at nociceptive nerve endings, and transmit a warning to the higher centres that the tissues are at risk of being damaged. Figure 4.1 shows the neural pathway by which pain signals are transmitted from the damaged tissue to the brain.

Pain fibres or nociceptors

Nerves have been classified according to what kind of message they carry, their size and the conduction rates of their fibres. Two of these pain fibres carry pain sensation and are the A-delta and C-fibres. The A-beta nerves carry other sensations that are not normally painful, for example warmth and touch.

A-delta fibres are myelinated neurons, which, because of their insulated sheath, when stimulated, transmit quickly resulting in the instant reflex response that will cause the rapid withdrawal of tissue from the pain stimulus. The pain experienced is instant, sharp and localised. The type of sensation carried by the A-delta fibres is called

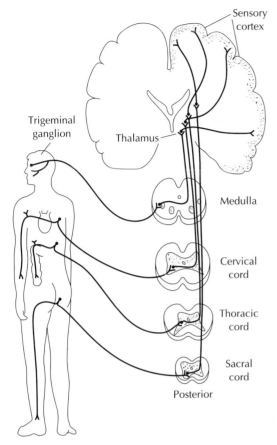

Figure 4.1　Diagram of neural pathways for pain impulses.

'first' or 'fast' pain. The larger the diameter of the myelinated A-delta nerve fibre, the sharper the pain sensation that is produced. An example is the pain of toothache, which produces an intense, jabbing sensation that cannot easily be ignored.

These fibres travel to the dorsal horn of the spinal cord, which is divided into layers of cells known as laminae, which are numbered according to their location. After terminating mainly in lamina 1, the nerves give off long fibres that cross to the other side of the cord and then travel to the thalamus and somatosensory areas of the brain cortex. As the A-delta fibres end in the 'thinking part' of the cortex, we are able to be reasonably accurate in localising pain.

These fibres do not have opioid receptors on their surface and they are responsible for pinprick sensation. Therefore, if a patient has received an opioid for post-operative pain, they will still react to the pain of an intramuscular injection. This 'first pain' remains intact as a protective mechanism to ensure that tissue is not exposed to further potential damage. Giving a nerve block or a general anaesthetic can eradicate this reflex.

Healthcare professionals who understand this aspect of pain transmission will not leave patients in pain because of the mistaken impression that analgesics will 'mask' the pain and make diagnosis more difficult. The tenderness and pain sensation carried by the A-delta fibres will not be affected by opioids. If an inflamed appendix is painful, morphine will make the patient more comfortable, but if the inflamed area is palpated during physical examination, the patient will still complain of pain.

The slowest, smallest, unmyelinated fibres are called C-fibres and are associated with 'second pain', the dull, burning, aching, throbbing, nauseous pain that is felt over a wide area usually after the sharp pain. C-fibres terminate in laminae 1 and 2 (the substantia gelatinosa) of the spinal cord and have short connecting fibres to lamina 5. They then generally follow the same pathway as the A-delta fibres but terminate over a wide area within the brain stem. No fibres project into the somatosensory cortex of the brain. C-fibre pain is almost always responsive to opioid analgesia.

A-beta fibres are not directly related to the transmission of painful stimuli since they only respond to mechanical or thermal stimuli. A-beta fibres are the largest and most rapidly conducting of the three fibres. They are multiple in number, are concentrated in the skin, and do not cross over to the other side of the spinal cord. These fibres have a role in aspects of pain suppression.

Following any tissue damage there results a volley of nociceptive impulses, which travel along small myelinated A-delta nerve fibres and unmyelinated C-fibres which then synapse with cells in the substantia gelatinosa of the dorsal horn of the spinal cord. If inhibitory impulses do not descend the spinal cord from the brain, the nociceptive impulses continue to ascend to the cortex, and pain is perceived. Figure 4.2 shows the types of nerve fibre involved in pain transmission.

Phantom limb pain

This is a disturbing pain disorder that is sometimes encountered in people who have undergone

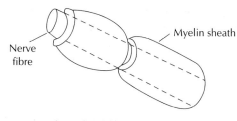

a. Large myelinated A-delta fibres transmit 'fast' precise pain signals

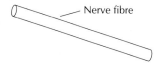

b. Small non-myelinated C-fibres transmit 'slow', burning pain signals

Figure 4.2   Types of nociceptive fibre.

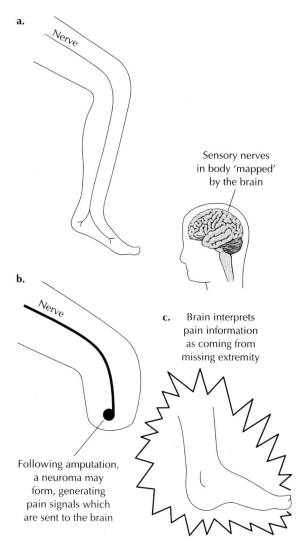

a.

Sensory nerves in body 'mapped' by the brain

b.

c.   Brain interprets pain information as coming from missing extremity

Following amputation, a neuroma may form, generating pain signals which are sent to the brain

Figure 4.3   Phantom limb pain.

previous limb amputation. Sensations that seem to originate in a part of the body that the individual knows has previously been removed surgically can be extremely disturbing. Phantom limb pain tends to occur as a result of previous surgical division of the nerve supply to the amputated extremity. The nerve fibre may partially regenerate, forming a neuroma, which then generates signals that ascend the spinal pain tracts to the sensory area of the brain. If the sensory area of the brain still has a 'map' of the amputated extremity, the perception is that there is pain or sensation originating from that area. Figure 4.3 illustrates how phantom limb pain develops.

Gate control theory

This theory was proposed by Melzack & Wall in 1965 and has been updated by later research (Wall & Melzack, 1994, 1999). Their theory provides an important explanation of aspects of the nature of pain, and reflects physiological, cognitive and emotional facets of the pain experience.

In the spinal cord, the nerve fibres of the dorsal columns (tracts) carry sensations from the periphery to the brain. The modifying mechanism in the spinal cord is called 'gate control' (Melzack & Wall, 1965). The mechanism may completely inhibit the upward transmission of pain impulses,

or may amplify them to make the pain more severe. Anxiety, excitement and anticipation may open the 'gate' and therefore increase the perception of pain. Conversely, cognitive activities such as distraction, suggestion relaxation, biofeedback and imagery tend to close the 'gate' and prevent the sensory transmission of pain (Melzack *et al.*, 1982). Activation of the faster transmitting A-beta fibres, with stimulation such as gentle massage on the affected area, can also close the 'gate'.

A child who falls and hurts her arm has the area 'rubbed better' by her mother. This action

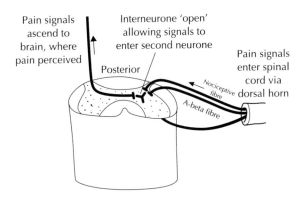

Pain signals ascend to brain, where pain perceived

Interneurone 'open' allowing signals to enter second neurone

Pain signals enter spinal cord via dorsal horn

Posterior

Nociceptive fibre

A-beta fibre

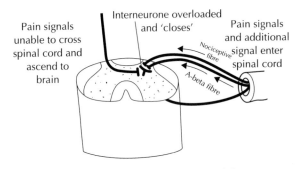

Pain signals unable to cross spinal cord and ascend to brain

Interneurone overloaded and 'closes'

Pain signals and additional signal enter spinal cord

Nociceptive fibre

A-beta fibre

Figure 4.4   The gate control theory of pain modulation.

stimulates the fast-acting A-beta fibres, which then feed into the dorsal horn of the spinal cord where they synapse in the same area as the pain-transmitting fibres (the substantia gelatinosa). If there are too many nerve fibres arriving at the same time, only the faster fibres taking the shortest route are likely to get through. The rubbing action produces heat and fewer pain sensations reach the brain. Also by distracting her daughter, the mother stimulates the cognitive features of the gate control mechanism higher up the CNS to help modulate the pain and reduce its impact on the child. Figure 4.4 summarises key features of the gate control theory of pain.

Nociception is transmitted towards the brain in various ascending tracts. Some tracts carry precise information about localisation of painful stimuli and others carry information about pain position and quality. Descending control from the brain can modify all nociceptive ascending transmission. Modification occurs mainly at spinal cord and brain stem levels and most pain impulses never reach conscious level. Modification involves the activation of inhibitory pathways and the release of inhibitory chemical transmitters. An example of this modification activity is when a hot dish of food is picked up. The sense of burning is felt, but the person realises that, if the reflex to drop the plate occurs, a carefully prepared meal will land on the floor. The ability to bear the pain and hold on to the hot dish until it can be put down safely is due to the modified response.

Each spinal cord mechanism has its own chemical transmitters including substance P, cholecystokinin and somatostatin. The spinal cord passes into the brain stem, which is responsible for processing and integrating pain sensations. The brain summates the sensory inputs and compares them to previous experiences to provide a basis for the rational behaviour of the individual. Parts of the brain exchange information between various parts of the body and formulate co-ordinated responses. Other parts convey information about the precise location and nature of noxious stimuli and influence the discriminative and motivational aspects of pain.

The processes of perception and response to pain are classified in four stages of nociception:

- *Transduction* – when the stimulus is detected by nociceptors
- *Transmission* – when the message is relayed from the receptors to the CNS
- *Modulation* – when the message is modified by other activity in the body, which may be activity of other peripheral nerves or may occur in the CNS
- *Perception* – when the brain perceives the sensation as painful

A key component of the four stages is the physiological 'gating' mechanism as described above. The amount of stimulation passing through the gate to produce pain is dependent on the response intensity in the conducting fibres and on descending influences from the brain which may reduce pain. The gate is thought to be situated in the dorsal horn of the spinal cord. When the amount of information passing through the gate reaches a certain level, it activates the neural areas responsible for pain experience and response. Pain perception can be modified by reducing or increasing the stimulation, i.e. 'closing' or 'opening' the gate, through ascending and descending neural mechanisms.

Wall & Melzack (1999) proposed that excitation of pain pathways can lead to a type of 'wind-up' phenomenon. In association with nerve injury, changes can occur in the neural mechanisms that lead to heightened excitation and the perception of pain long after the initial injury has ceased to be a causative factor. This explains why pain can continue long after the acute damage has occurred and become chronic.

Neuromatrix pain theory was developed from the gate control theory by Wall & Melzack (1999), and suggests that a neural system exists at brain stem level, which, when activated, results in a reduction in perceived pain. Specifically endogenous opioid neurotransmitters capable of reducing pain perception are released from brain tissue e.g. endorphins, enkephalins and dynorphins. So, not only does the body have natural pain-producing chemicals, it also has natural analgesic substances.

Opioid receptors are mainly found in the brain and spinal cord; opioids bind to one of the three different types of receptors, each receptor having a slightly different action. Opioids have the ability to lock onto the various receptors where they then enhance the natural receptor activity. Drugs that enhance a response at a receptor are called agonists. Although opioids can produce severe unwanted side-effects, such as respiratory depression, their activity can be reversed by administering an antagonist. An antagonist is a substance that can occupy the same receptor but has no biological activity, thus blocking the receptor against the biological active agonist. For example, if a patient is experiencing respiratory depression as a result of opioid administration and naloxone (an opioid antagonist) is administered, the unwanted side-effect is reversed and the patient's respiratory rate will increase. However, if too much naloxone is given, all analgesic effects are reversed.

Psychosocial aspects of pain

Pain has physical, emotional, cognitive, socio-cultural and spiritual factors and thus each pain event is a distinct and personal experience (Lemone & Burke, 2004). These factors account for some of the differences between people's perceptions of pain. Previous positive experiences may build confidence and empowerment whilst negative experiences may bring fear, uncertainty and helplessness, exacerbating the pain (Lemone & Burke, 2004). Stress and anxiety can both augment and result from pain. Negative psychological feedback can lead to defence mechanisms such as aggression, depression and withdrawal.

Our cultural background may influence every aspect of our experience of pain: how we react, what treatment we seek and the intensity and duration of the pain we tolerate; when we report pain and to whom, and what type of pain requires attention (Lemone & Burke, 2004). For example, patients of northern European ancestry are considered stoical and to value 'being a good patient' (Lemone & Burke, 2004). Western cultures also value the 'magic bullet remedy' in order to avoid the experience of pain, whilst eastern cultures tend to find a meaning for their pain (Carr & Thomas, 1997). Lemone & Burke warn, however, that behaviours within a culture vary greatly from generation to generation and that health professionals' own values and beliefs about pain will influence the way they assess and manage their patients' pain.

The effect of age upon pain perception is unclear: studies to date have proved inconclusive. Staff attitudes and behaviour may influence the management of pain in the older person with factors such as stoicism, communication and ageism shaping both patients' and nurses' attitudes (Brown, 2004).

Adverse effects of unrelieved pain

The effects of unrelieved acute pain have been studied and may be associated with post-operative complications and an increase in the length of hospital stay (Closs, 1990; Royal College of Surgeons and Anaesthetists, 1990; Justins & Richardson, 1991; Watt-Watson et al., 1999). Many of the effects are associated with the physiological stress response. Table 4.1 summarises the harmful effects of unrelieved pain in the post-operative patient. Because of the effects of unrelieved pain, patients need to be informed of the need to control their pain and encouraged if necessary to use the analgesia available to them. This will enable them to mobilise more quickly and avoid some of the complications associated with surgery.

Table 4.1   The harmful effects of unrelieved post-operative pain.

Cardiovascular	• Increased sympathetic nervous system (SNS) activity causes increase in heart rate, blood pressure and peripheral vascular resistance • As the workload and stress of the heart increase, owing to hypertension and tachycardia, the oxygen consumption of the myocardium also increases • When oxygen consumption is greater than oxygen supply, myocardial ischaemia (which, in the post-operative period, may be silent) will result and, potentially, myocardial infarction occur • Myocardial oxygen supply may be further compromised by the presence of any pre-existing cardiac or respiratory disease or by hypoxaemia due to impaired respiratory function
Respiratory	• 'Splinting' can occur whereby the patient limits the movement of the thoracic and abdominal muscles leading to respiratory dysfunction, reluctance to cough and sputum retention • Reduction in vital lung capacity, increased inspiratory and expiratory pressures; atelectasis and pneumonia may occur • Hypoxia may cause cardiac complications, disorientation and confusion as well as delayed wound healing
Gastrointestinal	• Increased SNS activity leads to temporarily impaired gastrointestinal function, delays in gastric emptying and reduced bowel motility with the potential for development of paralytic ileus • Stimulation of pain receptors in the CNS may lead to activation of the vomit centre in the brain causing vomiting to occur • Disturbance of the gastrointestinal tract can activate the release of the neurotransmitter 5-hydroxytryptamine ($5-HT_3$), which can also initiate vomiting
Renal	• Release of catecholamines, aldosterone, anti-diuretic hormone (ADH), cortisol, angiotensin II and prostaglandins causes retention of sodium and water, causing fluid overload, increased cardiac workload and hypertension
Musculoskeletal	• Involuntary responses to noxious stimuli can cause reflex muscle spasm at the site of tissue damage • Impaired muscle function and muscle fatigue can lead to immobility, causing venous stasis, increased blood coagulability, and an increased risk of DVT
Immunological	• Depression of the immune system may predispose the patient to wound infection, chest infection, pneumonia and sepsis.
Neuroendocrine	• Increased levels of catecholamine, cortisol, growth hormone, vasopressin, aldosterone and insulin can lead to hyperglycaemia • Increased fibrin and platelet activation may increase the risk of DVT and pulmonary embolism • Increased catabolism and a negative nitrogen balance may impair wound healing and immune function with a consequent decreased resistance to infection
Psychological and cognitive effects	• The stressor effects of unrelieved pain have the potential to increase anxiety levels and interfere with activities of living, such as eating, exercise, work or leisure activities and to interrupt normal sleep patterns • Distressing cognitive impairment, such as disorientation, mental confusion and a reduced ability to concentrate, may occur
Analgesic response	• Production of naturally occurring endogenous opioids (also known as encephalins and endorphins), found throughout the central nervous system, bind to opioid receptor sites • Release of neurotransmitters such as substance P is prevented causing inhibition of transmission of pain impulses, bringing about an analgesic effect • Unfortunately endogenous opioids degrade too quickly to be considered as useful analgesics

(Justins & Richardson, 1991; McCaffery & Pasero, 1999; Watt-Watson *et al.*, 1999)

Assessment of pain

Pain is a complex, subjective phenomenon and, by its nature, is difficult to assess. The patient's self-report of pain is the 'gold standard' in pain assessment, as only the patient can accurately describe his or her pain (Smeltzer & Bare, 2000). Pain assessment is also valuable as it provides patients with the means to verbalise their pain and takes account of their personal experience. If, following assessment, effective pain relief is provided, patients will have more confidence in the process.

Box 4.2   Examples of individuals who may be unable to describe their pain.

- Those with poorly developed language skills
- Those with cognitive impairment or dementia
- Patients who are unconscious
- Infants

Box 4.3   Behavioural signs of pain.

- Bodily posture – holding, protecting the affected site
- Vocalising – moaning, crying, shouting
- Immobility – keeping still, cautious on movement
- Rocking and rubbing the affected site
- Facial expressions – frowning, tension
- Irritability – noise intolerance, social withdrawal, impatience

However, some patients are unable to describe their pain (see Box 4.2) and in such circumstances it may be necessary to rely on physiological signs – such as increased heart rate or blood pressure – and behavioural signs (see Box 4.3). However, physiological and behavioural signs of pain are less reliable indicators and vary greatly between individuals (Smeltzer & Bare, 2000).

Wall & Melzack (1994) identify several main aims of pain assessment. Pain assessment should be performed frequently depending on the patient's condition, self-report and response to treatment. Continuous monitoring and recording of pain levels can indicate the effectiveness of treatment and identify when pain control needs adjustment. It is also helpful to monitor patient safety related to the administration of analgesia. However, despite the obvious benefits of pain assessment, it is

frequently not carried out effectively (Schafheutle et al., 2004), or not documented (Briggs & Dean, 1998). Table 4.2 identifies some barriers to effective pain assessment.

Pain assessment tools

Pain assessment tools aim to provide an evaluation by quantifying and describing objectively a subjective experience. A number of tools are available to measure pain. All have advantages and disadvantages and varying degrees of reliability and validity (Carr & Thomas, 1997); thus any data collected should be interpreted in the light of a particular tool's limitations.

Self-report measurement scales include numerical or descriptive (verbal) rating and visual analogue scales. A pain intensity score is a quick way of finding out the intensity of the pain for a given individual and evaluating the effectiveness of an intervention. Such scores are quick and simple to use, and most patients are able to understand them. However, the disadvantages of such scales include the fact that they are unilateral, measuring pain intensity only and giving neither a description of the pain or any additional relevant information (Brown, 2004).

Visual analogue scale

This scale consists of a 10 cm line, one end is labelled 'no pain at all' and the other end is labelled 'agonising pain' (see Figure 4.5). Patients are asked to mark on the line the point corresponding to their pain. A pain score is then obtained by measuring, usually in centimetres, the distance between 'no pain at all' and the patient's mark. This can then

Table 4.2   Barriers to effective pain assessment.

Patient	Nurses
<ul><li>Fear of addiction</li><li>Reluctance to report pain</li><li>Stoic, expect to suffer</li><li>Want to be a 'good patient'</li><li>Think professionals are the authority on their pain</li><li>Afraid that analgesia may mask symptoms</li></ul>	<ul><li>Poor knowledge of pain assessment</li><li>Afraid that analgesia may mask symptoms</li><li>Prefer to use own judgement</li><li>Assume the patient will ask for pain relief</li><li>Reliance on the presence of a pump (PCA or epidural)</li><li>Reliance on physiological and behavioural signs</li><li>Assume the pain is in one location and do not assess on movement</li><li>Nurses do not see it as a priority</li></ul>

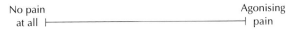

No pain
at all

Agonising
pain

Figure 4.5   Visual analogue scale.

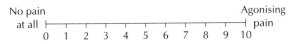

No pain
at all

Agonising
pain

0   1   2   3   4   5   6   7   8   9   10

Figure 4.6   Numerical rating scale.

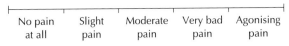

| No pain at all | Slight pain | Moderate pain | Very bad pain | Agonising pain |

Figure 4.7   Verbal rating scale.

give a precise figure and, when repeated later, can indicate small changes in pain intensity. This scale requires a patient to be able to concentrate. Some may have difficulty in understanding the concept, especially immediately post-operatively, or if they are cognitively impaired, in which case a numerical scale may be more appropriate.

Simple descriptive and numerical scales

These tools use words, numbers or a combination of both to indicate the intensity of the pain and the effectiveness of any pain-relieving measures (see Figures 4.6 and 4.7). They are easy to explain to the patient and can be asked as a simple question rather than requiring the patient to look at a scale. Patients are asked to describe their pain on a verbal scale giving predefined categories, or to assign a numerical value to their pain where 0 signifies no pain and 10 signifies the worst pain imaginable. Sometimes scales of 0–5 or 0–3 are used instead.

McGill pain questionnaire

The McGill pain questionnaire (MPQ) (Melzack, 1975, 1987) is a multidimensional pain assessment tool that addresses location, quality, duration and factors affecting the pain. Primarily developed for chronic pain assessment, it has been successfully used with acute pain sufferers. However, due to its lengthiness, its use in post-operative pain assessment is limited (Brown, 2004).

Pharmacological approaches to post-operative pain management

The causes of post-operative pain are multifactorial, therefore a variety of approaches to treating pain need to be considered. The site of surgery, the underlying disease and the patient's general health need consideration. The use of drugs is a major part of post-operative pain management so health professionals need to understand the properties and side-effects of the analgesia they administer and impart appropriate aspects of this knowledge to patients. This should help them to make informed decisions about their care and encourage patients to be active in reporting inadequate analgesia or side-effects. A multimodal approach using both opioid and non-opioid drugs is recommended for patients who have undergone major surgery (Cambitzi *et al.*, 2000; Pollok & Walsh, 2004).

Post-operative pain relief should start in the recovery area and will usually be in the form of intravenous opioids titrated until the patient is comfortable. Most hospitals now have acute pain teams or specialist nurses who assist with and advise on post-operative pain assessment and management. They also have an educational function to enable ward staff to better manage patients' pain.

Opioid therapy

Opioid drugs may either be weak or strong and, in their strongest form, act on several sites in the central nervous system involved in pain perception and block the transmission of pain signals by binding to the opioid receptors. Because they act directly on the parts of the brain where pain is perceived, opioids are the strongest analgesics and are therefore used to treat the pain arising from surgery and trauma. Their ability to produce a state of relaxation and euphoria is often helpful in relieving the stress that accompanies severe pain.

Strong opioids

Opioids are effective in controlling somatic and visceral pain and are partially effective in controlling neuropathic pain. Opioids produce analgesia by binding to receptors in the brain and spinal cord, thereby inhibiting or modulating nociceptive input. Morphine is frequently the opioid of choice in the management of post-operative pain and is metabolised in the liver and excreted by the kidneys. Others include diamorphine, pethidine and fentanyl. Fentanyl has a short onset and duration of action, but because it is lipophilic (having an affinity for fat), it may cause delayed sedation and respiratory depression with repetitive or continuous systemic administration. It is, however, widely used in epidural analgesia (Cambitzi *et al.*, 2000). The use of these powerful opioids is strictly controlled because the euphoria produced can lead to abuse and addiction. However, in short-term post-

operative use and when given under medical supervision, the risk of addiction is negligible.

Opioids can be administered via a variety of routes (see Chapter 2) and are frequently used in conjunction with non-opioid analgesia (see below) to obtain maximum pain relief. The route of administration affects the onset and duration of the drug's effect. In the immediate post-operative period, patients who have undergone major surgery are rarely able to tolerate oral medication and to gain maximum effect the intravenous or epidural routes tend to be used either by continuous infusion or patient-controlled analgesia (PCA) pumps (see

---

Box 4.4   Patient-controlled analgesia (PCA) administration.

Patient-controlled analgesia (PCA) is a mechanism that enables patients to administer and regulate their own intravenous or epidural analgesia. There are a variety of commercial devices available; however, the components of each type are similar with a pump, a remote demand button, an antisiphon and a backflow valve. There are also disposable and non-disposable devices.

The main principle of PCA is that patients self-administer an opioid, most commonly morphine, using a demand button according to the severity of their pain. The PCA is programmed according to a protocol or prescription that includes the dose and concentration, the lockout interval, duration of administration and the maximum dosage. Once the pump has been programmed it is locked and cannot be altered without use of a key.

A side-effect of morphine is nausea and vomiting so an anti-emetic is prescribed. Also, naloxone is prescribed to be administered in the event of decreased respiratory rate (< 8) and increased sedation level.

Advantages of PCA:

- The patient is in control of the analgesia administration and this can help to reduce anxiety
- The patient does not have to request analgesia or wait for it to be administered
- Regular small doses of analgesia are administered which help to maintain constant plasma concentration levels whilst reducing side-effects
- The patient is able to mobilise more quickly which contributes to a faster recovery
- There is a reduction in nursing time spent administering analgesia

The success of PCA is dependent on patient education pre-operatively, adequate prescription regimens and regular reviews by staff. Selection of patients is important from two perspectives: firstly, to be mentally capable

of understanding the concept of self-administration, and secondly, to be physically capable of pressing the button to deliver the analgesic dose.

Factors that may contribute to inadequate pain relief whilst using a PCA include:

- The patient is not adequately prepared in the use of the PCA pump and:
  - ○ Fears the adverse effects arising from opioids such as nausea and excessive sedation and consequently chooses to suffer the pain
  - ○ Fears addiction
- The patient has long periods of sleep and forgets to press the button
- The patient suffers acute confusional state post-operatively
- There is mechanical failure of the pump
- The nurse assumes that the PCA will provide adequate pain relief and fails to assess its effectiveness and offer adjuvant treatment

All patients with PCAs must have a patent intravenous cannula and be cared for in areas with full resuscitation equipment. During PCA administration the following must be recorded:

- Blood pressure
- Pulse
- Respiratory rate
- Pain score
- Sedation level
- Nausea and vomiting

The decision to discontinue the PCA should be discussed with the patient and members of the multidisciplinary team and adequate alternative analgesia prescribed and administered before removing the pump.

Boxes 4.4 and 4.5). It is important that pain is controlled before leaving recovery, particularly if a PCA device is used. A therapeutic plasma level of an opioid must be established because only small doses are delivered via the PCA; these are insufficient to manage pain without previous titration. Intramuscular injections are sometimes used but for major surgery they are only effective if given frequently and regularly (Pollok & Walsh, 2004).

Opioid side-effects include nausea and vomiting, reduced intestinal motility (possibly contributing to a post-operative paralytic ileus), sedation and respiratory depression, neuropsychological changes such as impaired cognitive function and slowed reactions. Nausea should be treated with prophylactic anti-emetics administered on a regular basis (see Chapter 3).

Sedation and respiratory depression are the most feared consequences of opioid use. Respiratory depression will reverse if the opioid dose is decreased or the infusion is stopped, and may respond to measures that support respiratory function such as airway clearance and oxygen administration. When necessary, naloxone, an opioid antagonist, is given incrementally, carefully titrated,

---

Box 4.5 Epidural analgesia administration.

This technique is performed by an anaesthetist under sterile conditions and involves injecting a local anaesthetic into the epidural space (see Figure 4.8). Epidural analgesia can be used either as an alternative to or in conjunction with a general anaesthetic and for post-operative pain relief in procedures involving the thorax, pelvic region or lower limbs. Providing the patient is suitable for an epidural it can be employed in a wide variety of surgical procedures but is commonly used in obstetric, general, urology and orthopaedic surgery. The site of injection will depend on the procedure. Positioning of the patient is important for this procedure and will involve either a lateral or sitting position; this allows for greater flexion of the spine and for this reason it is essential to have the co-operation of the conscious patient.

Epidural analgesia can either be by single injection or continuous infusion of local anaesthetic, usually bupivacaine, via an indwelling catheter. This can be administered as required by the anaesthetist or if prolonged pain relief is required then an epidural infusion pump may be attached, allowing the patient to self-administer the infusion (PCEA). The local anaesthetic is usually combined with an opiate such as fentanyl; however morphine and diamorphine may also be used. Once the initial dose of local anaesthetic has been injected, anaesthesia is usually obvious in 15–30 minutes and can last 3–6 hours with bupivacaine. The volumes of local anaesthetic injected are higher than that required for a spinal technique, and range from 8–30 mL depending on the surgical procedure (Green et al., 2003).

Contraindications to this method of analgesia have to be considered and these are some examples:

- Patient refusal
- Skin infection at the site of injection
- Hypovolaemia
- Tendency to bleed

- Anatomical abnormalities
- Cardiac disease

There are potential, though uncommon, major complications associated with epidural analgesia which can be avoided with regular assessment of the patient's condition. These include:

- Motor blockade of the intercostal muscles causing respiratory depression and arrest
- Injection of local anaesthetic into the epidural veins causing paraesthesia of the tongue and lips – this may also cause sudden loss of consciousness
- If the needle is advanced too far, accidentally puncturing the dura and entering the subarachnoid space, post-dural puncture headache can occur and sometimes breathing may cease
- Infection leading to epidural abcess

Mild and temporary side-effects of epidural analgesia include:

- Hypotension due to vasodilation (intravenous fluids are routinely administered to counteract this)
- Inability to pass urine
- Backache

Whilst administering epidural analgesia the following must be monitored:

- Blood pressure
- Heart rate
- Respiratory rate
- Sedation score
- Degree of motor block
- Urinary output

IV access is essential in any patient undergoing regional block procedures and patients will usually have received preload fluids.

to reverse respiratory depression. It is important to note that naloxone is short-acting and repeated injections may be required.

Weak opioids

Weak opioids include codeine, dihydrocodeine and tramadol, which are used to treat mild to moderate pain, usually in the later post-operative period and sometimes in conjunction with non-opioids such as non-steroidal anti-inflammatory drugs. In low dose, codeine (8 mg) is combined with paracetamol to form the compound co-codamol, whilst dihydrocodeine (10 mg) is combined with paracetamol to form co-dydramol (Cambitzi *et al.*, 2000). These drugs are given orally and side-effects include nausea and constipation. If patients are taking these regularly post-operatively they may have a reduced appetite and will often require an aperient to counteract the constipation.

Non-opioid analgesics

Non-opioid drugs are used in conjunction with opioids during the immediate post-operative period and later, either on their own, in combination with each other, or with weak opioids.

Paracetamol

Paracetamol acts by reducing the production of prostaglandins, which are known to be potent pain-producing substances, in the central nervous system. It does not usually irritate the stomach and allergic reactions are rare, but an overdose can cause severe and possibly fatal liver and kidney damage, whilst its toxic potential may be increased in heavy drinkers. Paracetamol is practically in-soluble and therefore is only administered via the oral and rectal routes (Cambitzi *et al.*, 2000). It is sometimes prescribed to be given regularly in combination with opioid analgesia or non-steroidal anti-inflammatory drugs (NSAIDs). Paracetamol is frequently present in compounds such as co-codamol, co-dydramol and cold remedies. Therefore when administering the drug it is wise to check that none of these drugs are being taken concurrently.

Non-steroidal anti-inflammatory drugs (NSAIDs)

Commonly used NSAIDs such as ibuprofen are good analgesics for somatic pain. NSAIDs block the generation of the original nociceptive fibres and cause inhibition of the enzyme cyclo-oxygenase (COX), thus inhibiting the production of prostaglandins. NSAIDs have analgesic, anti-inflammatory and antipyretic effects.

However, they also inhibit the production of prostaglandins, which have a protective effect on the stomach and small intestine, and some are involved in the maintenance of renal function and platelet adhesiveness (Cambitzi *et al.*, 2000). It is important, therefore, to undertake pre-operative screening of the patient's general health to ensure that post-operative analgesia will not exacerbate any pre-existing medical condition. Care should be taken when using NSAIDs post-operatively in fluid-depleted patients as there is a risk of causing renal impairment (see Chapter 3). Box 4.6 lists the adverse effects of NSAIDs.

Different NSAIDs are administered via different routes including the oral, intramuscular, rectal and intravenous routes. Used in conjunction with PCA they can significantly reduce the total dose of opioid administration (Pollak & Walsh, 2004). If one NSAID is ineffective, another can be used instead from a different chemical class. However, two types of NSAID must never be given together as this may result in serious side-effects.

Entonox

Entonox, a mixture of 50% oxygen and 50% nitrous oxide, is a useful adjunct in the management of

---

Box 4.6   Adverse effects of NSAIDs.

- Gastrointestinal – dyspepsia, gastric ulceration and bleeding. Ulceration may be caused by the production of mucosal ischaemia and by impairing the protective mucous barrier so that the mucosa is exposed to acid.
- Renal and hepatic impairment
- Bleeding due to inability of platelet function
- Peripheral oedema due to sodium and water retention
- Bronchospasm and skin rashes

post-operative pain. Nitrous oxide is an analgesic gas with a rapid onset and is excreted quickly from the body when no longer inhaled. It acts quickly because the tiny molecules cross the capillary walls in the lungs directly into the bloodstream.

Entonox is available in a portable cylinder, with a mask or mouthpiece and a patient-demand valve, meaning that the patient has control over the amount of gas received. Entonox is useful in procedures such as dressing changes, or to assist in the removal of drains following surgery. It is more effective when used with other analgesics.

Regional anaesthesia and analgesia

These are sometimes used by anaesthetists pre- and post-operatively to control pain and induce regional anaesthesia and involve the injection of local anaesthetics to block the passage of nerve impulses at the site of administration. Local anaesthetics are usually given by injection, for example into the subarachnoid space of the spinal cord (see Figure 4.8), or infiltrated into a wound at the end of an operation, but they can also be applied to the skin. They do not interfere with consciousness and can provide analgesia for several hours. Box 4.7 summarises the priorities of caring for patients who have received spinal anaesthesia.

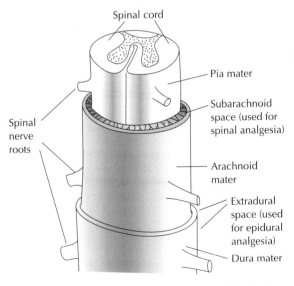

Figure 4.8 The spinal cord and meninges: sites for injection of analgesia.

Non-pharmacological approaches to post-operative pain management

Although pharmacological approaches to pain tend to be the mainstay of acute pain management they can be supplemented with non-pharmacological interventions such as relaxation techniques, distraction, assisting the patient into a comfortable position and touch. In a study of patients' experiences of post-operative pain, Carr & Thomas (1997) found the most utilised non-pharmacological strategy was distraction, whilst Roykulcharoen & Good (2004) concluded that the use of systematic relaxation substantially reduced the sensation and distress of pain in post-operative patients.

Self-test questions

1. Name three classifications of pain.
2. Briefly explain what is meant by somatic and visceral pain.
3. Which local chemicals are released following tissue damage?
   a. Prostaglandins, histamine, bradykinin, substance P and 5-hydroxytryptamine
   b. Prostaglandins, noradrenaline, substance P, serotonin and histamine
   c. Serotonin, acetylcholine, adrenaline, noradrenaline and prostaglandin
   d. Bradykinin, histamine, prostaglandin, adrenaline and serotonin
4. Which nerve fibres carry sensations of warmth and touch?
   a. A-delta fibres
   b. A-beta fibres
   c. Beta-delta fibres
   d. C-fibres
5. Which nerve fibres transmit fast pain?
   a. C-fibres
   b. Beta-delta fibres
   c. A-delta fibres
   d. A-beta fibres
6. Where do the A-delta fibres and the C-fibres synapse?
   a. In the brain stem of the spinal cord
   b. In the caudate nucleus
   c. In the substantia gelatinosa of the dorsal horn
   d. In the hypothalamus

Box 4.7   Spinal analgesia/anaesthesia.

This technique is performed by an anaesthetist and involves an injection through the epidural space, dura and arachnoid mater (Figure 4.8) until the needle reaches the subarachnoid space containing the cerebrospinal fluid (CSF). The aim is for the local anaesthetic to act on the cauda equina and spinal cord. Spinal anaesthesia is used for a wide variety of elective and emergency surgical procedures below the level of the umbilicus. Positioning of the patient is the same as for epidural; however the site of injection is usually below the region of L1/L2. Although the effects of the spinal block will not be complete for up to 25 minutes, the effects of motor and sensory loss will be present a few minutes after injection of the local anaesthetic. The effects usually last for about 2 to 3 hours.

Spinal anaesthesia is usually a single shot procedure and correct location of the subarachnoid space is confirmed by the appearance of CSF at the hub of the needle. The fact that this is a fluid-filled space is of significance and some points to note are identified below:

- Local anaesthetic solution used has to have a greater density or be heavier than the CSF to ensure that the solution does not travel upwards and potentially impair respiration
- The solution commonly used is called 'heavy' bupivacaine. This is because it has glucose added and therefore does not have the same density as CSF. This solution spreads in a very predictable way
- Adjusting the patient position following injection will affect the spread of the solution, the more upright the patient the less likely the spread upwards or, for

example, turning the patient laterally will encourage a spread in the direction of a fractured neck of femur
- Dosage is much less than that required for an epidural, usually about 2.5–3 mL

Contraindications are similar to those for epidural, as are the complications. However, post-dural puncture headache (PDPH) is a particular complication that may involve a further procedure:

- PDPH is related to the size of the needle used for injecting the local anaesthetic solution and is the result of a leakage of CSF through a hole in the dura
- Onset is usually within 24 hours of the procedure
- Patients complain of frontal and occipital headache that is present when lying flat but worsens on sitting up (Cambitzi et al., 2000)
- Treatment may involve a procedure known as a blood patch, whereby patients are given an injection of about 10 to 20 mL of their own blood back into the epidural space in an attempt to seal the hole through coagulation.
- Alternative treatment may involve bed rest, hydration and analgesics

Irrespective of the type of procedure it is essential that patient consent for the technique has been obtained and that a thorough but uncomplicated explanation of the procedure has been given. Patients can be frightened by the lack of feeling in their limbs and any associated side-effects, so information before and throughout the procedure is reassuring.

---

7. What is the importance of the gate control theory (Melzack & Wall, 1965)?
   a. It explains the aspects of the nature of pain
   b. It reflects physiological facets of the pain experience
   c. It reflects cognitive and emotional facets of the pain experience
   d. All of the above
8. Identify the four stages of nociception in the processes of perception and response to pain
   a. Transduction, transmission, perception and analysis
   b. Transduction, transmission, modulation and perception
   c. Transmission, perception, analysis and transport
   d. Transduction, modulation, transport and analysis

9. List the adverse effects of non-steroidal anti-inflammatory drugs

References and further reading

Briggs M & Dean K (1998) 'A qualitative analysis of the nursing documentation of post-operative pain management' *Journal of Clinical Nursing* 7(2): 155–163

Brown D (2004) 'A literature review exploring how healthcare professionals contribute to the assessment and control of postoperative pain in older people' *International Journal of Older People Nursing* in association with *Journal of Clinical Nursing* 13(6b): 74–90

Cambitzi J, Harries M & van Raders E (2000) 'Chapter 24 – Postoperative pain management' *in:* Manley K & Bellman L (eds) *Surgical Nursing – Advancing Practice.* Edinburgh: Churchill Livingstone

Carr ECJ & Thomas VJ (1997) 'Anticipating and experiencing post-operative pain: the patients' perspective' *Journal of Clinical Nursing* 6(3): 191–201

Closs SJ (1990) 'An exploratory analysis of nurses' provision of postoperative analgesic drugs' *Journal of Advanced Nursing* 15: 42–49

Green D, Ervine M & White S (2003) *Fundamentals of Peri-operative Management*. London: Greenwich Medical Media

Justins D & Richardson P (1991) 'Clinical management of acute pain' *British Medical Bulletin* 47: 561–583

Lemone P & Burke K (2004) *Medical Surgical Nursing: Critical Thinking in Client Care* (3rd edn). New Jersey: Pearson, Prentice Hall

McCaffery M (1979) *Nursing Management of the Patient with Pain*. Philadelphia: Lippincott

McCaffery M & Pasero C (1999) *Pain: Clinical Manual for Nursing Practice* (2nd edn). London: Penguin

Melzack R (1975) 'The McGill pain questionnaire: major properties and scoring methods' *Pain* 1: 277–299

Melzack R (1987) 'The short-form McGill pain questionnaire' *Pain* 30: 191–197

Melzack R & Wall PD (1965) 'Pain mechanisms: a new theory' *Science* 150: 971–979

Melzack R, Wall PD & Ty TC (1982) 'Acute pain in an emergency clinic: latency of onset and descriptor patterns related to different injuries' *Pain* 14(1): 33–43

Merskey H, Albe-Fessard DJ & Bonica JJ (1979) *in:* Cambitzi J, Harries M & van Raders E (2000) *op cit*

Pollok AJ & Walsh T (2004) *in:* Garden OJ, Bradbury AW & Forsythe J (eds). *Principles and Practice of Surgery* (4th edn). Edinburgh: Elsevier Churchill Livingstone

Royal College of Surgeons of England and the College of Anaesthetists (1990) *Commission on the provision of surgical service. Report on the Working Party on Pain after Surgery*. London: HMSO

Roykulcharoen V & Good M (2004) 'Systematic relaxation to relieve postoperative pain' *Journal of Advanced Nursing* 48(2): 140–148

Schafheutle EI, Cantrill JA & Noyce PR (2004) 'The nature of informal pain questioning by nurses – a barrier to post-operative pain management' *Pharmacy World and Science* 26(1): 12–17

Smeltzer SC & Bare BG (2000) *Brunner and Suddarth's Textbook of Medical-Surgical Nursing* (9th edn). Philadelphia: Lippincott

Wall PD & Melzack R (eds) (1994) *Textbook of Pain* (3rd edn). London: Churchill Livingstone

Wall PD & Melzack R (eds) (1999) *Textbook of Pain* (4th edn). Edinburgh: Churchill Livingstone

Watt-Watson JH, Clark AJ, Finley GA & Watson CP (1999) 'Canadian Pain Society position statement on pain relief' *Pain Research and Management* 4: 75–78

5 Psychosocial Aspects of Surgery

Fiona J McArthur-Rouse and Tim Collins

Introduction

Patients who require surgery experience a range of emotions that can influence their recovery and their interactions with staff and loved ones. It is important that staff caring for them understand their concerns and respond to them in a facilitative manner. This chapter discusses some of the psychosocial aspects of surgical care such as anxiety and stress, altered body image, sexuality and dying. Box 5.1 lists the aims of the chapter.

Anxiety and stress in the surgical patient

Being anxious is a natural response to being told that one needs to have a major operation. There are numerous sources of anxiety for the surgical patient, including fear of the unknown, separation from loved ones, fear of pain, illness and dying (see Box 5.2), although not all patients will find the same events anxiety provoking. The physiological effects of stress can influence healing processes in the body; however the overall impact on recovery remains debatable (Salmon, 1994).

Box 5.1 Aims of the chapter.

- Discuss the physiological effects of stress and anxiety on the individual undergoing surgery
- Identify potential sources of stress and anxiety for patients
- Discuss ways in which anxiety may be relieved for individual patients
- Discuss the effects of altered body image on an individual's self-esteem, identity and recovery from surgery
- Discuss ways in which sexuality may be affected by surgical treatment
- Discuss the challenges associated with caring for dying patients and their families in an acute surgical environment

---

Box 5.2 Causes of anxiety in surgical patients.

- Fear of dying, not 'waking up', pain, vomiting and the unknown
- Fear of being awake during the operation
- Loss of control of events and the environment
- Unfamiliarity of surroundings, procedures and routines
- Loss of dignity, privacy and identity
- Worry about serious illness, effects on future, loss of income
- Fear of cancer
- Anxiety about body image, sexuality, effects on relationships and coping
- Separation from loved ones

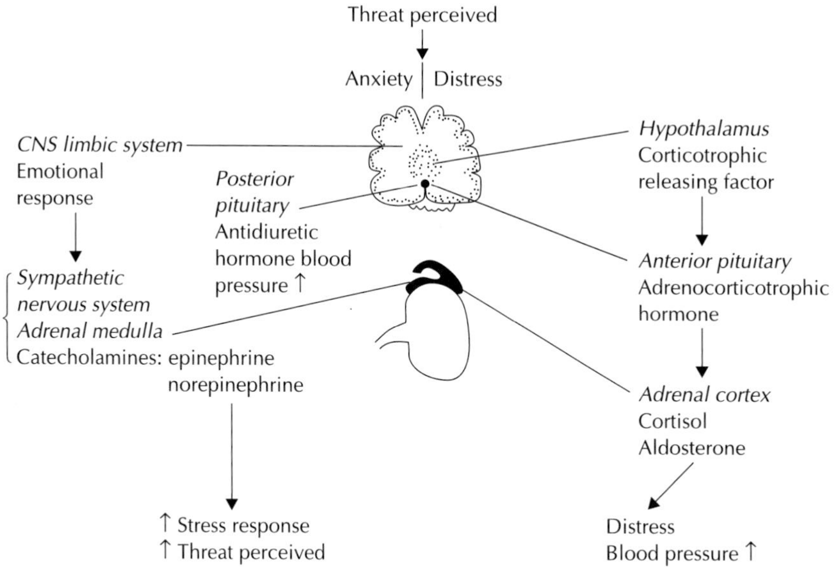

Figure 5.1   Physiological stress response.

Physiological effects of stress

When exposed to a 'stressor', whether physical or psychological, the body responds in order to maintain homeostasis. The stressor acts as a stimulus that causes the hypothalamus to initiate reactions that result in the release of the catecholamines adrenaline and noradrenaline and corticosteroids, in particular, cortisol (see Figure 5.1). The effects of these stress hormones on the body are summarised in Table 5.1.

Table 5.1   Effects of stress hormones on the body.

Catecholamines – adrenaline and noradrenaline:	Cortisol:
• Increased heart rate • Constriction of arterioles in skin and viscera • Increased blood pressure • Dilation of pupils • Inhibition of gastrointestinal function • Increased sweating • Increased rate and depth of respiration • Dry mouth	• Gluconeogenesis – mobilisation of amino acids from proteins (catabolism) • Hyperglycaemia • Immunosuppression

The catecholamine secretion leads to the 'fight or flight' response, which includes increased heart rate and blood pressure. However, this is not necessarily a negative response. A number of studies have found that raised catecholamines are indicative of increased effort and arousal in unfamiliar circumstances, and may be useful in dealing with the immediate surgical trauma (Salmon, 1994; Hibbert, 2000). The effects of cortisol are possibly more detrimental. Cortisol is particularly active in the fasted state and by breaking down protein in the process of gluconeogenesis may cause loss of muscle mass, delayed healing and increased risk of pressure ulcers. It has also been suggested that raised cortisol levels may contribute to immunosuppression and increase the risk of post-operative infection. These propositions need to be considered with caution, however, as there is still much debate regarding the relationship between stress and susceptibility to illness.

Anxiety and the surgical patient

Whether or not anxiety and stress cause detrimental physiological effects, most health professionals consider there to be a humanitarian need to relieve some of the anxiety for patients. Various ways of doing this have been attempted and range from simple reassurance to teaching relaxation techniques using guided imagery, music and aromatherapy. However, it has been suggested that simply trying to stop the patient from worrying is inappropriate because there are benefits to be gained from what has been termed the 'work of worry'. This theory suggests that 'worry' is an active process by which the patient thinks about the forthcoming surgery in such a way that the threat associated with it is reduced (Salmon, 2000).

Additionally, patients have various different coping strategies and what is right for one will not necessarily suit another. For example, traditionally practice has been based on the belief that giving information to patients pre-operatively has a positive effect on post-operative recovery. However, more recently it has emerged that for some patients, information giving can increase anxiety. This depends upon the patients' own coping strategies. Those who are 'vigilant copers' or 'monitors' are thought to benefit from information provision because their natural coping style is to seek out information about challenges; whereas those who are 'avoidant copers' or 'blunters' cope by ignoring information and may find being given too much information more anxiety provoking (Mitchell, 2000; Salmon, 2000). Information that is given to patients is typically procedural, sensory and behavioural (see Box 5.3); however, Salmon (1994) suggests it is not so much the information received that makes the patient feel less anxious, but the fact that its provision conveys some emotional support. The physical presence of an individual health professional, demonstrating 'intentional, compassionate caring', helps to reinforce the patient's own coping strategies (Salmon, 1994).

Another potential cause of anxiety in surgical patients is lack of choice and loss of control in a threatening situation. When admitted to hospital, patients often feel depersonalised and usually try to 'fit in' with the routine and behaviours expected

---

Box 5.3   Types of information.

Procedural – describes events and procedures, what will happen.
Behavioural – explains what the patient needs to do.
Sensory – describes how the patient will feel.

Box 5.4   Behavioural manifestations of anxiety.

- Anger
- Tearfulness
- Withdrawal
- Gregariousness
- Aggression
- Depression
- Inappropriate joviality

---

of them as patients. Those who do not may sometimes be labelled as 'difficult'. Anxiety is manifested in many different ways (see Box 5.4) and it is important that staff caring for anxious patients can interpret their behaviours and respond to them in a supportive manner. Giving patients the perception of choice and control over decisions about their treatment has shown increased efficacy and adherence to treatment in some studies. However, not all patients appreciate being given choice and prefer the healthcare professionals to provide direction. Salmon (2000) suggests that most patients realise that in fact they have very little choice or control, but appreciate having their feelings of autonomy and dignity acknowledged when receiving information and giving consent. Figure 5.2 summarises the reasons for providing patients with information and opportunities for control.

Body image

Schilder (1935) is one of the earliest writers to acknowledge both physical and psychological dimensions of body image and defines it as the picture that individuals form in their minds of their own bodies. Body image is influenced by a number of factors such as age, mood, health, fashion, social norms and relationships and is closely related to self-image and self-esteem. When asked to describe themselves, individuals may describe what they look like (short, tall, blonde, brunette); their roles in life (mother, father, nurse, student); or aspects of their personality (cheerful, bubbly, strong-willed). However, often it will be a combination of all three. This illustrates how one's body image, role function and personality are closely related and how changes in one will often extend to the other two.

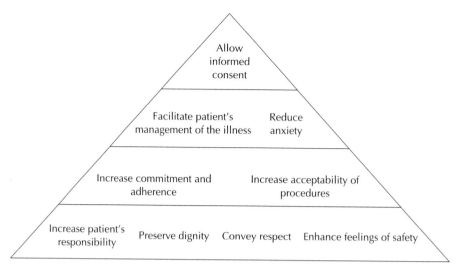

Figure 5.2   Information and involvement: the 'needs iceberg'.
Providing patients with information and the opportunity to be involved in decisions meets different needs. The most obvious is the medico-legal requirement for informed consent. However, there are many other psychological needs that are met in this way. (*Psychology of Medicine and Surgery – a guide for psychologists, counsellors, nurses and doctors*, p. 197, Salmon (2000) ©John Wiley & Sons Limited. Reproduced with permission.)

Surgical intervention inevitably causes temporary or permanent changes in the individual's body image and function, and although some major procedures such as mastectomy or stoma formation are generally associated with body image disruption, the degree of disruption is not necessarily proportional to the amount of scarring or tissue damage because individuals attribute significance differently to different parts of their bodies. For example, two women may undergo a vaginal hysterectomy and have no visible changes to their bodies. One of the women may be relieved at the removal of her uterus because of the pain and problems it has caused her, whereas the other may experience severe body image disturbance due to the loss of her fertility and perceived femininity. This example illustrates how individuals assign different significance to different parts of their bodies and how body image, function, self-esteem and self-image are inextricably linked (see Box 5.5).

Unless specifically asked, patients tend not to inform healthcare staff directly of their body image concerns because they feel embarrassed or concerned that staff will consider them vain or ungrateful for the treatment they have received. Also, during the immediate post-operative period, the patient's energies are usually directed at

> **Box 5.5**   Reflective point.
>
> How would you describe yourself (looks, role, personality)?
> What aspects of your body do you like and dislike?
> Which surgical procedure would you least like to undergo and why?
> What are your feelings towards having cosmetic surgery?

recovering from the surgery, so it is often towards the end of their hospital stay that concerns about body image emerge. It is important, therefore, to give patients the opportunity to discuss their concerns, not only pre-operatively, but again during the recovery phase. Opportunities for such discussions often arise during a dressing change or wound inspection when patients can be asked if they have looked at the wound and how they feel about it. The patient's feelings can be assessed by observation of their behaviour, body language and attitude towards the wound, stoma or affected body part (Box 5.6). It is important to remember that during dressing changes and wound inspections the patient will often be observing the reaction of the health professional towards the wound or body

Box 5.6   Manifestations of altered body image.

- Social withdrawal
- Refusal to look at the wound or affected body part
- Behaviour towards affected part (ignoring, naming)
- Language used to describe the affected part or wound (positive/negative terms, language associated with feelings of loss – 'I'm not the same person')
- Relatives' reporting on patient's mood, behaviour and coping methods
- Immobility
- Disinterest
- Depression
- Anger

part. If staff show disgust or aversion the patient will feel it deeply.

Learning to adapt to an altered body image can be a difficult and painful process. In a first person account of his loss and grief reactions following bowel surgery and stoma formation Kelly (1985), a senior lecturer in sociology, uses language power-fully to illustrate how his self-concept and identity were affected by his recent stoma formation:

'. . . I doubt whether any amount of counselling could have prepared me for the shock of seeing my new stoma uncontrollably pouring out liquid excrement . . . I thought that the possession of a stoma would not only be stigmatizing, but would be the dominant element in my life . . . I knew the bodily mutilation could be concealed and kept secret. What really alarmed me were the physiological consequences, especially the incontinence and the smell. These, I believed, would become the defining characteristics of my social identity and everything about me, my rela-tionships, the ways others viewed me, would be conditioned by these.'

(Kelly, 1985, p. 521)

Although published 20 years ago, the feelings Kelly describes remain relevant today. With refer-ence to Parkes' (1972) model of bereavement, he goes on to analyse the process of adaptation, acknowledging the need to work through the grief.

It is important for staff working in surgical wards to remember that many patients will experience feelings of loss and grief associated with their surgery. This may be directly related to the loss of

a limb in the case of an amputation; or indirectly related to the loss of self-image or identity that can result from less obviously mutilating surgery. Although the process of adaptation may only just be starting when the patient is discharged from hospital, recognising these emotions can assist staff in understanding the patient's behaviours and moods and enable them to treat them sensitively.

Recognising the need for successful adaptation to an altered body image, a number of authors have developed models for body image care and 're-imaging' (Price, 1990; Norris et al., 1998), which attempt to assist the individual in coming to terms with their new self-image. Price (1995) defines altered body image as:

'. . . a state of personal distress, defined by the patient, which indicates that the body no longer supports self-esteem, and which is dysfunctional to individuals, limiting their social engagement with others. Altered body image exists when coping strategies . . . are overwhelmed by injury, disease, disability or social stigma.'

Whilst this definition is rather long, it does acknowledge the individual nature of altered body image and the interrelation between body image, self-esteem, social engagement and coping strat-egies. Price (1990) developed a model for body image care, which comprises three components (Box 5.7) presented in diagrammatic form as an equilateral triangle, illustrating the tension and balance required to sustain a satisfactory personal body image. He argues that through the use of appropriate coping strategies and social support networks, patients can be helped to adapt to their new body image (Price, 1990).

Norris et al. (1998) propose a framework for re-imaging following alteration of body appearance or function. They discuss how reimaging occurs in

Box 5.7   Price's model for body image care (1990).

Body reality – how the body really is when it is described objectively.
Body ideal – how we would like our bodies to look and perform – influenced by societal norms.
Body presentation – the way we present ourselves to the outside world. It is employed because we recognise that our body reality does not meet our ideal, and includes the way in which we dress, walk and talk.

Table 5.2   A grounded theory of reimaging.

Phases:	Processes:
1. **Body image disruption** – surprise, shock, attempts to minimise awareness, denial, grieving	**Assimilation** – 'taking in' that life will not be the same (occurs mostly during the first and second phases)
2. **Wishing for restoration** – idealisation; efforts to mobilise personal resources, maximise efforts to improve healing, appearance and function	**Accommodation** – the realisation that life has changed prompts the accommodation of the self or the environment to facilitate living with the changes (occurs in all three phases)
3. **Reimaging the self** – replacement of idealised expectations with more realistic views of the self and capabilities	**Interpretation** – the individuals' perceptions of themselves and of other people's reactions to them influence their feelings and overall adjustment in each phase

(Norris *et al.*, 1998)

response to developmental or situational changes. Developmental changes that happen in response to normal ageing are gradual and shared with peers; whereas situational changes occur in response to illness, injury or surgery, and are sudden, unexpected and individual (Norris *et al.*, 1998). It is suggested that situational changes disrupt the individual's role, appearance and function and therefore easily influence self-image and self-esteem.

The basic social process of reimaging occurs in response to changes in physical appearance or function. Norris *et al.* (1998) explain that, although overall it involves forward movement, the pace and direction varies between individuals. Reimaging involves three phases and three active ongoing processes (Table 5.2), the outcomes of which are reconciliation and normalisation. Reconciliation may be positive or negative and may take up to a year or more. It is indicated by an acceptance of the new image within the self-concept – 'this is who I am now'. A positive or negative evaluation of the new self-concept can potentially influence self-esteem for the better or worse. Normalisation involves learning to live with the limitations or losses of the changed body (Norris *et al.*, 1998). The conflicting emotions that patients experience throughout the phases can be distressing for them and their families. Understanding that a process of reimaging is expected can help patients feel less isolated and embarrassed.

Sexuality

Expressing sexuality is an integral part of our personalities and our daily lives and is closely related to the concepts of body image, self-esteem and self-concept. Thus a positive self-concept and body image are important factors in the maintenance of healthy sexuality. The World Health Organization (WHO, 1975) defines sexuality as:

'. . . the integration of the somatic, emotional, intellectual and social aspects of sexual beings in ways that are positively enriching and that enhance personality, communication and love.'

Attitudes towards sexuality and sexual expression are influenced by experiences throughout our lives, starting in early childhood. Some families have very open attitudes towards sexuality, nakedness and bodily functions, whereas others will rarely mention them. These attitudes will influence an individual's ability to discuss issues of sexuality in relation to health and illness and applies equally to healthcare staff and patients.

A number of studies have identified that patients frequently have unanswered anxieties and questions about sexual matters related to their illness and surgical treatment (Burke, 1996; Clifford, 1998; Wilmoth *et al.*, 2000). Thus this aspect of care is frequently omitted, disregarded or acknowledged only cursorily. Possible reasons for this are identified in Box 5.8. Healthcare professionals cannot assume that patients will ask for information about how their surgery will influence them sexually as many patients will be too embarrassed to raise the issue. Therefore the onus is on the staff caring for these patients to offer them the opportunity to discuss such issues and to acknowledge the legitimacy of their concerns.

Many major surgical procedures affect the patient's sexuality and sexual function either

Table 5.3   Effects of surgery on sexuality and sexual function.

Physiological	Psychological
<ul><li>Surgical procedures that directly affect reproductive organs leading to impotence and dyspareunia (e.g. urological and gynaecological procedures – see Chapters 10 and 11)</li><li>Nerve and vasculature disruption within the pelvis causing changes in sensation, quality of orgasm and possible impotence (e.g. pelvic surgery and stoma formation)</li><li>Surgical procedures that cause physical disability (e.g. amputation, cardiac surgery)</li><li>Effects of illness, pain, discomfort, fatigue and loss of desire</li></ul>	<ul><li>Surgical procedures that leave visible mutilating scars causing alterations in body image and perceived attractiveness (e.g. mastectomy, facial surgery, stoma formation)</li><li>Surgical procedures that cause alteration in self concept and role function (e.g. hysterectomy)</li><li>Illness or surgical procedures that result in major lifestyle changes, loss of independence and reduction in social engagement</li></ul>

Box 5.8   Reasons why sexuality is not addressed.

- Poor training or education in sexuality and sexual health
- A lack of relevant nursing experience
- Religious beliefs, culture or personal views on sexuality
- Interventions to support healthy sexuality are not seen as a priority, particularly in an acute ward environment
- Embarrassment or lack of confidence

(Royal College of Nursing (2000) *Sexuality and sexual health in nursing practice: an RCN discussion and guidance document for nurses who want to develop their nursing practice in the field of sexuality and sexual health.* London: RCN).

Box 5.9   The P-LI-SS-IT model.

Permission – the patient is given 'permission' to discuss issues relating to sexuality, legitimising concerns and providing reassurance that their concerns are 'normal'. This involves creating an environment that facilitates private, uninterrupted discussion, possibly involving the partner.

Limited information – involves non-expert intervention in which the healthcare professional provides factual information to clarify concerns and eliminate myths.

Specific suggestions – at this level of intervention specialist training may be required. Specific advice is given regarding strategies for enhancing sexual expression.

Intensive therapy – when in-depth counselling is required, the patient may be referred to a psychosexual therapist.

(Annon, 1976)

---

physiologically or psychologically (see Table 5.3) and therefore these issues should be discussed. However, staff frequently have difficulty initiating such conversations either due to embarrassment or a belief that they will not be able to respond to the patient's queries. One model that can be used to facilitate discussion is the P-LI-SS-IT model (Annon, 1976), which identifies four distinct but interconnected levels of intervention (see Box 5.9). Most healthcare professionals working in a surgical speciality should be familiar enough with the surgical procedures to understand the possible impact on the patient's sexuality. Therefore most staff should be able to offer permission and limited information to patients in need of sexuality-related care. However, in order to do so, the staff member needs to be comfortable with his or her own sexuality and that of others. See Borwell (1997) and Heath & White (2002) for further reading on this subject.

Caring for the dying patient in an acute surgical environment

Whilst the majority of patients undergoing surgery have positive outcomes, there are times when this is not the case. Surgical intervention carries a number of risks and complications, which can ultimately lead to death. Additionally, some patients are admitted as emergencies and require immediate interventions in an attempt to save their lives. Others may be admitted in such a debilitated condition or with disease that is so advanced that surgery is inappropriate or not feasible. Caring for the dying patient in an acute surgical environment presents particular challenges (see Box 5.10). The purpose of this section is not to explore theories

> **Box 5.10** Challenges of caring for dying patients and their families in the acute surgical environment.
>
> - Conflicting priorities – balancing the needs of the dying patient and his/her family with the needs of acutely ill and post-operative patients
> - Lack of resources, facilities, staff, skills and time
> - Inappropriate environment
> - Ambiguity regarding resuscitation status
> - Issues associated with witnessed resuscitation
> - Breaking bad news
> - Supporting relatives who may be dealing with sudden death
> - Issues relating to organ and tissue donation

of dying and bereavement (the reader is directed to specialist texts for further information on this), but to discuss these challenges and suggest some ways in which they may be addressed.

Balancing the needs of the dying patient and his or her family with the needs of acutely ill and post-operative patients is often difficult for those working in an acute surgical ward. Whilst staff may wish to spend time with the dying patient and his or her relatives, the competing needs of patients requiring admission and discharge, close observation and monitoring, and escorting to and from theatre, mean that the care of the dying patient may be delegated to a junior member of staff. Additionally, staff working in acute wards rarely have specific training and education in caring for dying patients and their families. If the patient has a malignant disease, they will normally be supported by a Macmillan or hospice team who will advise on suitable palliative treatment regimens and offer

some counselling to the patient and relatives. However, if surgical nurses are not familiar with the pumps, drugs and treatment regimens prescribed, there may be delays in their administration, causing distress for all concerned. If the patient's condition permits it, transfer to a local hospice may be arranged. However, for various reasons this may not be possible and the death may occur in the surgical ward.

The fast-paced, often noisy ward environment is rarely conducive to enabling and supporting a 'good death'. Few surgical wards have facilities for relatives such as a 'quiet room' or tea- and coffee-making facilities. Patients and their relatives may be offered privacy by moving them into a single room if available, or by drawing the curtains around the bed. However, this may cause them to feel isolated and neglected. Culturally, death is not often discussed in the UK, and the presence in a ward of a dying patient and their family is felt deeply by all patients who are reminded of their own mortality. Those caring for these patients need to be aware of this and help them express their fears and emotions.

Some of the problems identified above can be relieved by the identification of a particular member of staff to care for and support the dying patient and his or her family during a shift. This should be an experienced individual who is comfortable talking to the patient and relatives and who has the time to devote to their particular needs. This enables a rapport to be built up between the patient, family and nurse, which may help those involved in coming to terms with their situation.

Clarity regarding the patient's resuscitation status is essential to enable him or her to be treated

Table 5.4 Advantages and disadvantages of witnessed resuscitation.

Advantages	Disadvantages
- The process can assist relatives in coming to terms with the reality of death avoiding prolonged denial - Relatives can speak to the patient believing they may still hear them - They are not distressed by being separated from their loved one - The relative may have given CPR at the scene or witnessed paramedics doing this, so why not allow them to see this in hospital? - Due to the popularity of medical dramas, the public are more aware of what happens during a resuscitation - It is possible for the relative to see that everything possible was done for the dying patient - They can speak to or touch the deceased person whilst the person is still warm	- The attempt may prove too distressing for some relatives - Staff could be physically or emotionally hindered during the resuscitation attempt - Relatives may be disturbed by the memory of events - Staff may feel threatened by being observed during CPR with fear of litigation - The resuscitation team's performance may be affected if they know they are being observed

with honesty and dignity. A resuscitation policy is usually invoked which involves discussing the issue with the patient and their family. Many healthcare workers have difficulty initiating such conversations; however, patients are often philosophical about these issues. Careful documentation and communication of the outcome is essential so that all members of staff are aware of the patient's resuscitation status.

If a patient's condition deteriorates suddenly, for example in an emergency situation, cardiopulmonary resuscitation (CPR) may be required (see Chapter 13). This can be a traumatic event not only for the patient, but for staff, other patients in the ward and, if they are present, the affected patient's relatives. Traditionally in such situations the relatives have been shepherded out of the area to enable the resuscitation team to carry out their work. However, recently it has been suggested that relatives may benefit from observing the resuscitation attempt, a practice known as witnessed resuscitation (RCN, 2002). The advantages and disadvantages of this are identified in Table 5.4.

Following a death in the surgical ward, it is the remit of a member of staff, usually the nurse, to inform the relatives of the death. Breaking bad news is one of the most difficult aspects of healthcare work, particularly when the death is sudden or unexpected and the relatives have been unable to prepare themselves or say goodbye. A variety of reactions may be evident including anger and the need to blame someone. This task can be easier if the nurse has had the opportunity to develop a relationship with the family. McLauchlan (1996) suggests that breaking bad news should be tailored to the situation and to the particular relatives. Box 5.11 identifies some key points to follow when breaking bad news.

Box 5.11   Key principles for breaking bad news.

Preparation
- Death pronounced
- Remove plastic aprons, stethoscopes and clinical equipment
- Be familiar with the patient's name, past medical history and cause of death
- Temporarily give pager to another member of staff to answer/cover
- Ensure the practitioner is familiar with the family
- Ensure the practitioner has sensitivity and effective interpersonal skills
- Do not deliver bad news at the bedside or in a corridor
- Select a private and quiet room
- Ensure the room has enough chairs for relatives to sit on and that tissues are available
- Ensure a telephone is available to enable relatives to make outside calls to family members; however, ensure that the phone is transferred whilst breaking bad news to prevent interruptions

Communication
- Initially confirm that the correct relatives are being addressed
- Introduce yourself to the relatives
- Sitting down to talk to relatives gives the impression that you are not in a rush to leave
- Do not stand. Maintain same eye level; if no additional chairs are available, kneel on the floor
- Do not obstruct the doorway, as a family member may wish to leave the room

- During the breaking of bad news it may be natural to touch or hold the hand of the bereaved relative
- Getting to the point quickly is important
- When providing information and answering questions, be honest, direct and avoid medical 'jargon'
- Use phrases such as 'dead' or 'died' as they are unambiguous. Giving the news thoughtfully and showing concern will enable relatives to understand that the death is a reality. 'I am very sorry but _____ has just died'
- Avoid euphemisms such as 'we have lost him', 'he has passed on', 'has slipped away' or 'gone to a better place'
- Do not rush the process, allow time for silence whilst the reality is absorbed, but re-emphasise the situation if appropriate
- Be prepared for a variety of emotional responses or reactions. Remember that these responses are not the fault of the bearer of bad news, but are a reaction to the news itself
- Offer the relatives the opportunity to view the body
- Explain the role of the family liaison officer for the relatives following them leaving the hospital
- Explain all the necessary paperwork and how to register the death

Remember
- It does not have to be a senior person as long as they display the above skills
- Families gain support from being aware that you may also feel their grief

(McLauchlan, 1996; Dolan & Holt, 2000)

Another consideration following a death in the surgical ward is the possibility of broaching the subject of tissue donation with the relatives. Collins (2005) states that the majority of patients who die in hospitals may be eligible for tissue donation; however, relatives are infrequently asked for consent because nursing and medical staff are either unaware of tissue donation, or they are inadequately prepared to obtain donation consent. Many patients and relatives feel reassured that the tissues they have donated improve the quality of life for another individual following their own or their loved one's death (Stocks *et al.*, 1992; Pelletier, 1993; UK Transplant, 2005). Organ transplantation has proven to be an effective treatment for end-stage organ failure and tissue donation has been shown to significantly improve the quality of life for patients awaiting a tissue transplant (Cantwell & Clifford, 2000). Most organs such as the heart, lungs, liver and kidneys come from patients who have been certified brain-stem dead whilst in intensive care, as a result of a sudden injury or cerebral insult (Collins, 2005). However, it is possible for ward patients to donate tissues up to 48 hours following death; these tissues include corneas, heart

valves, skin, bone and tendons (Collins, 2005; UK Transplant, 2005).

There are several contraindications to tissue donation, which are identified in Box 5.12. The patient's relatives or the patients themselves may approach the nurse to offer consent for tissue donation; or alternatively, healthcare professionals

---

Box 5.12   Contraindications for tissue donation.

Main contraindications for tissue donation (UK Transplant, 2005)

- High-risk groups, e.g. IV drug users, prostitutes
- Hepatitis B and C, HIV
- Alzheimer's disease, Creutzfeldt–Jakob disease (CJD), dementia
- Significant systemic infection
- Auto-immune diseases
- Active tuberculosis (TB)
- Carcinomas, excluding primary brain tumours
- Recent tattoos

If you are in doubt about any contraindications or patient suitability for tissue donation you should always contact your regional transplant co-ordination service via your hospital switchboard.

Box 5.13   Key points to consider when approaching a family for tissue donation consent.

When?
- Death pronounced
- Relatives informed
- Relatives understand the cause of death

Where?
- Not at the bedside or in a corridor
- Private and quiet room
- Speak at the same level

Who?
- A practitioner who is familiar with the family
- A practitioner with sensitivity and effective interpersonal skills

It does not have to be a senior person or medical staff as long as they display the above skills.

Phrases that help
- 'I know this is a very difficult time, but I have some important information for you to consider'
- 'Do you know if _____ carried a donor card?'
- 'It may be possible for _____ to donate if you think that is what s/he would have wanted to do'
- 'Did you ever talk about organ donation as a family?'

Remember
- It cannot get any worse for the family; there is no harm in asking as relatives may gain relief in their bereavement by being given the option
- If relatives refuse consent respect their wishes and just say this was an option for them to consider

may ask a bereaved relative for donation consent. There is evidence that, if undertaken appropriately, asking for tissue or organ donation consent does not further distress bereaved relatives and helps in the grieving process (Randhawa, 1998; Bires, 1999; British Transplantation Society, 2003). Most hospitals have guidelines available on how to approach families for tissue donation consent and Box 5.13 identifies some key points to consider when undertaking this difficult task. If a potential patient is to be referred for tissue donation, or if specific organ or tissue donation advice is required, it is usually possible to contact the local transplant co-ordinator via the hospital switchboard. Transplant co-ordinators are usually critical care nurses who have undertaken specialised training in organ and tissue transplantation and they aim to provide expert advice for healthcare staff on donation issues.

Self-test questions

1. Which of the following statements is **true**?
   a. Pre-operative stress causes delayed wound healing
   b. Pre-operative stress causes post-operative infection
   c. Pre-operative stress causes post-operative pressure sores
   d. The link between pre-operative stress and post-operative recovery is uncertain
2. What is thought to be the benefit of the 'work of worry'?
3. Giving detailed information pre-operatively is thought to benefit:
   a. Avoidant copers
   b. Vigilant copers
   c. Blunters
   d. All patients equally
4. Information that describes how the patient will feel pre- and post-operatively is referred to as:
   a. Procedural
   b. Behavioural
   c. Sensory
   d. Intentional
5. Which of the following may be indicative of an altered body image?
   a. Social withdrawal
   b. Anger

   c. Depression
   d. All of the above
6. List three possible reasons why patients' anxieties related to sexuality are often not addressed.
7. Give three reasons why it is important to address sexuality issues with surgical patients.
8. Identify three challenges associated with caring for dying patients in an acute surgical ward.
9. Identify three tissues that can be donated following death.
10. Which of the following statements is **true**?
    a. Only patients who die in intensive care units can be tissue donors
    b. Only doctors should break bad news and approach relatives for tissue donation consent
    c. All tissues have to be donated immediately after death
    d. Contraindications for tissue donation include recent tattoos, dementia and Alzheimer's disease

References and further reading

Annon J (1976) *in*: Heath H & White I (2002) *The Challenge of Sexuality in Health Care*. Oxford: Blackwell Science

Bires M (1999) 'Comparison of consent rates between hospital-based designated requestors and organ procurement co-ordinators' *Journal of Transplant Co-ordination 3*: 177–180

Borwell B (ed.) (1997) *Developing Sexual Helping Skills – a guide for nurses*. Maidenhead: Medical Projects International

British Transplantation Society (BTS) (2003) *Standards for solid organ transplantation in the United Kingdom*. London: BTS

Burke LM (1996) 'Sexual dysfunction following radiotherapy for cervical cancer' *British Journal of Nursing 5*(4): 239–244

Cantwell M & Clifford C (2000) 'English nursing and medical students' attitudes towards organ donation' *Journal of Advanced Nursing 32*(4): 961–968

Clifford D (1998) 'Psychosexual awareness in everyday nursing' *Nursing Standard 12*(39): 42–45

Collins T (2005) 'Organ and tissue donation: a survey of nurses' knowledge and educational needs in an adult ITU' *Intensive and Critical Care Nursing 21*(4): 226–233

Dickenson D, Johnson M & Samson Katz J (2000) *Death, Dying and Bereavement* (2nd edn). London: Sage

Dolan B & Holt L (2000) *Accident and Emergency: Theory into Practice.* London: Baillière Tindall

Heath H & White I (eds) (2002) *The Challenge of Sexuality in Health Care.* Oxford: Blackwell Science

Hibbert A (2000) 'Chapter 8 – Stress in surgical patients: a physiological perspective' *in*: Manley K & Bellman L (eds) (2000) *Surgical Nursing – Advancing Practice.* London: Churchill Livingstone

Kelly MP (1985) 'Loss and grief reactions as responses to surgery' *Journal of Advanced Nursing 10:* 517–525

McLauchlan C (1996) 'Handling distressed relatives and breaking bad news' *in*: Skinner D, Driscoll P & Earlam R (eds) *ABC of Major Trauma* (2nd edn). London: BMJ

Mitchell M (2000) 'Nursing intervention for pre-operative anxiety' *Nursing Standard* 14(37): 40–43

Norris J, Kunes-Connell M & Stockard Spelic S (1998) 'A grounded theory of reimaging' *Advances in Nursing Science* 20(3): 1–12

Parkes CM (1972) *in*: Kelly MP (1985) 'Loss and grief reactions as responses to surgery' *Journal of Advanced Nursing 10:* 517–525

Pelletier M (1993) 'The needs of family members of organ and tissue donors' *Heart and Lung 22*: 25–30

Price B (1990) 'A model for body image care' *Journal of Advanced Nursing 15*: 585–593

Price B (1995) 'Assessing altered body image' *Journal of Psychiatric and Mental Health Nursing 2*: 169–175

Randhawa G (1998) 'Specialist nurse training programme: dealing with asking for organ donation' *Journal of Advanced Nursing* 28(2): 405–408

Royal College of Nursing (2000) *Sexuality and sexual health in nursing practice: an RCN discussion and guidance document for nurses who want to develop their nursing practice in the field of sexuality and sexual health.* London: RCN

Royal College of Nursing (2002) *Witnessing Resuscitation.* London: RCN

Salmon P (1994) 'Chapter 10 – Psychological factors in surgical recovery' *in*: Gibson HB (ed.) (1994) *Psychology, Pain and Anaesthesia.* London: Chapman & Hall

Salmon P (2000) *Psychology of Medicine and Surgery – a guide for psychologists, counsellors, nurses and doctors.* Chichester: John Wiley & Sons Ltd

Schilder P (1935) *Image and Appearance of the Human Body.* London: Kegan Paul

Stocks L, Cutler J, Kress T & Lewino D (1992) 'Dispelling myths regarding organ donation: the donor family experience' *Journal of Transplant Co-ordination 2:* 147–152

UK Transplant Organization (2005) (online). www.uktransplant.org.uk/ (Accessed 22.12.06)

Wells D (ed.) (2000) *Caring for Sexuality in Health and Illness.* London: Churchill Livingstone

Chamberlain Wilmoth M & Spinelli A (2000) 'Sexual implications of gynecologic cancer treatments' *Journal of Obstetric, Gynecologic and Neonatal Nursing* 29(4): 413–421

Wilton T (2000) *Sexualities in Health and Social Care – a textbook.* Buckingham: OUP

World Health Organization (1975) *Education and Treatment in Human Sexuality: the training of healthcare professionals.* Geneva: WHO

Part 2

Surgical Specialities

6

Head and Neck Surgery

Tracey Sharpe and Carma Harnett

Introduction

This chapter discusses some of the major head and neck procedures, such as laryngectomy and tracheostomy, which may be seen in surgical wards. It includes thyroidectomy and a brief discussion of other endocrine conditions. Box 6.1 identifies the aims of this chapter.

Tracheotomy and tracheostomy

It is important from the outset to be clear about the terms tracheotomy and tracheostomy. A tracheotomy is an opening in the trachea; this procedure is temporary in nature and performed for a variety of reasons (Box 6.2). A tracheostomy is a surgical opening in the anterior wall of the trachea linking

> **Box 6.1** Aims of the chapter.
>
> - To discuss the management of patients requiring a tracheotomy/tracheostomy
> - To discuss the different types of tracheostomy tube and their management
> - To discuss the priorities of care for patients requiring a laryngectomy
> - To discuss the pathophysiology, assessment and management of patients requiring thyroidectomy

> **Box 6.2** Indicators for tracheotomy.
>
> - Airway obstruction (congenital, trauma, infection, tumour, vocal cord paralysis)
> - Protection of upper respiratory tract (aspiration of secretions, laryngectomy, neurological insult, trauma to face and neck, reduced conscious states)
> - Ventilator support (reduction in dead space – decreased work of breathing, weaning from ventilator, secretion aspiration, comfort)

the trachea to the surface of the skin resulting in a stoma. This procedure may be permanent as when used to maintain an airway following total laryngectomy (the removal of the larynx), undertaken as treatment for carcinomas (Serra, 2000). The stages of a cancer determining this form of treatment are graded on a tumour-nodes-metastases staging grid (TNM), ranging from a T1 and T2 tumour that can be successfully treated in most cases with radical radiotherapy, to a T3 and T4 tumour that is normally treated with a total laryngectomy. T1 and T2 tumours are generally limited to the affected area and have not spread to other areas, remaining confined to the vocal cords and not involving the larynx or pharynx. T3 and T4 tumours generally have extended further and have spread to other areas often invading the larynx, pharynx and thyroid cartilage (Burton, 2003).

Tracheostomy may also be undertaken to reduce the volume of dead space in the respiratory passages. This diminishes the work of breathing for patients with restrictive respiratory problems. In these cases, the mechanics of breathing are impaired, creating a risk of asphyxia. Examples of restrictive conditions which may require tracheostomy to maintain respiratory function include paralysis of the respiratory nerves or conditions in which the normal mobility of the chest wall is diminished.

Tracheotomy procedure

A tracheotomy should, where possible, be performed in a controlled environment. The patient is positioned in the supine position with the shoulder rolled back to extend the neck. The surgeon then identifies landmarks such as the thyroid notch, the sternal notch and the cricoid. An incision is made in the skin two fingerbreadths above the sternal notch. Adrenaline can be injected into the wound to reduce blood flow and improve the surgeon's vision. The strap muscles are separated in the midline and an incision is then made between the second and fourth tracheal rings. Sometimes it is necessary to divide the thyroid isthmus, as this can obscure the trachea (Lalwani, 2005).

The space below the cricoid cartilage (first ring) should be avoided where possible, as there is an increased incidence of stenosis of the larynx using this approach. The access of choice is the space between the third and fourth rings, with the front segment of the ring removed to facilitate the insertion of a tracheostomy tube (Cherry, 1997), the cuff on the tube is then inflated to provide a secure airway. The skin around the site is then closed with sutures.

Percutaneous tracheotomy is an alternative option favoured by intensivists, as the procedure is one of dilatation following a small incision; the procedure has to be planned, as the dilatation process is time consuming and therefore not appropriate for emergency situations. A small incision is made in the skin of the throat using the normal landmarks and a tunnel in the tissues is made which is enlarged by dilatation. The trachea is punctured and a guide wire is inserted to guide the placement of the chosen tracheostomy tube. Care has to be taken not to puncture the posterior wall of the trachea – to prevent this occurrence some surgeons choose to perform this procedure with concurrent bronchoscopy.

Post-operative management

Careful post-operative management of the tracheotomy patient enhances recovery. The patient should be nursed in an upright position, with the neck well supported at all times. Tracheostomy tube ties help secure its position. The tapes are fastened using a reef knot at each side of the neck. It is important that the nurse securing the ties checks for tension and comfort, by sliding a little finger between the skin and the tube tapes. Easy insertion should be established but no more than one small finger space should exist. Occasionally, the surgeon sutures the flange of the tracheostomy tube to the neck skin, thus making it almost impossible for the tube to be dislodged or expelled. This is usually performed when difficulty in replacing the tube if accidentally expelled is anticipated (Serra, 2000). The tube holders or ties should be checked and changed at least once every 24 hours.

Suctioning is necessary to maintain and clear the airway of secretions that could potentially block the airway. An aseptic technique should be adopted for this to reduce the risk of infection. Using a sterile catheter no more than half the size of the tube's inner diameter and only touching the inside of the tube, suctioning should be undertaken only on withdrawal of the suction catheter and not on insertion (Alexander et al., 1995). It is important to remember that whilst suctioning, the patient loses the ability to breathe and for this reason, suctioning should be undertaken for no longer than 10–15 seconds. The patient should then be given the opportunity to recover, should it be necessary to repeat the procedure. Secretion quantity and consistency should be monitored to observe for signs of infection and trauma. Initially post-operatively blood-streaked secretions may occur as a direct result of the surgical procedure.

In normal breathing, inspired air is warmed, filtered and moistened by ciliated epithelial cells in the nose and upper airway. A tracheostomy tube bypasses these natural mechanisms and can cause physiological changes such as crusting, thickening

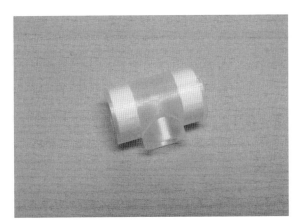

Figure 6.1 Heat moisture exchange device (HME).

of secretions, 'plugging' of the tube and, possibly, infection.

A 'heat moisture exchange' device (HME) mimics the natural mechanisms of the upper airway and should be worn whenever humidified oxygen therapy is not in use. It should be checked at least every four hours and changed if soiled to prevent resistance to breathing and increased work of breathing leaving the patient exhausted (Figure 6.1).

There has been much debate over the correct method of cleaning around a tracheostomy and whether it is appropriate to adopt an aseptic technique for this procedure. Harris (1984) supports the use of a clean rather than aseptic technique. The tracheal stoma will require regular cleaning and dressing to prevent encrustation, infection, pressure sores caused by the tube and excoriation of skin caused by secretions expelled.

Potential post-operative complications

Complications of a tracheostomy can be divided into 'early', 'delayed' and 'late' categories, as set out below.

Early complications (see Box 6.3)

The potential for haemorrhage in the immediate post-operative period is reduced by the use of a cuffed tube that applies direct pressure to bleeding points; it can also prevent aspiration of blood and clots. Despite this, there is still the potential for haemorrhage from the innominate artery. The nurse needs to observe the tube for pulsation that suggests that the tube is resting on the artery. In such cases, the medical staff should be informed immediately.

Observation of vital signs and visualisation of the stoma site are necessary to detect cardiovascular instability, respiratory compromise and bleeding from around the tube and out of the stoma site.

Displacement of the tube presents in two ways. Either the tube is visibly displaced out of the stoma and can be seen resting on the neck's surface, or the tube becomes dislodged from the trachea but remains inside the pre-tracheal tissues of the neck; both are as a direct result of the tube ties being secured incorrectly. Complete displacement of the tube is easily seen. Dislodgement into the pre-tracheal tissues is characterised by respiratory distress normally in the form of stridor (noisy laboured breathing). If the patient is able to speak without a speaking valve or obvious tube occlusion, it suggests that the tube has slipped into the soft tissues. Medical assistance must be sought immediately whilst the tube is removed and the airway is maintained with tracheal dilators until a new tube is inserted.

Pneumothorax is rare, however there is potential during the procedure to puncture the pleura at the apex of the lung. If this happens, the patient will experience a sudden onset of respiratory distress characterised by a rise in the respiratory rate, increased work of breathing and a fall in the oxygen saturation (SaO_2). Some patients may exhibit cyanosis if the pneumothorax is not relieved rapidly. Urgent medical assistance is necessary as decompression is required and a chest drain may be needed. The tracheostomy tube should be left in situ.

Subcutaneous emphysema is an abnormal presence of air in the tissues; this is as a result of poor suturing techniques, where the sutures are pulled too tightly, thus preventing the dissipation of trapped air. This air is then forced into the tissues causing swelling and a distinctive 'crackle' when the skin surface is touched. Following medical examination, the emphysema can be relieved by the removal of the sutures.

Recurrent laryngeal nerve damage is rare but can occur when the nerve is not identified at the time of the procedure and it is either traumatised or displaced.

Delayed complications (see Box 6.4)

Tube blockages and occlusion are usually caused by crusting of secretions or plugs of mucus, secondary to poor humidification techniques as described earlier in this chapter. Tube obstruction is characterised by noisy breathing, continued coughing and increased respiratory effort. In some cases there will be a significant drop in the SaO_2; however, some patients may not exhibit this as they are able to breathe around the tube if it is not cuffed. The initial treatment will be suction of the tube and nebulisation with 5 mL of normal saline. For patients with a two-piece tube, changing the inner tube will immediately resolve this complication. If the occlusion persists after suction and nebulisation, the tube must be removed, whilst maintaining the airway with tracheal dilators. Medical assistance must be sought to replace the tube.

Infection will occur as a direct result of a poor cleaning technique. As previously highlighted, there are different schools of thought regarding the use of an aseptic technique when cleaning the tracheal stoma site, changing the tube or suctioning. Infection can be identified when odour, pyrexia, redness or inflammation are present. Medical advice and rigorous skin care are necessary. The use of topical antimicrobials may be required and with

some infections systemic antibiotics may be needed. Due to their nature and location, tracheal stomas have been at high risk of infection by organisms such as *Staphylococcus aureus* and *Pseudomonas aeruginosa*. Recent advances in wound care have led to silver-impregnated dressings being used to reduce the risk of infection.

Mucosal ulceration is caused by asymmetrical inflation of the cuff, excessive cuff pressures or tube migration due to inadequate securing of the tube, resulting in reduced perfusion of tracheal mucosa (St George's Healthcare Trust, 2000). Nowadays, the risk of this occurring is reduced by using high-volume, low-pressure softer cuffs, which reduce pressure trauma although not completely eradicating it. Symptoms may include bleeding and discomfort, but diagnosis is usually made through nasoendoscopic examination by a member of the medical team. Damage to the tracheal mucosa may also be caused through a poor suction technique, where the suction catheter inserted exceeds the length of the tube and causes tracheal damage. As previously discussed, care must be taken when selecting the size of the suction catheter and insertion into the tube should always be undertaken with care and caution.

Late complications (see Box 6.5)

Tracheal stenosis describes a narrowing of the trachea through granulation tissue developing on the anterior tracheal wall. This then leads to bleeding and possible obstruction. It may develop up to five years after the procedure. Symptoms include increased dyspnoea on exertion, a cough and retained secretions. Immediate medical assistance needs to be sought resulting in surgical removal of the stenosed area.

Scar formation is most frequently caused by the vertical skin incision used on formation of the tracheotomy. It is unsightly and distressing for the patient. The risk of scarring is reduced dramatically

---

Box 6.4   Delayed complications of tracheotomy (1–14 days).

- Tube blockage/occlusion
- Infection
- Mucosal ulceration/tracheal necrosis

Box 6.5   Late complications of tracheotomy (> 14 days).

- Tracheal stenosis
- Scar formation
- Tracheo-esophageal fistula

in those patients for whom it is possible to remove the tube sooner, rather than later.

The complication of a tracheo-esophageal fistula is usually fatal and can be directly linked to an overinflated cuff causing severe pressure necrosis. This causes erosion through the posterior and anterior wall of the oesophagus; this in turn results in pneumonitis secondary to aspiration through the formed fistula. The patient will present with repeated chest infections and altered secretion production. There may also be pyrexia present.

Decannulation

Removal of a tracheostomy tube is known as decannulation. Occasionally the tube can be removed without any preliminaries (Alexander *et al.*, 1995).

More frequently, however, the patient is gradually weaned off the tube in a strict and closely observed procedure. A tube is never removed without first being occluded for at least 24 hours to determine the patient's ability to breathe with a closed tracheostomy. It also enables the patient to become psychologically and physically accustomed to 'normal' breathing.

When it is decided to decannulate, a patient's tube is changed to a smaller and fenestrated one, thus allowing a patient to breathe through the tube and through the larynx. This can be done in the community with close outpatient monitoring if the patient has already been discharged. Once comfortable and stable with the smaller fenestrated tube, the patient is usually admitted to hospital (if not already an inpatient) for the external tube opening to be blocked off by a decannulation plug. This is usually done for varying and increasing lengths of time until the patient has maintained a period of at least 24 hours with the tube being occluded and good oxygen saturation maintained. Once this is established, the tube can be removed and an airtight dressing applied, so that the patient breathes through his nose and mouth. The patient can then be discharged home with instructions to community nursing staff to continue airtight dressings. The stoma should then shrink rapidly and close off in a short length of time. The patient is at potential risk of respiratory distress during this procedure, so staff need to ensure that a small tube and tracheal dilators are available at the bedside.

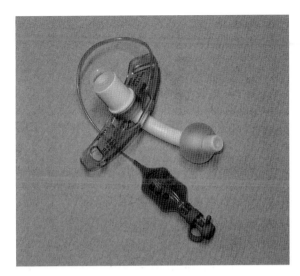

Figure 6.2   Cuffed tracheostomy tube.

Tube types

Cuffed tracheostomy tubes (Figure 6.2)

These are usually the first tubes inserted in theatre during the immediate post-operative phase, or when a tracheostomy is required in an emergency. Patients are assessed following surgery for their ability to protect their own airway and the cuff deflated. The modern day cuffed tube-cuff is of low pressure and high volume thus reducing the risk of pressure trauma, although that risk is not completely eliminated. The inflated cuff permits ventilation by providing a seal in the trachea as it prevents air escape around the tube during mechanical ventilation. Airflow is then via the tracheostomy tube and totally bypasses the upper airway. The cuffed tube reduces the likelihood of aspirate entering the lungs.

The inflated cuff, however, does impair the ability to swallow due to cuff pressure on the oesophagus. It also reduces laryngeal elevation and anchors the larynx. Due to the nature of the cuff, it is unsuitable for use with speaking valves as the airflow is unable to pass over the vocal cords and thus prevents phonation. For this reason, a patient call system and nursing vigilance are needed.

It is also important to note that cuff pressure may cause damage to tracheal mucosa, thus leading to erosion. It is important that care is taken not to overinflate the cuff.

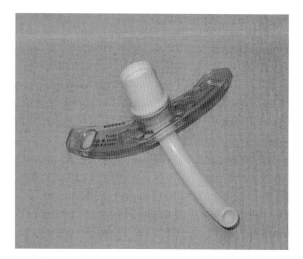

Figure 6.3   Uncuffed tracheostomy tube.

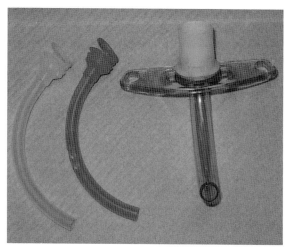

Figure 6.4   Two-piece tracheostomy tube.

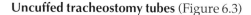

Uncuffed tracheostomy tubes (Figure 6.3)

These are more suitable for long-term use and are often chosen when a tracheostomy tube is still required to maintain the individual's airway. Often it is introduced seven days post-operatively, when the first tube change is required. In the event of a blocked tube, patients are still able to breathe around the tube, as there is no cuff to obstruct tracheal airflow. Patients are also able to speak with an uncuffed tube using a one-way speaking valve. Air is allowed into the tube opening on inhalation but not exhaled through the tube route. Instead it is redirected back down to the tube tip and up into the larynx on exhalation. This then creates a voice.

One of the disadvantages of these tubes is that there is no cuff to prevent the aspiration of oral or gastric contents, making the tube unsuitable for patients who have impaired swallowing. The absence of a cuff also makes these tubes unsuitable for patients requiring mechanical ventilation as the air/oxygen will leak backwards past the outside of the tracheostomy tube, rather than descending the air passages to inflate the lungs.

Two-piece tracheostomy tubes (Figure 6.4)

These tubes have an inner tube that fits into the outer tube; this inner cannula can be changed frequently to reduce the risk of occlusion. The correct size inner cannula must be used for each tube. An oversized inner cannula will protrude through the tip of the tracheostomy tube and erode the soft mucosa of the trachea. If it is too small, secretions will build up between the inner cannula and outer lumen. The presence of an inner cannula also enables less frequent tube changes. Due to secretion collection reducing the internal lumen diameter over time, inner tube changes need to be frequent. Recommendations for frequency of change are unsupported by literature, but good practice guidelines recommend that a tube without an inner cannula should be changed every 7–14 days. This in itself can cause trauma to the stoma site. By using tubes with an inner cannula, tube changes can be reduced to 30 days (EEC Directive, 1993). It is important to note that the presence of an inner cannula reduces the internal diameter of the inner lumen by 1–1.5 mm and can initially increase the patient's effort of breathing.

Fenestrated tracheostomy tubes (Figure 6.5)

These are available for both cuffed and uncuffed tubes. They consist of either a large hole or collection of small holes on the outer cannula and inner cannula. They allow air to pass through the fenestration and up past the vocal cords, allowing vocalisation. They are provided with both a fenestrated and non-fenestrated inner cannula. It is important to remember that the non-fenestrated tubes are worn overnight and when suctioning to

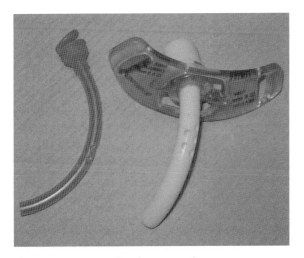

Figure 6.5   Fenestrated tracheostomy tube.

prevent trauma. As these tubes assist with redirecting airflow past the oral/nasal pharynx, it assists the patient's return to normal breathing. Often, these tubes are used when helping to wean patients from temporary tubes. Risk of aspiration is greater with these tubes and they should not be used for high-risk patients.

Adjustable flange tracheostomy tubes
(Figure 6.6)

These are specifically designed for patients who have deep-set tracheas; obese patients or patients with distorted anatomy within the neck following inflammation, trauma or oedema. These tubes can be adjusted to the desired length according to the individual's anatomy. They also allow for patients with granulation tissue to have the tube rotated back and forth to prevent granulation tissue build-up.

   These tubes have no inner tubes and are not available in the two-piece option, therefore making the wearer at greater risk of crusting and potential 'blocking off' of the tube. They can also be easier to dislodge. The length of tube sitting on the outside of the patient's neck is far greater than in other types of tube. This, coupled with equipment such as HME filters, ventilation tubing and suction apparatus, may lead to considerable torque on the tracheostomy tube, increasing the risk of displacement.

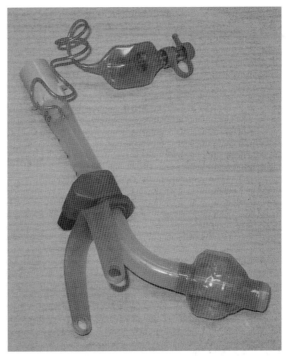

Figure 6.6   Adjustable flange tracheostomy tube.

Silver Negus tracheostomy tubes (Figure 6.7)

These tubes are suitable for long-term use to maintain the individual's airway. They come as a set with a built-in speaking valve tube and plain inner tube. They protrude far less than disposable alternatives. Speaking attachments are built into their inner tubes, preventing the need for prominent speaking attachments. These tubes can help those patients who require a long-term tracheostomy overcome the anxiety of altered body image. When worn with a Buchanan foam filter protector they can be easier to disguise.

Neoplastic disease of the head and neck

Benign head and neck tumours are rare. Benign tumours generally arise as a result of voice abuse or overuse. These tumours are usually attached to the vocal cords and can vary considerably in size. These nodules can be resolved through voice rest and intensive speech therapy. Occasionally surgical intervention is necessary in larger-sized nodules.

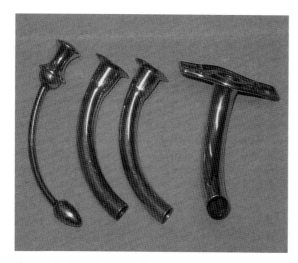

Figure 6.7   Silver Negus tracheostomy tube.

Box 6.6   Neck lumps unrelated to neoplasia

- Thyroid masses
- Glandular fever
- Tuberculosis
- Parotitis
- Branchial cyst

There are many other causes of neck lumps that are not associated with cancers of the head and neck. These can be broken down into different categories as detailed in Box 6.6.

Lymphomas are increasing in incidence. There is a large quantity of lymphatic tissue within the head and neck. Lymphoma is classified under two headings – Hodgkin's lymphoma or non-Hodgkin's lymphoma. The classification of these is determined by the presence or absence of cells known as Reed–Sternberg cells (Burton, 2003). These patients are usually biopsied within the ear, nose and throat (ENT) department and referred to a specialist in lymphoma management.

Most malignant tumours involving the larynx and pharynx are squamous cell carcinomas. Often, tumours in this area present to the specialist at an advanced stage, due to their 'silent' behaviour. Most patients do not develop any symptoms until the later stages of disease. Patients will quite often ignore the early warning signs of hoarseness for some time. The two main aetiological factors that most laryngeal carcinoma sufferers share are tobacco smoking and high alcohol consumption. However, laryngeal cancer does occur in non-smokers.

Symptoms of a laryngeal carcinoma are a progressively hoarse voice, stridor (noisy breathing), dysphagia (the inability to swallow) and pain. The patient sometimes complains of associated ear pain also known as otalgia.

Laryngectomy

Laryngectomy is the surgical removal of the larynx. It is a radical procedure with severe consequences for future communication. It is performed for cancers of the larynx that are too advanced for successful treatment with radiotherapy (T3 and T4 tumours) as discussed earlier in the chapter. Surgery involves creating a permanent opening into the pharynx. Following laryngectomy surgery, the trachea terminates as a permanent and irreversible stoma on the skin surface. In some cases, severely advanced tumours may be considered inoperable and the only option left is palliative radiotherapy given in the attempt to slow down the rapid progression of disease. These patients are sometimes given a tracheostomy to aid breathing and alleviate symptoms associated with airway occlusion caused by tumour.

Post-operative care of the patient with a laryngectomy (a laryngectomee) very much mirrors the post-operative care of the tracheostomy patient. Additional post-operative considerations include nutrition and communication.

Nutrition is provided either nasogastrically or via a puncture site through the posterior wall of the trachea into the oesophagus (tracheo-oesophageal puncture) and a catheter is passed through this during surgery. Feed can then be delivered via the catheter straight into the oesophagus. The patient remains nil-by-mouth for approximately 14 days or until wound healing has occurred. A barium swallow is usually performed to assess this prior to the commencement of any oral nutrition. Once the successful commencement of oral nutrition is established, the transoesophageal puncture site is then used to aid future communication for the patient.

The loss of the voice is often the most devastating consequence of a total laryngectomy.

Traditionally, patients were taught to develop oesophageal voice by swallowing air and then expelling it in short gulps – so causing the pharynx to vibrate and produce sound (Burton, 2003). Approximately one-third of patients can produce a satisfactory voice in this way. Alternative oesophageal speech has also been developed using an external electronic vibrator that produces a mechanical and poor quality voice.

There have been recent developments in surgical voice restoration, enabling the use of the tracheo-oesophageal puncture site to utilise a one-way valve inserted into the puncture site once the catheter for feeding is no longer required. The valve prevents any risk of aspiration but also allows the redirection of airflow from the lungs into the pharynx. This then causes the neopharynx to vibrate. This produces sound that is converted into speech by mouthing the words as in normal speech. This technique allows over 80% of total laryngectomy patients to achieve satisfactory speech (Burton, 2003).

An additional post-operative consideration for the management of the laryngectomee is care of the neck and suction drains. The patient will usually return to the ward environment with bilateral wound drains. It is important to observe these for evidence of saliva, which may indicate the formation of a fistula and excessive drainage. Wound closure is usually achieved using fine sutures around the stoma site itself and clips on the remaining neck incision. These are usually covered with a clear dressing or left exposed so that the wound site can be closely observed.

Potential post-operative complications

As with the tracheostomy patient, the laryngectomy patient is at risk of severe post-operative complications (see Box 6.7).

Box 6.7 Potential post-operative complications of laryngectomy

- Blockage of the trachea
- Stenosis of the tracheostomy
- Wound breakdown
- Fistula formation

Blockage of the trachea is a potentially life-threatening complication and can occur at any time post-operatively. It is caused by inadequate humidification causing secretions to thicken, creating a mucous plug that occludes the airway. Staff should ensure that the importance of humidification is taught when educating the patient to care for the laryngectomy site. This is particularly important, as this problem tends to occur when patients have returned home (Alexander *et al.*, 1995).

Stenosis of the tracheostomy is similar to a blockage. It is once again life threatening and most commonly presents in the community patient. Poor patient education and neglect result in crust formation around the stoma. As with the risk of blockage, patients need to be taught stringent care of the stoma. Careful toilet of the stoma should prevent its occurrence. Wearing a tube for a part of the day can also help prevent crust formation.

For patients receiving radiotherapy, there is a risk of wound breakdown due to the intensity of the therapy. Careful wound observation throughout the course of treatment can assist in the early detection and management of this problem.

A final significant post-operative complication is when the pharyngeal repair performed during surgery breaks down, allowing food and saliva to leak from the incision. This then leads to excoriation of the skin and potential infection. Once a fistula develops, it may take several weeks to heal and often requires antibiotic therapy during this time. Patients are kept nil-by-mouth and nutrition provided nasogastrically or through other enteric feeding methods such as PEG (percutaneous endoscopic gastrostomy) feeding. This complication is most common following radiotherapy and, in some cases, further surgery may be necessary in order to assist a slow-healing fistula by removing devitalised tissue.

Surgery of the thyroid gland

Applied physiology

Disorders of the thyroid gland may be associated with swelling of the neck. The thyroid is an H-shaped structure situated in front of the trachea and below the larynx (Figure 6.8). It is situated in

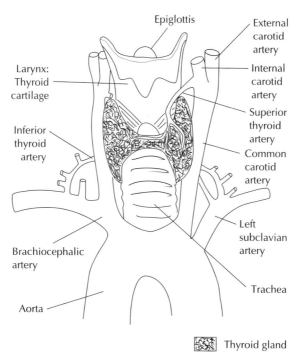

Epiglottis

External carotid artery

Internal carotid artery

Superior thyroid artery

Common carotid artery

Larynx: Thyroid cartilage

Inferior thyroid artery

Brachiocephalic artery

Aorta

Left subclavian artery

Trachea

Thyroid gland

Figure 6.8   Thyroid gland – anatomical relations and blood supply.

close proximity to the recurrent laryngeal nerve and, like all endocrine organs, has an extensive blood supply. The thyroid secretes thyroxin and calcitonin. Microscopically, the thyroid tissue comprises cells arranged into hollow spherical follicles into which thyroid hormone is secreted. Thyroid hormone controls metabolic rate and consists of two different compounds: thyroxin (T_3) and tri-iodothyronine (T_4), which are made by the thyroid from thyroglobulin and iodine. The major physiological effects of thyroid hormone can be seen in Box 6.8. Figure 6.9 shows the microscopic structure of thyroid tissue.

Calcitonin is produced by parafollicular cells within the thyroid tissue. The role of this hormone is to regulate blood calcium by increasing uptake into bone and increasing excretion of calcium and phosphate ions by the kidney. Calcitonin therefore reduces plasma calcium levels. In the case of both thyroid hormone and calcitonin, secretion is controlled by a rapid negative feedback mechanism according to the hormone levels in the bloodstream.

Box 6.8   Major effects of the thyroid hormones.

Increases:
- Metabolic rate
- Oxygen consumption
- Calorie usage and appetite
- Cerebral activity and anxiety
- Body temperature
- Pulse rate and blood pressure
- Gut motility

Situated on the posterior aspect of the thyroid are the four parathyroid glands, small collections of cells embedded within the thyroid tissue. The parathyroids secrete parathormone, which raises plasma calcium levels. This is achieved by reducing renal excretion of ionised calcium, increasing intestinal uptake of dietary calcium, and by stimulating osteoclasts to resorb bone, which releases stored calcium from the skeleton into the bloodstream.

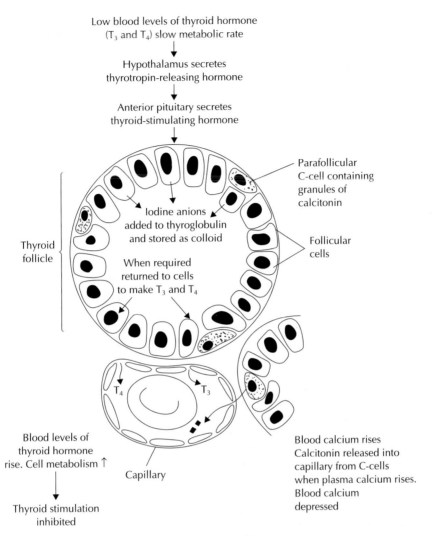

Low blood levels of thyroid hormone
(T_3 and T_4) slow metabolic rate

↓

Hypothalamus secretes
thyrotropin-releasing hormone

↓

Anterior pituitary secretes
thyroid-stimulating hormone

Parafollicular
C-cell containing
granules of
calcitonin

Iodine anions
added to thyroglobulin
and stored as colloid

Follicular
cells

Thyroid
follicle

When required
returned to cells
to make T_3 and T_4

T_4 T_3

Blood levels of
thyroid hormone
rise. Cell metabolism ↑

Capillary

Blood calcium rises
Calcitonin released into
capillary from C-cells
when plasma calcium rises.
Blood calcium
depressed

Thyroid stimulation
inhibited

Figure 6.9   Microscopic structure of the thyroid gland and production of hormones.

Calcium ions are important for nerve conduction, muscle contraction and blood clotting, so maintenance of appropriate plasma levels takes precedence over maintenance of normal bone mass.

Thyroid disorders

Surgery to the thyroid gland may be required because the gland has become overactive, causing hyperthyroidism. The levels of circulating plasma thyroid hormones increase the metabolic rate, produce heat intolerance and make the tissues more sensitive to sympathetic nervous system stimulation. The pulse rate increases and tachyarrhythmias such as atrial fibrillation may be present. The patient may experience weight loss and increased appetite and diarrhoea, and the skin may be thin and moist. Anxiety and irritability may be present and the blood pressure may be elevated due to the sympathetic effect upon the cardiovascular system. Severe hyperthyroidism is termed thyrotoxicosis and requires medical stabilisation by antithyroid drugs such as carbimazole and sympathetic

> **Box 6.9** Effects of inadequately treated hyperthyroidism upon recovery from surgery.
>
> - Impaired healing (thinner skin)
> - Impaired rehabilitation (loss of muscle mass and strength)
> - Cardiovascular instability
> - Nutritional deficits leading to catabolic state
> - Poor compliance (anxiety/irritability)

beta-blockers before surgery. Some of the effects of inadequately controlled hyperthyroidism upon surgical recovery are shown in Box 6.9. Hyperthyroid patients may have exopthalmos: protruding eyeballs giving a characteristic staring expression. This occurs because of accumulated fibrous and fatty tissue behind the eye and can predispose to corneal abrasion and ulceration in severe cases where the eyelids can no longer close fully over the eyes. Nutritional and cardiovascular status as well as careful psychological handling may need to be addressed pre-operatively.

Hyperthyroidism may result from a small area of thyroid tissue being overactive (a 'hot spot') or a generalised increased mass and activity of a large area of tissue. In the latter, goitre (swelling of the anterior neck) may be noticeable. If the patient is a male who wears a shirt and tie, this may be detected relatively early due to his becoming unable to fasten the shirt collar. A woman may seek help because the goitre has developed sufficiently to produce an unsightly swelling.

Not all goitres are associated with thyroid overactivity, some occur because of a lack of dietary iodine impairing thyroid function and causing the gland to enlarge in compensation. Thyroid overactivity may be the result of an autoimmune reaction against the thyroid cells. Sometimes, hyperthyroidism results from a disorder of either the hypothalamus or the pituitary, so the patient may be investigated to identify the prime cause of the disorder to ensure the correct treatment is initiated. Plasma thyroid releasing factors (hypothalamus) and thyroid stimulating hormone (anterior pituitary) may be measured pre-operatively. Hyperthyroidism may also be the result of thyroid carcinoma. If the patient is not suitable for surgery, the pathological thyroid function may be suppressed by the use of radioactive iodine.

Surgical treatment

The common surgical management for hyperthyroidism is a subtotal thyroidectomy, leaving sufficient thyroid tissue to maintain metabolic homeostasis and preserving the parathyroids to ensure continued calcium homeostasis. The surgery involves a transverse incision across the neck, which the surgeon usually positions so that, after healing, the scar is virtually indistinguishable from the natural skin folds. The major considerations are to stabilise the thyroid function pre-operatively to minimise peri-operative cardiovascular risk; to deal with blood loss owing to the vascularity of the tissues; and to observe for other complications. As well as assessment of the thyroid status, peri-operative screening may include electrocardiography.

Following recovery from anaesthesia, the patient will be nursed in a semi-recumbent position, and there will be surgical suction drains from the operative site. Sitting propped up will decrease the risk of haemorrhage and will promote wound drainage. Patients commonly recover uneventfully following thyroidectomy, but there are some potentially life-threatening complications. There is a risk of haematoma formation which could press upon the trachea impeding respiration, so it is important to observe the rate of drainage and to observe the wound for swelling. For this reason, thyroidectomy wounds are commonly closed with surgical staples or clips, which, apart from leaving no extra scarring, are also rapidly removed in an emergency. Staple/clip removers are kept at the bedside for this purpose.

On rare occasions, thyroid surgery results in a sudden outpouring of thyroid hormones into the bloodstream, causing a potentially catastrophic rise in the pulse and blood pressure. This is termed a thyroid crisis. Another hazard is that, if the parathyroid glands were not easily visualised during the operation, they could have been accidentally removed. This would result in hypocalcaemia, which, if untreated, could result in cardiac arrest. As a warning sign, increased neuromuscular irritability would be present. The patient should be observed for tetany: complaints of tingling in the fingers or around the lips and cramp-like muscular pains and spasms should be taken seriously. In tetany, the facial muscles may exhibit twitching if the side of the face is tapped (Chvostek's sign), or

---

Box 6.10 Effects of hypothyroidism.

- Reduced metabolic rate
- Reduced body temperature
- Weight gain
- Reduced appetite
- Slowed thought processes
- Bradycardia and hypotension
- Facial oedema, thinning of hair
- Raised plasma cholesterol and triglycerides
- Reduced activity, coma and death in severe cases

---

the hand may go into spasm if a sphygmomanometer cuff is inflated on that arm (Trousseau's sign). If tetany develops the treatment is to give intravenous calcium as a matter of urgency.

One more potential risk is damage to the recurrent laryngeal nerve. If a branch of this is accidentally divided, the vocal cord on the affected side will be paralysed and will project into the airway. The patient must be observed post-operatively for the return of normal breathing and speech quality. Damage may produce laryngeal stridor, difficulty with swallowing and hoarseness, which may be permanent.

In the longer term, there is a risk of hypothyroidism if a significant amount of thyroid tissue has been excised. Over a period of time, the thyroid secretions become insufficient to produce normal metabolic control and, possibly years after the thyroidectomy, the person may exhibit signs of thyroid underactivity (see Box 6.10). These signs develop slowly, so may be noticed first by someone who has not seen the patient for a period of time. Following diagnosis, treatment is replacement therapy with thyroxine.

Other endocrine conditions

Surgical treatment of pituitary or adrenal conditions is usually undertaken in specialist units so will be mentioned only briefly. Pituitary tumours may present in a variety of ways, from dysfunction of target organs controlled by the pituitary (for example adrenal overactivity resulting in Cushing's disease), to headaches or loss of visual fields caused by local pressure within the cranium. Hypophysectomy (removal of the pituitary gland) would

require neurosurgical facilities, and the patient would need careful pre-operative stabilisation and lifelong post-operative replacement of the pituitary hormones. Pituitary tumours may also be treated with radiotherapy to reduce the tumour mass, as they are sometimes difficult to remove completely.

Tumours of the adrenal gland may occur. Phaeochromocytoma is a tumour of the adrenal medulla resulting in excessive production of epinephrine and norepinephrine (adrenaline and noradrenaline). Hypertension and tachyarrhythmias are commonly present, in addition to signs of sympathetic nervous system overstimulation. As far as possible, the condition must be stabilised pre-operatively and monitored with great care during and after the surgery.

Corticosteroids and surgery

It is important to discover whether a patient has been taking corticosteroids for any reason before any surgical procedure is undertaken. Sudden cessation of this medication in association with the physiological demands of surgery may cause adrenal insufficiency: the blood pressure may fall as the body is unable to respond to the extra demands encountered. Additional corticosteroids may need to be given to maintain cardiovascular haemostasis.

Surgical treatment of disorders of the gonads is discussed respectively in Chapter 10 (male reproductive system) and Chapter 11 (women's health).

Self-test questions

Circle the correct answer(s). There may be more than one correct answer.

1. True or false? Tracheostomy may be performed:
   a. To improve respiratory function
   b. To increase dead space
   c. Following laryngectomy
   d. For multiple rib fractures
2. A patient returns from theatre with a newly formed tracheostomy. Which of the following statements are true?
   a. A silver tube with a speaking valve will be in situ

b. The patient should be nursed sitting upright with the neck supported

c. Suction apparatus should be by the bedside

d. Tracheal dilators should be on the locker

3. Which of the following are hazards following formation of a tracheostomy?
   a. Ulceration of the tracheal mucosa
   b. Dysphagia
   c. Airway obstruction
   d. Respiratory infection

4. Which of the following statements about a post-operative patient with a tracheostomy are true?
   a. A humidifier or a heat moisture exchange device should be used
   b. A call system and pencil and paper should be available for the patient
   c. Tracheostomy tapes should be changed at least daily
   d. The stoma site should be cleaned daily using aseptic technique

5. Laryngeal carcinoma is commonly associated with which of the following symptoms?
   a. Lump in the neck
   b. Stridor
   c. Dysphagia
   d. Hoarseness

6. True or false? Following laryngectomy, the patient:
   a. Will be nil-by-mouth for about two weeks
   b. May be fed via a tracheo-oesophageal tube
   c. Requires high-calorie nutrition
   d. May have a barium swallow X-ray before resuming oral diet

7. Which of the following are serious complications following laryngectomy?
   a. Tracheal occlusion with crusted mucus
   b. Infection with *Pseudomonas aeruginosa*
   c. Aspiration of diet
   d. Breakdown of the wound

8. Which of the following risks to post-operative recovery can occur as a result of inadequate control of an overactive thyroid?
   a. Hypothermia
   b. Respiratory obstruction
   c. Impaired wound healing
   d. Tachyarrhythmias

9. **True** or **false**? Following thyroidectomy, which of the following observations should be reported as a matter of urgency?
   a. Signs of haematoma accumulation at the wound site
   b. Hoarseness of the voice
   c. Hypertension
   d. Tingling around the mouth and muscle cramps

10. Which of the following statements are **true**?
    a. Following thyroidectomy, weight gain, cold intolerance and drowsiness may develop years later
    b. Goitre always indicates an overactive thyroid
    c. In the early post-operative stage, plasma calcium may rise due to loss of para-thyroid tissue
    d. In the early post-operative stage, plasma calcium may fall due to loss of para-thyroid tissue

References and further reading

Alexander M, Fawcett J & Runciman P (eds) (1995) *Nursing Practice Hospital and Home: The Adult*. London: Churchill Livingstone

Buglass E (1999) 'Tracheostomy care: tracheal suction and humidification' *British Journal of Nursing* 8(8): 500–504

Burton M (2003) *Diseases of the Ear, Nose and Throat* (15th edn). London: Churchill Livingstone

Cherry J (1997) *Ear, Nose and Throat Surgery*. London: Cavendish Publishing

Dhillon R & East C (2001) *Ear, Nose, Throat and Head and Neck Surgery* (2nd edn). London: Churchill Livingstone

EEC Directive – Class 11A, Rule 7 (1993) Council Directive Concerning Medical Devices, 93/42EEC

Gavaghan M (1997) 'Surgical Treatment of Pheochromocytomas' *AORN Journal* 65(6): 1039, 1041, 1044

Harris RB (1984) 'Clean vs sterile tracheostomy care and pulmonary infection' *Nursing Research* 33(2): 80–85

Lalwani A (2005) *Current Diagnosis and Treatment in Otolaryngology – Head and Neck Surgery*. New York: Lange Medical Books

Schori-Ahmed D (2003) 'Thyroid Disease' *RN* 66(6): 38–44

Seay S & Gay S (1991) 'Problems in tracheostomy patient care' *ORL Head and Neck Nursing* 15(20): 10–11

Serra A (2000) 'Tracheostomy Care' *Nursing Standard* 14(42): 45–52

St George's Healthcare NHS Trust (2000) *Guidelines for the Care of Patients with Tracheostomy Tubes*. Kent: Sims Portex

To EW, Tsang WM, Lai ECH & Chu MC (2002) 'Retrospective study on the need of intensive care unit admission after major head and neck surgery' *ANZ Journal of Surgery* 72(1): 11–14

Williams M (1998) 'Disorders of the adrenal gland' *Seminars in Perioperative Nursing* 7(3): 179–185

7

Vascular Surgery

Ann M Price

Introduction

The incidence of vascular surgical cases is increasing in numbers and complexity due to the ageing population and advances in surgical techniques. These patients can be critically ill after surgery. The National Confidential Enquiry into Perioperative Deaths (NCEPOD, 2001) noted that some patients did not have access to an appropriate critical care bed post-operatively after major surgery. This inevitably puts more pressure on surgical beds within the ward setting and requires medical and nursing staff to have the knowledge and skills to manage patients appropriately (NCEPOD, 2001). An increase in risk factors for cardiovascular disease is also occurring (Wolf *et al.*, 1999) so vascular problems are increasing (Lakatta & Levy, 2003). Box 7.1 identifies the aims of this chapter.

Box 7.1 Aims of the chapter.

- To discuss assessment of the vascular patient including main investigations
- To identify risk factors for vascular disease
- To discuss the vessels dysfunction associated with vascular disease
- To discuss the main surgical techniques used and their complications
- To highlight the priorities of care for the vascular patient

---

Common vascular pathophysiological conditions

Peripheral vascular disease (PVD)

This refers to disease of blood vessels outside the heart and brain and usually involves narrowing of the vessels. The American Heart Association (2004) discusses 'functional' PVD as causing spasm in the blood vessels (such as Raynaud's disease), which can be triggered by cold temperatures, vibration and smoking. 'Organic' PVD is a result of structural changes within the vessel, such as inflammation, tissue damage and atherosclerosis: peripheral arterial disease is an example of this.

Cardiovascular disease (CVD)

Cardiovascular disease has similar causes to PVD but refers to the heart and systemic vessels. PVD and CVD are often closely related in the patient population, leading to complex and multiple health problems. Grundy *et al.* (2004) identified the clinical signs associated with cardiovascular disease as involving abdominal obesity (waist circumference of above 40 inches in men and more than 35 inches in women), elevated triglyceride levels, reduced high-density lipid cholesterol levels, hypertension and raised fasting blood sugar.

Peripheral arterial disease

Sometimes the terms peripheral vascular disease (PVD) and peripheral arterial disease (PAD) are used virtually interchangeably, which can be confusing (Mohler, 2003). However, peripheral arterial disease (PAD) refers to the accumulation of atheromatous plaques within the arteries. The plaques cause hardening of some parts of the vessels and can partially occlude vessels (stenosis) leading to poor blood flow beyond the occlusion (Mohler, 2003) (see Figure 7.1). The development of PAD is thought to be due to hypertension, hyper-lipidaemia, poor blood sugar control (diabetes mellitus), tobacco smoking (Pedrini, 2003) and lack of exercise; there is some discussion about the role of familial tendency and insulin resistance (Grundy et al., 2004). Ischaemic heart disease and hypertension may result in further damage, and stress the vascular system. PAD is not an isolated disease and can lead to cerebrovascular complications and other organ damage (Mohler, 2003). Inflammation is thought to contribute to the development of PAD as inflammatory markers have been shown to be present in plaque deposits (Eckel et al., 2002).

Vascular occlusion

Atherosclerotic plaques are thought to rupture in susceptible people. The contents irritate the vessels and can encourage clot formation in the affected area. This can lead to total or partial occlusion, either from the narrowing of the vessel or from thrombosis formation. Vascular stenosis (partial occlusion) is a major cause of vascular disorders as it restricts the blood flow to vital organs (such as brain and limbs), leading to ischaemic damage of the affected area.

Arterial insufficiency

This occurs when vascular disease is so severe that blood flow (usually to the limbs) is reduced. This leads to ischaemia of the affected area and arterial ulcers. Diabetic patients are particularly prone to arterial ulcers because of concurrent neuropathy (the reduction of sensation in the extremities such as fingers and toes). Tissue damage is not felt, so the source of injury, such as poorly fitting shoes, is not removed (Sieggreen & Kline, 2004).

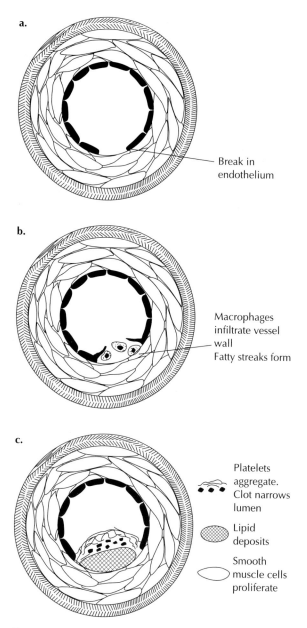

a.
Break in endothelium

b.
Macrophages infiltrate vessel wall
Fatty streaks form

c.
Platelets aggregate. Clot narrows lumen
Lipid deposits
Smooth muscle cells proliferate

Figure 7.1 Formation of atheroma.

PVD and diabetes mellitus

Atherosclerosis formation seems to be increased in patients with diabetes mellitus. This is due to changes in the endothelial cells of the artery caused by a combination of hyperglycaemia, increased fatty acids and lipoproteins, and other metabolic changes that are common in diabetic patients

(Eckel *et al.*, 2002; Creager *et al.*, 2003). The damage to the endothelial cell barrier allows fatty deposits to be laid down more swiftly as fatty streaks. The plaques can have a lipid core which may rupture and spill into the vessel causing thrombosis, or a stable plaque may develop that causes stenosis.

Eckel *et al.* (2002) and Grundy *et al.* (2004) note that hyperglycaemia is associated with increased PVD and CVD, thus controlling blood sugars within normal limits is important. However, the role of lipoprotein changes in diabetes may also be a significant factor affecting the development of atherosclerosis in this patient population (Eckel *et al.*, 2002). Recognising the patient at risk of developing diabetes mellitus and commencing interventions early can delay the onset of full diabetes and may reduce or delay the worsening effects of PVD (Grundy *et al.*, 2004).

Hypertension is another common complication of diabetes mellitus, which is known to be a factor in PVD development and should be controlled (Luscher *et al.*, 2003). The hypercoagulation that is evident in diabetic patients may add to the risk of thrombosis development, exaggerating the effects of PVD (Eckel *et al.*, 2002). Thus the effects of diabetes mean that this patient group is more likely to suffer adverse effects of PVD and require interventional surgery. Additionally, patients with diabetes are more at risk of post-operative complications such as infection and hyper- or hypoglycaemia.

PVD and the older person

PVD progressively worsens with increasing age (Lakatta & Levy, 2003). Thus, patients presenting with vascular problems are likely to be over 50 years old and often have cardiovascular disease or other health problems. The worsening of PVD in older people may be due to longer exposure to the known risk factors or may be due to degenerative changes in the arterial wall. PVD can vary significantly between people and an undefined genetic factor may also be implicated.

Arterial wall thickening and dilatation occurs with age and this may increase the risk of atherosclerosis developing (Lakatta & Levy, 2003). Stiffening of the arterial walls with age leads to hypertension, which is difficult to bring under control. PVD is particularly debilitating for this patient population as it affects their independence,

social contact and psychological well-being. Also, the older person has degeneration of other body systems and is more susceptible to complications such as infection, particularly in wounds and the respiratory system.

Development of aneurysms

An aneurysm results when dilatation of a blood vessel occurs. The vessel wall progressively weakens and the aneurysm enlarges; as the vessel dilates the risk of spontaneous rupture increases (Bick, 2000; Thompson, 2002). Atherosclerosis is thought to be the underlying cause of most aneurysms as the vessel wall degenerates and becomes prone to dilatation (Bick, 2000). However, other risk factors have been recognised including connective tissue disorders (such as Marfan's syndrome), familial tendency and infection. Other lifestyle factors that are associated with cardiovascular disease are also evident in this patient population and cigarette smoking seems to be linked to the increased incidence and rate of aneurysm development (Bick, 2000).

The aneurysm affects the aortic artery and its related branches. Arteries that may be involved in an aneurysm include inferior phrenic, coeliac arteries (which supply the liver, stomach and spleen), renal arteries (supplying the kidney) and mesenteric arteries (supplying the colon); thus a ruptured aneurysm can affect other organs due to lack of blood flow. Figure 7.2 highlights the areas affected by thoracic and abdominal aortic aneurysms. (The reader may find it useful to carry out Activity 7.1 to locate the vessels discussed in this chapter.)

Four main forms of aneurysm have been described (Bick, 2000) (see Figure 7.3).

- *Fusiform* – This is the most common type of aneurysm – it encircles the artery leading to a circumferential dilatation of a segment.

Activity 7.1   Identifying arteries and veins within the body.

Either use an anatomy and physiology book or look at this website to find the arteries and veins that are discussed in this chapter.

www.innerbody.com/image/cardov.html

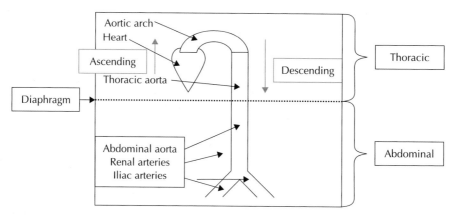

Figure 7.2   Thoracic versus abdominal aneurysm position (with main associated structures that may be involved in aneurysm).

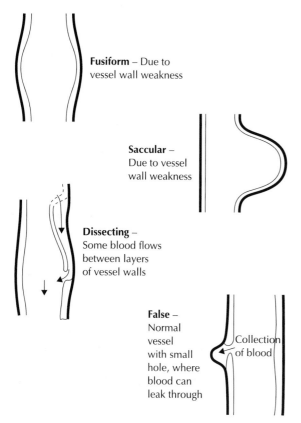

Figure 7.3   Types of aneurysm.
(based on Bick, 2000)

- *Saccular* – This occurs when a small area of the vessel wall becomes thin and stretches to form a pouch.
- *Dissecting* – This type results from a small tear in the inner wall of the artery. Blood seeps between the layers of the artery wall forming the dilatation.
- *False* – A false aneurysm develops from an injury affecting all three layers of the artery wall. Blood leaks from the artery and forms a clot outside the arterial wall; connective tissue is then deposited around the clot to form the 'false' aneurysm. 'True' aneurysms occur because of vessel wall dilatation; this does not occur in a false aneurysm.

Small aneurysms can develop in minor arteries and veins with the same pathophysiological basis as aortic aneurysms. These can sometimes cause problems with blood flow to distal areas and may need surgical intervention although rupture is less common.

Investigations and assessment of vascular disease

The aim of specialised investigations is to enable accurate assessment of the vascular disease and to aid planning for appropriate management (including surgery where indicated) (Dawson, 2000). Box 7.2 explains common investigations used to assess vascular disease.

Assessing and monitoring the patient with vascular disease

The underlying cause of atherosclerosis is difficult to assess overtly but signs, symptoms and risk

Box 7.2 Common investigations used in the assessment of vascular disease.

Arteriography/venograms – These are used to outline the blood vessels and aid in the assessment of blood flow to a particular area and the extent of any occluded vessels (Dawson, 2000). Usually radio-opaque dyes are used to highlight the vessels and enhance the problematic areas.

Aortogram/aortography – Similar to arteriography but examines the aorta and attached vessels.

Computed tomography (CT) – CT scans enable an in-depth evaluation of parts of the body. For vascular surgery this can help with the assessment of the size, position and extent of the vascular problem.

Magnetic resonance imaging (MRI) – Sometimes used to assess neurological deficits in the vascular patient.

Ultrasound – Ultrasound uses high frequency sound waves to image internal organs. Its usefulness in vascular diagnosis is more limited because of the advancement in other techniques. However, it may be useful when other methods are unavailable and Pedrini (2003) believes that it is helpful to identify the best treatment option in aorto-iliac, femoral and tibial arterial disease.

Ankle brachial index (ABI) – This is a simple technique that involves inflating a blood pressure cuff over an artery and deflating whilst assessing for systolic blood pressure (SBP) and also assessing blood flow return via a Doppler ultrasound device; a normal ABI is 1–1.3. Normally ankle SBP should be slightly greater or equal to brachial SBP. In peripheral vascular disease ankle SBP falls below brachial SBP and results in an ABI < 1 (Mohler, 2003) (see Table 7.1 for ABI significance).

ABI is unreliable in patients who have calcified incompressible arteries, as a falsely high reading is obtained; patients with diabetes are prone to this problem (Mohler, 2003). However, Mohler (2003) suggests that ABI is a useful predictor of long-term morbidity and mortality from ischaemic stroke, myocardial infarction and other vascular complications.

Exercise tolerance – This is a useful tool to assess some patients' suitability for surgery (Malster & Parry, 2000) and identifies the severity of the disease in some vascular patients. It involves walking the patient on a treadmill and assessing their tolerance to speed and duration in relation to pain and symptoms experienced. It can be used in conjunction with ABI to confirm or discount peripheral vascular disease as the cause of the patient's symptoms (Mohler, 2003).

Digital subtraction angiography (DSA) – This is felt to be the best diagnostic tool in peripheral vascular disease (Pedrini, 2003). This method usually uses femoral catheterisation, often using contrast dye, and involves a variety of views using different spatial resolutions to obtain images.

Doppler – Colour flow and power Doppler are useful to pick up flow in small blood vessels (Pedrini, 2003); duplex ultrasound can also be used (Mohler, 2003).

Magnetic resonance (MR) angiography – May replace DSA as the diagnostic tool of choice in the future (Pedrini, 2003).

Electrocardiograph (ECG) – Vascular patients have a high incidence of cardiovascular disease and routine ECG is used to exclude myocardial infarction and other cardiac disorders.

Blood tests – Assessing the coagulability of blood is important in vascular surgery. Hypercoagulability can increase the risk of vascular occlusion in some cases. Equally prolonged clotting times can increase the risk of post-operative bleeding. Other blood tests are also important to assess for co-existing disease that may affect recovery, such as renal impairment and diabetes mellitus.

Table 7.1 Significance of ankle brachial index (ABI).

ABI	Disease status
1.0–1.3	Normal
0.7–0.9	Mild disease
0.4– < 0.7	Moderate disease
< 0.4	Severe disease

(cited in Mohler, 2003)

factors related to ischaemic heart disease are common. Thus the following findings may be suspicious of disease and further investigation may be needed. The more common signs and symptoms of specific conditions are also discussed.

Vital signs

Hypertension is a common finding. Sometimes the patient may suffer from angina pectoris or abnormal heart rhythms. Thus assessment and monitoring of pulse, blood pressure and respiration are vital. Skin colour and temperature are also useful to monitor the effectiveness of the circulation (Mohler, 2003).

Peripheral signs

Patients may have poor or absent peripheral pulses, particularly in feet and ankles. They may have cool or cold limbs and get changes in sensation and pain at times. A grading system from 0 to 2

Table 7.2 Grading for presence of pulse.

Grade of pulse	Description of pulse type
0	Absent
1	Diminished
2	Normal

can be used to assess the pulse (see Table 7.2). Mohler (2003) suggests that the femoral, popliteal, posterior tibial and dorsalis pedis pulses should be compared with radial and ipsilateral pulses (see Activity 7.1). Bruits (sounds caused by turbulent blood flow) are sometimes present in affected pulses and are assessed by auscultation. In severe disease, limb pain and difficulty in walking are often the key features of the disease getting worse. Intermittent claudication (limb pain due to poor blood flow) on exercise may progress to pain at rest and critical limb ischaemia leading to gangrene, ulceration and tissue damage (Pedrini, 2003). Limb extremities should be inspected for tissue damage and poor nail growth. Impotence and atrophy of lower extremities may be present. Capillary refill can be tested by pressing firmly on the finger or toe for three seconds and then releasing. The skin tone should look pale but return to normal within two seconds – if it does not, then blood flow to the extremities is reduced (Sieggreen & Kline, 2004).

Blood glucose

Diabetes mellitus is common and may be un-diagnosed in some patients. Therefore patients' blood sugar levels should be assessed (usually by fasting blood sugar) and appropriate investigation and treatment commenced if found to be high.

Abdominal signs

On abdominal examination a pulsating mass may be found in the patient with an abdominal aortic aneurysm. This may be found accidentally while the patient is being examined for other conditions.

Neurological signs

Transient ischaemic attacks (TIAs) are a feature in carotid vascular occlusion, causing brief lapses in conscious level or alertness. This is due to the blood flow being limited to the brain, particularly if the head is moved from side to side. Some patients complain of dizziness too. Cerebrovascular accidents (CVA or strokes) are a complication of vascular disease and can be the first indication that the patient has a problem. Therefore assessment of neurological status is important.

Pain

The site of the vascular disorder will affect the type and intensity of pain experienced. In the early stages of the disease process the patient is often asymptomatic but, as the disease progresses, pain is likely to intensify. The patient should be asked about the position and type of pain; for example, someone with a thoracic aneurysm may experience chest pain. An abdominal aneurysm may cause abdominal pain, a person with carotid stenosis may have headaches and people with peripheral vessel problems may experience limb pain (claudication). The patient should be asked if the pain is associated with activity or at rest and asked to describe the pain so that other possible causes (such as myocardial infarction) can be excluded.

Table 7.3 identifies the priorities of care for patients undergoing surgery for vascular disease and should be referred to alongside the rest of this chapter.

Management of abdominal aortic aneurysms

Abdominal aortic aneurysms (AAA) account for approximately 10 000 deaths per year in the UK and are more common in males than females, particularly in the over 60 years age group (Bick, 2000). Awareness of the disease seems to have increased and improved diagnosis is leading to earlier detection, thus more patients are being reviewed for possible surgical intervention. The difference between aortic and thoracic aneurysms is highlighted in Figure 7.2.

Patients with AAAs are usually asymptomatic until the aneurysm begins to leak. They are sometimes discovered incidentally when the patient is being investigated for other problems, such as urinary disorders. A leaking aneurysm is suspected

Table 7.3 Priorities of care for patients undergoing surgery for vascular disease.

Issue	Care considerations
Cardiovascular stability	Control of hypertension, maintenance of ischaemic heart disease, control of arrhythmias, encourage smoking reduction or cessation, anti-platelet therapy and exercise rehabilitation (Mohler, 2003).
Infection control	MRSA has been identified as a major concern and post-operative problem for vascular patients (NCEPOD, 2001). Infection leads to wound breakdown but can have serious consequences for vascular patients when grafts become infected. Therefore, adhering to strict infection control precautions and aseptic technique is vital.
Fluid balance and renal function	Inadequate monitoring of fluid intake and output, vital signs, CVP and urine output can lead to the seriousness of the patient's condition being overlooked. Early warning signs scoring systems have been developed as a method of identifying patients early in an acute stage of illness (see Chapter 13) and they include measures for blood pressure, heart rate, urine output and respiratory rate. These factors all can indicate fluid imbalance and are an essential component of assessment.
Neurovascular observation	Vascular procedures have the potential to cause clot formation within the veins and arteries, which can lead to cerebral embolism and vascular occlusion. Thus, monitoring to detect changes in neurological function and vascular integrity is important. Neurological function can be assessed using the Glasgow Coma Score, which is a useful tool in the initial post-operative stages to monitor acute changes.
Blood products	A variety of blood products are often used to manage vascular patients. Blood loss can be a problem during some procedures and replacement is necessary. Clotting disturbances can be present and products such as platelets, cryoprecipitate and fresh frozen plasma may be used. All blood products carry a risk of adverse reactions and infection transmission and, therefore, should only be administered if clear clinical indications are present. Monitoring during transfusion of any blood product is vital to detect changes in heart rate, blood pressure, temperature and respiratory rate as well as looking for skin reactions and difficulty in breathing (see Chapter 3).
Nutrition	The ageing population and nature of illness in vascular patients can predispose patients to effects of malnutrition. Patients with diabetes mellitus are particularly prone to some vascular disorders and, therefore, controlling blood sugar levels and nutritional advice is important to limit vascular damage. It is also important that appropriate nutrition intake is maintained; hyperlipidaemia is associated with some vascular disorders and a low-fat diet may be required. A balanced diet should promote wound healing and improve well-being for this susceptible group of patients.

when the patient presents with abdominal and back pain and a tender, pulsating mass may be evident on abdominal examination (Bick, 2000). Diagnosis in the obese patient can be difficult and abdominal X-ray, computed tomography (CT) scan and/or ultrasound may be used to confirm provisional diagnosis (see Box 7.2). Hall (2003) notes that ultrasound is the diagnostic tool of choice and is superior to physical examination alone. Patients with acute rupture of the aneurysm suffer massive haemorrhage and will present in a collapsed state with hypotension and tachycardia. Mortality is high in acute rupture with many patients dying before they reach hospital. Figure 7.4 shows an aortic aneurysm.

The prognosis for AAA is improved if the patient is treated under elective surgical conditions before rupture occurs. A screening programme using ultrasound is suggested for high-risk patients (Earnshaw *et al.*, 2004). Medical management is considered suitable for patients with asymptomatic aneurysms of less than 5.5 cm in diameter who undergo ultrasound examination every six months (Thompson, 2002). Medical management involves blood pressure control (usually using beta blockers or antihypertensive medication), control of blood sugar in diabetes mellitus, help with giving up smoking, assessment for related cardiovascular disorders and regular screening.

Patients with aneurysms larger than 5.5 cm in diameter should be considered for surgical intervention. If the aneurysm is thought to be expanding rapidly or becomes symptomatic, then surgery should be urgently undertaken (Hall, 2003). Ruptured aneurysms require emergency surgical repair.

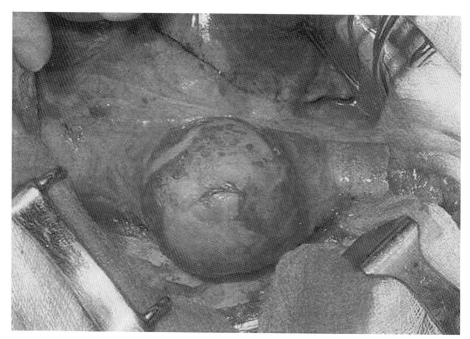

Figure 7.4 Aortic aneurysm.
(Reprinted from *Clinical Surgery*, p. 501, Cuschieri *et al.* (2003) with permission from Blackwell)

Operative procedures

Two main operative procedures are used: repair of the aneurysm using a graft or stabilising the aneurysm through inserting an endovascular stent.

Graft surgical repair

This involves a midline incision in the abdominal wall. The aorta is clamped above and below the aneurysm site to reduce bleeding and the aneurysm will be opened and any thrombus will be removed. A Dacron or woven graft (synthetic) is then inserted (see Figure 7.5); straight grafts are used in the aorta but 'trouser' grafts are available if the aneurysm involves the iliac arteries (Bick, 2000). Once the graft is sutured into place, the clamps are removed and the anastomoses are observed for signs of bleeding. In elective cases heparin is often used to reduce clot formation post-operatively to avoid occlusion of the graft during the recovery period. Graft occlusion can lead to sudden loss of peripheral pulses and cold legs.

Complications of graft surgical repair are numerous and close observation in an intensive care or high-dependency area is usually required for 24–48 hours post-operatively. Bleeding from the anastomosis and renal failure due to restricted blood flow to renal arteries are common complications (Bick, 2000) and early warning signs such as tachycardia, hypotension, reduced urine output, increasing abdominal distension and increasing confusion should be monitored closely. Patients usually have co-existing cardiovascular disease, which increases their risk of myocardial infarction. They may require inotropic support in the post-operative period.

Respiratory complications are related to the large abdominal incision, which restricts breathing and promotes atelectasis. Many patients have a history of chronic respiratory conditions or smoking, which increases the risk of pneumonia. Pain control is often achieved using epidural analgesia, which can improve depth of breathing without increasing drowsiness or respiratory depression.

Less common complications include paralytic ileus, bowel infarction and impotence (Bick, 2000).

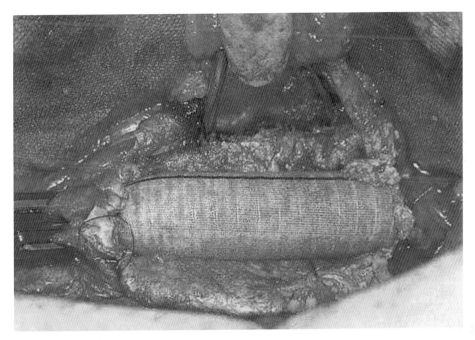

Figure 7.5   Aortic aneurysm graft.
(Reprinted from *Clinical Surgery*, p. 505, Cuschieri *et al.* (2003) with permission from Blackwell)

Rare complications from surgery are spinal cord ischaemia, which can lead to paralysis; and graft infection, which can lead to anastomosis breakdown.

Endovascular stent

This is a less invasive technique that is particularly suitable for high-risk surgical patients (Hall, 2003). Abdominal aortic and pelvic angiograms may be performed to assess the patient's suitability for endovascular stent and to provide more detailed data about the patient's anatomy. Endovascular stents are most suitable for straightforward aneurysms of the aorta with limited risk to associated arteries. The procedure can be performed under general or local anaesthetic.

Endovascular systems available include a graft that attaches to the aorta and iliac arteries via a balloon implantation that hooks into the artery walls. A self-expanding device is also available which is made of graft material and attaches to the vessel wall when exposed to body heat (Hall, 2003) (see Figure 7.6).

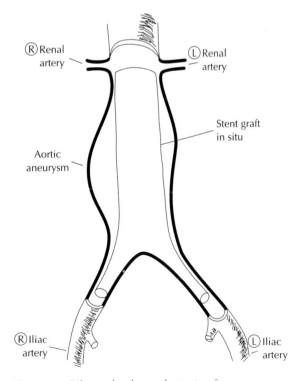

Figure 7.6   Bifurcated endovascular stent graft.

Table 7.4 Complications of AAA repair.

Abdominal AAA repair	Endovascular stent repair
• Bleeding	• Bleeding
• Renal failure	• Graft occlusion
• Myocardial infarction	• Endoleaks (can occur after many months)
• Respiratory distress	• Graft infection
• Graft infection	• Anastomosis breakdown
• Anastomosis breakdown	
• Paralytic ileus	
• Bowel infarction	
• Impotence	
• Spinal cord ischaemia	

Box 7.3 Complications of thoracic aneurysm repair.

• Bleeding
• Heart failure
• Spinal cord ischaemia and paralysis
• Respiratory depression/difficulty
• Pain
• Cardiac arrhythmias
• Graft infection
• Anastomosis breakdown
• Multi-organ failure

The stent is inserted via the femoral artery through an introducer needle and guide wire system. Both femoral arteries are exposed and the guide wire inserted in one side and the graft via the other side (Hall, 2003). The stent is put in place and positioning is checked via fluoroscopy to ensure that branching arteries are not occluded and an aortogram is undertaken to ascertain if there are any leaks present.

Complications of endovascular stent insertion include endoleaks, where blood leaks from the stent into the aneurysm sac. This can occur immediately post-operatively or after many months. Post-operatively, patients need to be monitored in an intensive care or high-dependency area for signs of bleeding such as hypotension and tachycardia, or increased pain. In the longer term, patients need to be monitored for endoleaks at one month, six months, one year and then annually after insertion (Hall, 2003). The National Institute for Health and Clinical Excellence (2003) felt that more evidence about the safety and efficacy of endovascular stents in this patient group was needed. Table 7.4 summarises the complications of these two methods of AAA repair.

Thoracic aneurysm

Thoracic aneurysms are much rarer than abdominal ones but have a similar pathophysiology and treatment. They occur above the level of the diaphragm (see Figure 7.2) in the ascending or descending aorta. Age, chest trauma, penetrating injury or connective tissue disorders (such as

Marfan's syndrome) are the most common causes (Cuschieri et al., 2003). Thoracic aneurysms are often discovered by accident on chest X-ray showing widened mediastinum and confirmed with other tests such as CT scan (see Box 7.2). Pain in the chest, neck and back are the main symptoms and management can be medical or surgical. Surgery requires the thoracic cavity to be opened and chest drain(s) will be inserted (see Chapter 8) but the repair strategies are similar to AAA. The main complications of thoracic aneurysms are highlighted in Box 7.3.

Care is aimed at maintaining haemodynamic stability through monitoring and observation, particularly looking for sudden deterioration in blood pressure and tachycardia. Usually patients will be managed in an intensive care unit immediately post-operatively. Antihypertensive drugs, blood products or inotropic drugs may be required to achieve stability. Pain needs to be treated and epidural analgesia may be used post-operatively. Patients may experience anxiety both pre- and post-operatively as this condition is life threatening; therefore, psychological support for the patient and family is vital. A period in the intensive care unit post-operatively adds to patients' concerns and they will require close cardiovascular monitoring on return to the ward.

Varicose veins

Varicose veins occur when the saphenous veins become elongated and dilated due to incompetent valves. They are present in up to 40% of the population (Crane & Cheshire, 2003). Most surgery is for aesthetic reasons, although venous incompetence can lead to venous ulceration (Simpson, 1998). Treatment is usually by surgically stripping the veins through small incisions in the leg. However, Crane & Cheshire (2003) note that endovenous obliteration (using radio frequency and ultrasound to occlude affected veins) may be an alternative. Post-operative complications are few but haemorrhage and haematoma should be monitored. Post-operatively, patients need to wear supportive bandages and/or stockings depending on the surgeon's preference. When patients return home they should be advised to elevate their legs when sitting and keep legs moving when standing to reduce reoccurrence.

Peripheral vascular disease in limbs

Peripheral vascular disease (PVD) in the limbs, and particularly the legs, can be asymptomatic or can lead to intermittent claudication (pain usually associated with exercise) or pain at rest in the lower limbs, eventually leading to critical limb ischaemia (see amputation, below) (Pedrini, 2003). The Fontaine Classification describes PVD in stages (Pedrini, 2003) (see Table 7.5). Treatment varies with the site of the occlusion and severity of the disease. Commonly affected vessels are the femoral and iliac veins.

Non-surgical management

Percutaneous transluminal angioplasty (PTA)

PTA is used for occlusions under 3 cm in length and is particularly useful in iliac artery disease to improve limb blood flow. The technique involves inserting a balloon and dilating the diseased vessel. Stents are sometimes inserted to hold open the occlusion with good effect in the majority of cases (Pedrini, 2003). This technique can be effective in common iliac artery disease, but surgery is still considered superior for most patients (Sieggreen & Kline, 2004).

Thrombolysis

This is used when the occlusion is thought to be a result of thrombosis, such as deep vein thrombosis. Thrombolytic drugs aim to disintegrate the clot (thrombus) more quickly and so improve blood flow to the affected limb(s). Although not a common cause of occlusion in vascular disorders, it may need to be considered in some circumstances.

Surgical management

Atherectomy

This involves an arteriotomy or percutaneous method of removing atherosclerotic plaque deposits by a device that shaves or pulverises and removes the plaque (Simpson, 1998). This reduces the blockage in the affected vessel(s).

Endarterectomy

This involves opening the artery and removing the plaque deposits to improve blood flow to the affected area.

Patchplasty

This is often preformed in conjunction with endarterectomy as a prosthetic patch is applied to the affected area to expand the occlusion or repair the vessel and promote blood flow to the affected area.

Bypass surgery

There are a number of different bypass surgical techniques employed, depending on where the occlusion occurs. Femoral to tibial (anterior or posterior) artery is the most common procedure.

Table 7.5 Fontaine Classification of PVD.

Stage	Symptom(s)
I	Asymptomatic
II	Claudication
III	Rest pain
IV	Gangrene or ulceration

(based on Pedrini, 2003)
(NB: III and IV are often termed 'critical ischaemia')

Bypass from femoral to dorsalis pedis or common plantor/lateral plantor or popliteal arteries may be required, often in diabetic patients with gangrene or infection (Pedrini, 2003). Aorto-femoral or bi-femoral bypass may be required in severe iliac disease where endarterectomy or angioplasty are inappropriate or have failed. Bypass surgery has been demonstrated to be effective at reducing the need for amputation, particularly in elderly patients (Eskelinin *et al.*, 2003).

Grafts are usually prosthetic above the knee but the saphenous vein may be more suitable below the knee (Pedrini, 2003). However, Berglund *et al.* (2005) suggested that femoro-popliteal bypass above the knee using saphenous vein had better long-term results in preventing reocclusion. Bifurcated tube-grafts ('trouser' graft) can be used where both iliac arteries are involved (see Figure 7.7). All the techniques have potential for post-operative occlusion for thrombosis or graft malfunction; thus pulses and peripheral blood flow should initially be monitored closely.

Arterial insufficiency leading to amputation

Pedrini (2003) noted that about 2% of patients with PVD will require a major amputation (including a limb) and others will require minor amputation (such as a toe). About one-fifth of patients who develop critical limb ischaemia (Fontaine Classification stage III and IV, see Table 7.5) will require amputation (Pedrini, 2003). Men are more prone to critical limb ischaemia than women and the risk of amputation is increased in diabetic patients and those who continue to smoke tobacco.

Sieggreen & Kline (2004) state that arterial insufficiency in limbs is recognised by pale colour, claudication and development of foot and leg ulcers, usually without limb oedema. Ischaemic tissue can become mottled and purple in appearance and will eventually turn black due to cell death. The ankle brachial index (ABI) and pulse will be reduced in the affected limb. Diabetics are prone to ulceration as they often suffer peripheral neuropathy, which means that they lack pain sensation and can injure extremities (such as the foot) inadvertently (Sieggreen & Kline, 2004). The resulting tissue damage cannot heal because of the poor blood supply and may progressively worsen (see Figure 7.8). Surgical intervention such as bypass surgery is the most effective treatment (see above); however, some patients are unsuitable for surgery and Sieggreen & Kline (2004) suggest that these patients can try an intermittent compression device.

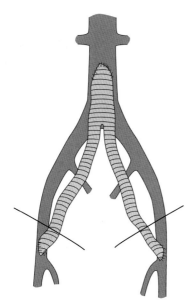

Figure 7.7   Bifurcated tube-graft.
A bifurcated tube-graft has been inserted from the aorta to the femoral arteries, bypassing the diseased lower aorta and iliac arteries.
(Reprinted from *Clinical Surgery*, p. 490, Cuschieri *et al.* (2003) with permission from Blackwell)

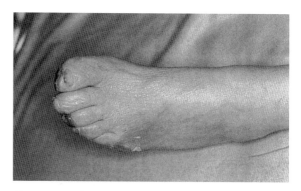

Figure 7.8   Ischaemic foot.
Note patches of dry gangrene over pressure points in foot.
(Reprinted from *Clinical Surgery*, p. 485, Cuschieri *et al.* (2003) with permission from Blackwell)

This simulates walking while patients are sitting to improve blood flow to the popliteal artery. The compression starts at the foot and progresses up the ankle to the calf in a cyclic pattern; benefits should be seen within two weeks but maximum effect may take three months. Bosiers *et al.* (2005) suggest that laser-assisted angioplasty may also be useful in patients with critical limb ischaemia who are a high operative risk. However, this research involved only a small group of patients and further studies are needed.

Amputation is indicated in patients with a severe infection in an arterial ulcer wound, severe pain or tissue loss that is so extensive that regrowth or tissue coverage using other means is not feasible (Sieggreen & Kline, 2004). The patient needs to be assessed for his or her suitability to use a prosthetic limb and likelihood of successful rehabilitation. Sometimes toe amputation is sufficient, although healing is not guaranteed. Below-knee amputation is better for mobility using a prosthetic limb but some patients will require above-knee amputation. Sieggreen & Kline (2004) noted that above-knee amputations seem to heal more easily, although below-knee amputation is more desirable for most patients' functional state. Box 7.4 identifies aspects of post-operative care of patients undergoing lower-limb amputation.

Patients require extensive support to ensure wound healing post-operatively, including good nutrition and cessation of smoking. They also need psychological and social support to adjust to the amputation; especially as many are elderly, may lack motivation and suffer concurrent health problems. Many patients require intensive rehabilitation to use prosthetic limbs effectively. Counselling may be required regarding future expectations as Dillingham *et al.* (2005) found that 26% of patients who had toe or foot amputations needed further, more extensive amputation surgery within 12 months.

Carotid endarterectomy

Carotid artery stenosis is linked to cerebrovascular accidents (CVA or stroke) and transient ischaemic attacks (TIAs). Between 15 and 25% of CVAs are due to narrowing of the carotid artery (Bick & Imray, 2001). Blood flow to the brain is provided mainly by the internal carotid artery, thus occlusion can lead to ischaemia. Table 7.6 summarises the signs and symptoms associated with carotid artery stenosis. Bick & Imray (2001) note that patients who may benefit from carotid endarterectomy are often not referred to a vascular surgeon for treatment. Other causes of CVA include cardiogenic causes (such as atrial fibrillation) and haematological causes (such as hypercoagulation). These must be excluded as part of the assessment process.

The use of selection criteria for carotid endarterectomy is controversial (Cundy, 2002). The American Heart Association suggests that immediate surgical intervention is beneficial for symptomatic patients with ipsilateral (single-sided) stenosis of 70–90% and a recent neurological event that was not disabling (Cundy, 2002). The benefits for symptomatic patients with 30–60% stenosis are uncertain and for symptomatic patients with 0–29% stenosis no benefit is proven (Cundy, 2002). The surgical procedure itself is risky and the known benefits compared to risk of surgery need to be carefully considered. The American Heart Association (2004) recognises that surgical techniques have improved and complication rates are reducing.

The surgical incision is made either vertically and parallel to the anterior border of the sternocleidomastoid muscle or horizontally along a neck

---

Box 7.4   Post-operative considerations for lower-limb amputation.

Stump wound – risk of abrasion and infection. Difficult to secure dressings and asepsis can be difficult to maintain (especially if the patient is incontinent).

Limb contractions – need physiotherapy to maintain stump in the correct position to enable use of prosthetic devices.

Phantom limb pain – feeling that the limb is still there; can cause severe pain in some patients. Need involvement of pain team and psychological support.

Change in body image – this can be devastating for some patients depending on the social and work issues involved (see Chapter 5).

Mobility – the lack of mobility can be demotivating, especially if mobility was difficult before the amputation. This can lead to added problems of pressure sores.

Table 7.6   Signs and symptoms associated with carotid artery stenosis.

Neurological signs	Severity of carotid artery disease
Asymptomatic	Identified on routine physical examination by carotid bruit or vibration on palpation. Bruits may be absent in severe stenosis or can be caused by other factors (such as aortic valve disease)
Transient ischaemic attacks (TIAs)	Symptoms vary but TIAs last from a few seconds up to 24 hours Temporary hemiparesis Temporary blindness (amaurasis fungas)
Cerebrovascular accident (CVA/stroke)	Neurological deficit that never returns to normal – often permanent hemiparesis May fluctuate or progress Deficit becomes stable and lasts more than 24 hours Usually confirm diagnosis by CT or MRI scans

(adapted from Bick & Imray, 2001; Cundy, 2002)

Box 7.5   Complications of carotid endarterectomy.

- Hoarseness due to laryngeal nerve damage
- Difficulty in swallowing due to hypoglossal nerve damage
- Bradycardia/hypotension intra-operatively due to vagal nerve stimulation
- Stroke due to fragments of atherosclerotic plaque dislodging
- Myocardial infarction due to pre-existing PVD
- Haematoma at surgical site may restrict trachea and breathing
- Hyper/hypotension
- Neurological dysfunction such as seizures, intracranial bleeding
- Vomiting post-operatively needs to be avoided as this stresses the suture site

---

crease and oblique to the carotid artery; the second option is more aesthetically pleasing (Cundy, 2002). Careful surgical technique is needed to avoid some of the possible complications (see Box 7.5). Anticoagulation is usually achieved intra-operatively by the use of heparin (Cundy, 2002). An intra-arterial shunt may be used during the procedure to bypass blood to the brain past the surgical site. The atherosclerotic plaque is removed and debris irrigated.

The vessel may have a prosthetic patch applied to widen the vessel and reduce reoccurrence of stenosis (Cundy, 2002), or a vein can be used (Bick & Imray, 2001). Blood flow through the carotid artery is re-established and usually confirmed with ultrasound. Protamine may be used to reverse the anticoagulation and drains may be inserted (Cundy, 2002). Payne *et al.* (2004) have suggested that anti-platelet therapy post-operatively may prevent the complication of stroke but further research is needed. Patients usually spend between 2 and 24 hours in a post-operative high-dependency area to ensure stable neurological and cardiovascular status (Bick & Imray, 2001; Cundy, 2002). Patients can usually be discharged home the following day if no complications develop. Following discharge patients need advice about how to prevent reoccurrence of the disease (see Table 7.7).

Carotid angioplasty and stenting are becoming more commonly used methods to enlarge and maintain carotid artery patency in stenosis. Bettman *et al.* (1998), as detailed by the American Heart Association, believe that the benefits of these methods are not proven although surgeons are becoming more adept at the techniques. Further research is in progress into the benefits over carotid endarterectomy and LaMuraglia *et al.* (2004) felt that carotid endarterectomy was still the treatment of choice at present, even in high-risk surgical patients (Boules *et al.*, 2005).

Conclusion

Patients with PVD can reduce the reoccurrence of disease and its complications by making lifestyle changes and simple medical interventions. Table 7.7 highlights the main recommendations for limiting and preventing the disease process (Wolf

Table 7.7   Reducing the risk of PVD – recommendations of the American Heart Association

Risk factor	Recommendation
Hypertension	<ul><li>Control with lifestyle changes or drug therapy</li><li>Aim systolic BP < 140 mmHg</li><li>Aim diastolic BP < 90 mmHg</li></ul>
Smoking	<ul><li>Promote stopping smoking</li><li>Support with replacement therapies and counselling strategies</li></ul>
Diabetes mellitus	<ul><li>Control blood sugar levels with diet, oral drugs or insulin regime</li></ul>
Lipids	<ul><li>Use low fat diet</li><li>Promote exercise and weight reduction</li><li>Drug therapy</li></ul>
Alcohol	<ul><li>At most two units per day</li></ul>
Exercise	<ul><li>Walking, cycling, jogging, aerobic exercise</li><li>30–60 minutes three to four times per week</li><li>For high-risk patient a structured programme is needed</li></ul>
Weight control/reduction	<ul><li>Aim for body mass index of < 25</li><li>Diet and exercise, structured programme with dietician if clinically obese</li></ul>
Risk of thrombosis	<ul><li>Consider anti-platelet therapy</li></ul>

(Wolf *et al.*, 1999)

et al., 1999). The importance of these strategies needs to be explained to the patient and processes to aid the patient in attaining these goals may be needed.

Self-test questions

1. Explain the development of atherosclerosis and its effects on the vascular system.
2. Why are diabetic and older patients more prone to the development of peripheral vascular disease?
3. What should you assess when considering vascular problems with a patient?
4. What are the differences between fusiform, saccular and dissecting aneurysms?
5. Explain the difference between an arterioplasty and an endarterectomy.
6. Explain the different effects you would expect to see between a patient with carotid artery stenosis and one with femoral artery stenosis.
7. What are the major complications you should be observing for following vascular surgery?
8. What advice would you give to a patient who wanted to reduce their risk for peripheral vascular disease?
9. What advice would you give a diabetic patient to reduce complications of peripheral vascular disease?
10. What psychological issues may need considering with vascular surgery?

References and further reading

American Heart Association (2004) *What is Peripheral Vascular Disease?* Texas: AHA

Berglund J, Bjorck M & Elfstrom J, on behalf on SWED-VASC Femoro-popliteal study group (2005) 'Long-term results of above knee femoro-popliteal bypass depend on indication for surgery and graft material' *European Journal of Vascular Endovascular Surgery* 29: 412–418

Bettman MA, Karzen BT, Whisnant J, Brant-Zawadzki M, Broderick JP, Furlan AJ, Hershey LA, Howard V, Kuntz R, Loftus CM, Pearce W, Roberts A & Roubin G (1998) 'Carotid Stenting and Angioplasty: A statement for healthcare professionals from the councils on cardiovascular radiology, stroke, cardio-thoracic and vascular surgery, epidemiology and prevention and clinical cardiology' American Heart Association. *Circulation 97*: 121–3 (online). http://circ.ahajournals.org/cgi/content/full/97/1/121 (Accessed 03.01.07)

Bick C (2000) 'Abdominal aortic aneurysm repair' *Nursing Standard 15*(3): 47–52, 54–56

Bick C & Imray C (2001) 'Carotid endarterectomy' *Nursing Standard 16*(3): 47–55

Bosiers M, Peeters P, Elst FV, Vermassen F, Maleux G, Fourneau I & Massin H (2005) 'Excimer laser-assisted angioplasty for critical limb ischemia: results of the LACI Belgium Study' *European Journal of Vascular Endovascular Surgery 29*(6): 613–619

Boules TN, Proctor MC, Ahmad BS, Upchurch GR, Stanley JC & Henke PK (2005) 'Carotid endarterectomy remains the standard of care, even in high-risk surgical patients' *Annals of Surgery 24*(2): 356–363

Cuschieri A, Grace PA, Darzi A, Borley N & Rowley DI (2003) *Clinical Surgery.* Oxford: Blackwell Publishing

Crane J & Cheshire N (2003) 'Recent developments in vascular surgery' *British Medical Journal 327*(7420): 911–915

Creager MA, Luscher TF, Cosentino F & Beckman JA (2003) 'Diabetes and vascular disease: pathophysiology, clinical consequences and medical therapy: part 1' *Circulation 108*(12): 1527–1532

Cundy JB (2002) 'Carotid artery stenosis and endarterectomy' *AORN 75*(2): 309–310, 314–324, 326, 328–332

Dawson (2000) 'Principles of Pre-operative Preparation' *in*: Manley K & Bellman L (eds) *Surgical Nursing: Advancing Practice.* London: Churchill Livingstone

Dillingham TR, Pezzin LE & Shore AD (2005) 'Reamputation, mortality and health care costs among persons with dysvascular lower-limb amputations' *Archives of Physical Medicine and Rehabilitation 86*: 480–486

Earnshaw JJ, Sahw E, Whyman MR, Poskin KR & Heather BP (2004) 'Screening for abdominal aortic aneurysms in men' *British Medical Journal 328*(7448): 1122–1124

Eckel RH, Wassef M, Chait A, Sobel B, Barrett E, King G, Sopes-Virella M, Reusch J, Ruderman N, Steiner G & Vlassara H (2002) 'Prevention Conference IV: Diabetes and Cardiovascular Disease. Writing group II: pathogenesis of atherosclerosis in diabetes' *Circulation 105* (online). http://circ.ahajournals.org/cgi/content/full/105/18/e138/ (Accessed 03.01.07)

Eskelinin E, Luther M, Eskelinin A & Lepantalo M (2003) 'Infrapopliteal bypass reduces amputation incidence in elderly patients: A population-based study' *European Journal of Vascular Endovascular Surgery 26*: 65–68

Grundy SM, Hansen B, Smith SC, Cleeman JI & Kahn RA (2004) 'Clinical Management of Metabolic Syndrome:

report of the American Heart Association/National Heart, Lung and Blood Institute/American Diabetes Association Conference on scientific issues related to management' *Circulation 109*: 501–556

Hall SW (2003) 'Endovascular repair of abdominal aortic aneurysms' *AORN 77*(3): 630–643, 645–648

Lakatta EG & Levy D (2003) 'Arterial and cardiac aging: major shareholders in cardiovascular disease enterprises: part 1: Aging arteries: a set up for vascular disease' *Circulation 107*(1): 139–146

LaMuraglia GM, Brewster DC, Moncure AC, Dorer DJ, Stoner MC, Trehan SK, Drummond EC, Abbott WM & Cambria RP (2004) 'Carotid endarterectomy at the millennium: what interventional therapy must match' *Annals of Surgery 240*(3): 535–544

Luscher TF, Creager MA, Cosentino F & Beckman JA (2003) 'Diabetes and vascular disease: pathophysiology, clinical consequences and medical therapy: part II' *Circulation 108*(13): 1655–1661

Malster M & Parry A (2000) 'Day surgery' *in*: Manley K & Bellman L (eds) *Surgical Nursing: Advancing Practice.* London: Churchill Livingstone.

Mohler ER (2003) 'Peripheral arterial disease: identification and implications' *Archives of Internal Medicine 163*(19): 2306–2314

National Confidential Enquiry into Perioperative Deaths (NCEPOD (2001) *The 2001 Report of the National Confidential Enquiry into Perioperative Deaths* (online). www.ncepod.org.uk (Accessed 03.01.07)

National Institute for Health and Clinical Excellence (2003) *IPG010 Stent-graft placement in abdominal aortic aneurysm.* September (online). www.nice.org.uk/page.aspx?o=85719 (Accessed 03.01.07)

National Institute for Health and Clinical Excellence (2005) *IPG127 Endovascular stent-graft placement in thoracic aortic aneurysms and dissections – guidance.* June (online) www.nice.org.uk/guidance/IPG127 (Accessed 03.01.07)

Payne DA, Jones CI, Hayes PD, Thompson MM, London NJ, Bell PR, Goodall AH & Naylor AR (2004) 'Beneficial effects of clopidogrel combined with aspirin in reducing cerebral emboli in patients undergoing carotid endarterectomy' *Circulation 109*(12): 1476–1481

Pedrini L (2003) 'Critical ischaemia of the lower limbs: diagnostic and therapeutic strategies' *Foot and Ankle Surgery 9*: 87–94

Sieggreen MY & Kline RA (2004) 'Arterial insufficiency and ulceration: diagnosis and treatment options' *Nurse Practitioner: the American Journal of Primary Health Care 29*(9): 46–52

Simpson P (1998) 'Vascular surgery' *in*: Simpson PM (ed.) *Introduction to Surgical Nursing.* London: Arnold

Thompson RW (2002) 'Detection and management of small aortic aneurysms' *New England Journal of Medicine* 346(19): 1484–1486

Wolf PA, Clagett GP, Easton JD, Goldstein LB, Govelick PB, Kelly Hayes M, Saccs RL & Whishart JP (1999) 'Preventing ischemic stroke in patients with prior stroke and transischemic attacks: A statement for health professionals from the Stroke Council of the American Heart Association' (online). Available at: http://stroke.ahajournals.org/cgi/content/full/30/9/1991 (Accessed 03.01.07)

8

Upper Gastrointestinal Surgery

Ian Felstead

Introduction

The upper gastrointestinal tract extends from the mouth to the pylorus of the stomach and incorporates the oesophagus, stomach, gallbladder and pancreas. The aims of this chapter are to provide information for nurses working on surgical wards that care for patients who have undergone upper gastrointestinal surgery (Box 8.1). Information will firstly be presented on the common pathophysiological conditions detailing the diagnostic investigations. The major surgical procedures will then be addressed, including the specific pre-operative assessment, monitoring and preparation required, the operative procedure and the specific post-operative management and care. This section will include acute pancreatitis management as this is considered to be a surgical diagnosis.

Chapter 1 has discussed the general principles of pre-operative assessment and preparation of the patient for surgery. Patients who are to undergo upper gastrointestinal surgical procedures also require some specific assessment and preparation, as detailed within this section. Patients undergoing upper gastrointestinal surgery will require the same general post-operative care as those patients undergoing other major surgical procedures. The overall principles of post-operative management have been discussed in Chapter 3 and these should be considered alongside the information presented within this section.

Oesophageal disorders

Applied pathophysiology

Achalasia

This is a relatively rare condition whereby the passage of food slows down in the oesophagus due to dilatation and muscular hypertrophy above the lower sphincter (Henry & Thompson, 2005). Long-standing disease can lead to the development of a malignancy, probably due to the inflammation of

---

Box 8.1 Aims of the chapter.

- To introduce the reader to the most common pathophysiological conditions in the upper gastrointestinal tract
- To discuss the common investigations and diagnostic tests performed on patients with the common conditions
- To discuss the major surgical procedures undertaken on the upper gastrointestinal tract with regards to specific pre-operative assessment, monitoring and preparation; the surgical procedure and post-operative care and management

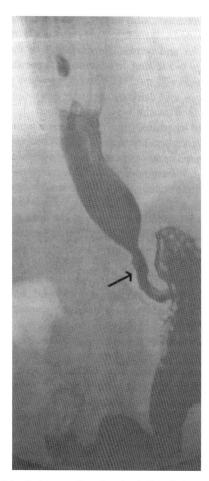

Figure 8.1   Barium swallow showing early achalasia.
(Reprinted from *Clinical Surgery*, p. 292, Cuschieri *et al.*
(2003) with permission from Blackwell)

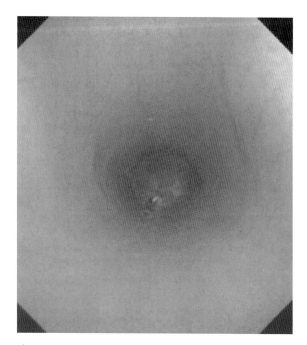

Figure 8.2   Normal oesophagus.
(from Gastrolab.net – reproduced with permission)

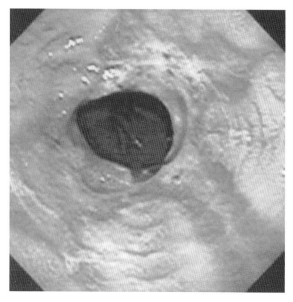

Figure 8.3   Reflux oesophagitis.
(from Gastrolab.net – reproduced with permission)

the oesophageal mucosa from food stasis. Dysphagia develops over time and initially the patient will only have an increased food transit time. Eventually patients will develop dysphagia and present with symptoms of regurgitation, weight loss and pain behind the sternum. Figure 8.1 is a barium swallow X-ray showing early achalasia.

Oesophageal strictures

Benign oesophageal strictures most commonly occur in the distal oesophagus as a result of gastro-oesophageal reflux disease (GORD) or oesophagitis. Chronic GORD results in inflammation and formation of scar tissue, which in advanced cases can involve the full thickness of the oesophageal wall (compare normal appearance in Figure 8.2 with reflux oesophagitis in Figure 8.3). This can result in oesophageal shortening, although most oesophageal strictures are less than 1 cm in length.

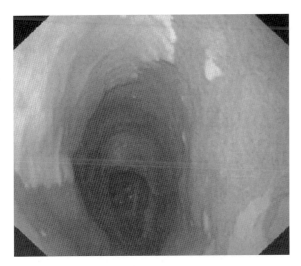

Figure 8.4   Barrett's oesophagus.
(from Gastrolab.net – reproduced with permission)

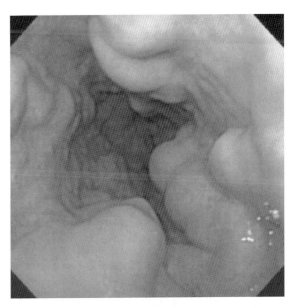

Figure 8.5   Oesophageal varices.
(from Gastrolab.net – reproduced with permission)

In those patients who develop a stricture, the lower oesophageal sphincter pressure, oesophageal motility and gastric emptying are more severely impaired than in those patients with GORD who have not developed this complication. Patients with an oesophageal stricture usually present with dysphagia that is often confined to solids. In advanced cases dysphagia to liquids may occur. Symptoms usually develop slowly and the degree of weight loss seen in patients with malignant strictures is not often seen.

Chronic oesophagitis may be treated with intraluminal oesophageal dilatation followed by treatment of the underlying cause of the reflux (Walsh, 2002). Failure to treat could lead to the development of Barrett's oesophagus, a condition in which the normal squamous epithelium lining the oesophagus is replaced by columnar epithelium (see Figure 8.4). This is usually asymptomatic (Walsh, 2002) but predisposes the patient to a 50-fold increase in the incidence of adenocarcinoma (Lattimer *et al.*, 2002).

Oesophageal varices

This is a serious condition associated with cirrhosis of the liver (see Figure 8.5). Any disorder, such as cirrhosis of the liver, that obstructs the flow of blood through the portal venous system results in portal hypertension. Portal hypertension is abnormally high blood pressure in the portal venous system (McCance & Huether, 2002). This is the part of the vascular system that carries blood to the liver from the gastrointestinal tract, pancreas and spleen. High pressure in the portal veins causes collateral vessels to open between the portal veins and the systemic veins, in which the blood pressure is considerably lower (McCance & Huether, 2002). If this pressure is maintained for long, the collateral veins dilate and develop into varices, most commonly in the oesophagus and stomach as they are very close to the surface here. Eventually one may rupture, causing massive blood loss through haematemesis, melaena or both (Walsh, 2002). Treatment options include intravariceal sclerotherapy (injection of an irritant solution into the varices causing thrombophlebitis and eventual development of scar tissue), banding via endoscopy or the use of a compression balloon (balloon tamponade – see Figure 8.6). Drug therapy includes the administration of vasopressin or, more commonly, glypressin. Glypressin is similar to antidiuretic hormone (ADH) and is a potent vasoconstrictor thus reducing portal vein pressure by limiting blood flow to the area.

Oesophageal cancer

Most oesophageal tumours are squamous cell in origin and the majority occur in the mid to lower

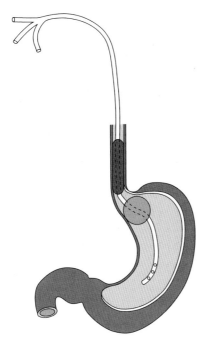

Figure 8.6   Balloon tamponade.
(Reprinted from *Clinical Surgery*, Cuschieri *et al.* (2003),
p. 336, with permission from Blackwell)

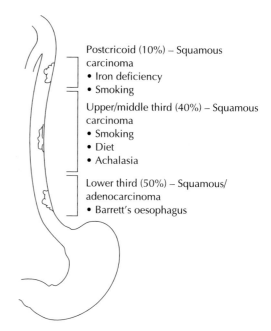

Postcricoid (10%) – Squamous
carcinoma
• Iron deficiency
• Smoking

Upper/middle third (40%) – Squamous
carcinoma
• Smoking
• Diet
• Achalasia

Lower third (50%) – Squamous/
adenocarcinoma
• Barrett's oesophagus

Figure 8.7   Oesophageal carcinoma distribution.
(Reprinted from *Surgery at a Glance*, p. 86, Grace & Borley
(2002) with permission from Blackwell)

region of the oesophagus. The small numbers of adenocarcinomas that occur are located in the lower third of the oesophagus and at the gastro-oesophageal junction (see Figure 8.7). Adeno-carcinomas are usually secondary to infiltration by a gastric carcinoma or to the presence of Barrett's oesophagus (McCance & Huether, 2002). Almost all lesions are a combination of narrowing and ulceration (Henry & Thompson, 2005) although the extent of each varies. Tumours develop due to alterations in the structure and function of the oesophagus, ulceration due to gastric reflux and long-term exposure to irritants such as smoking and alcohol. These, in combination with nutritional deprivation, result in an altered mucosal lining that is susceptible to cancerous changes (McCance & Huether, 2002).

Investigations and diagnosis

All patients complaining of dysphagia should have a plain chest X-ray and barium swallow. An endoscopy is undertaken to detect any oesophageal disorders – particularly in elderly patients where the risk of invasive malignancy is greater (Henry & Thompson, 2005). If it is suspected that the patient has a malignant tumour, this can be confirmed by an oesophagoscopy where histological biopsies may be taken. An endoscopic transluminal ultrasound is sometimes performed to identify if there is any local invasion of the tumour into the surrounding tissues. The depth of penetration of the tumour is a vital prognostic indicator. If it is suspected that the bronchus may be involved, a bronchoscopy can be performed and a computer-aided tomography (CT) scan is often carried out to highlight any distant metastases. Box 8.2 summarises the investigative and diagnostic procedures for this condition.

Staging laparoscopy

The patient may undergo a laparoscopy to assess whether there is any liver or peritoneal involvement. A laparoscopy is an examination of the abdominal structures by means of a laparoscope. Following an injection of carbon dioxide into

---

Box 8.2   Oesophageal investigative and diagnostic procedures.

Chest X-ray
- A chest X-ray will indicate any lung disease or metastases from a primary oesophageal carcinoma for example

Barium swallow
- This procedure is simple, relatively inexpensive, provides an accurate determination of the site of any strictures. However, it does not indicate if the stricture is malignant and is often not carried out in favour of an endoscopy

Computed tomography
- Usually performed on the abdomen and thorax to identify any metastases or tumour invasion

Oesophagoscopy
- An endoscopic examination of the oesophagus performed using a flexible tube (an endoscope)
- The patient should not be given food for 6–8 hours pre-procedure to allow the stomach to empty

- Any loose-fitting teeth/dentures must be removed pre-procedure
- The patient will usually receive intravenous sedation and local anaesthetic will be sprayed to the back of the throat
- The endoscope will be carefully passed through the mouth and into the oesophagus where small tissue samples may be taken from any abnormal areas (biopsy)
- The procedure usually takes between 10 and 20 minutes
- There is a small risk of perforation following the procedure, so careful monitoring of the patient's blood pressure, pulse and temperature is vital

Endoscopic transluminal ultrasound
- An endoscopy is performed with a specially designed ultrasound probe to allow for an internal ultrasound scan of the oesophagus
- This allows accurate staging of any local tumour spread as any invasion will be noted

---

the abdomen to inflate the abdominal cavity, the laparoscope is passed through a small incision in the abdominal wall. This enables the surgeon to see if there are any peritoneal seedling metastases on the anterior abdominal wall. This procedure is useful for spotting small nodules of disseminated disease not evident on ultrasound, CT and magnetic resonance image (MRI) scanning. Staging laparoscopy is performed before surgery so that the surgical risks can be weighed against the benefits.

Pre-operative assessment, monitoring and preparation for oesophagectomy

Dysphagia/swallow assessment

Dysphagia, or difficulty in swallowing, is one of the primary symptoms in a patient with oesophageal cancer. It is important to determine how long the patient has had difficulty swallowing and whether it affects all foods or if the patient is able to tolerate fluids. Other information can also be obtained regarding how long it takes for food to be swallowed and whereabouts the patient feels it sticks. The dysphagia/swallow assessment should be completed along with a nutritional assessment

to ascertain information regarding any nutritional deficit.

Nutritional status

It is likely that the patient will have a reduced nutritional status on admission and, if they can take them, high-calorie drinks form part of the pre-operative management. Often patients will require full nutritional management pre-operatively and occasionally a fine-bore feeding tube is inserted to provide a high-protein liquid feed. Patients should be fasted for 4–6 hours to ensure an empty oesophagus and stomach during the surgery, and intravenous fluids are given to reduce the risk of dehydration. The patient is likely to have a reduced transit time within the oesophagus, making appropriate pre-operative fasting even more important. All patients scheduled for surgery require an adequate level of hydration and nutrition as these contribute to effective post-operative recovery.

Tumour staging

Oesophageal cancers are staged using the tumour–nodes–metastases (TNM) system (see Table 8.1). Full staging of the tumour should take place

Table 8.1   TNM staging system for oesophageal cancer.

Primary tumour (T)

TX	Primary tumour cannot be assessed
T0	No evidence of primary tumour
Tis	Tumour in situ
T1	Tumour invades lamina propria or submucosa
T2	Tumour invades muscularis propria
T3	Tumour invades adventitia
T4	Tumour invades adjacent structures

Regional lymph nodes (N)

NX	Regional lymph nodes cannot be assessed
N0	No regional lymph node metastasis
N1	Regional lymph node metastasis

Distant metastasis (M)

M0	No distant metastasis
M1	Distant metastasis
	Tumours lower oesophagus
	M1a Coeliac nodal metastases
	M1b Other distant metastases

Stage grouping

Stage	T	N	M
I	1	0	0
IIA	2	0	0
	3	0	0
IIB	1	1	0
	2	1	0
III	3	1	0
	4	Any	0
IV	Any	Any	1

Box 8.3   Contraindications to oesophagectomy.

- Aged 75+ years
- Myocardial infarction within the last six months
- Diagnosis of chronic heart failure or cirrhosis of the liver

following pathological diagnosis using the TNM system. This usually includes a barium swallow, endoscopy, CT scan, bronchoscopy, endoscopic ultrasound and staging laparoscopy. Patients scheduled for surgery should have satisfactory cardiopulmonary function and mobility, as these are a prerequisite to successful recovery from oesophageal resection. An electrocardiogram is performed to check for any ischaemic changes; an echocardiogram checks left ventricular function. Spirometry and arterial blood gas analysis are also performed.

In the majority of centres, curative resection is thought to be contraindicated in patients aged 75 years and over, and those who have had prior myocardial infarction (within the previous six months) and a diagnosis of chronic heart failure or cirrhosis of the liver (Box 8.3). In these patients the

risks of surgery outweigh the potential benefits and resection may not be offered. The bowel may be prepared pre-operatively as occasionally the blood supply to the stomach is lost during surgery and the stomach can quickly become necrotic. In this case part of the colon will need to be used to anastomose the bowel to the remaining oesophagus as the stomach must be resected. With regards to pre-operative respiratory function, the patient should be advised to stop smoking in the weeks prior to surgery to encourage a complication-free recovery.

Partial and total oesophagectomy

As with most solid tumours, surgery offers the best option for cure, and all patients without evidence of distant metastases who are clinically fit should be considered. The surgical approach may be through the thorax and abdomen, through the thorax alone, or through the abdomen and an incision in the neck. Knowledge of surgical approaches is vital for safe management post-operatively. Patients will have wounds in various sites and drainage systems requiring different nursing care.

The Ivor Lewis approach (left oesophago-gastrectomy)

This approach is performed for tumours of the lower oesophagus and stomach. A thoraco-laparotomy approach allows the surgeon access to the oesophagus and the upper abdomen. Once the stomach has been mobilised and the diaphragmatic hiatus has been enlarged via laparotomy, the abdomen is closed and the patient is placed onto their left side for a right thoracotomy incision. This allows mobilisation of the oesophagus. The stomach is then brought through the diaphragmatic hiatus and the tumour is resected along with partial or total removal of the stomach if there is localised tumour invasion. The remaining portion of the oesophagus is anastomosed with the stomach, usually in the chest.

If the patient has had previous gastric surgery or the tumour is so extensive that a total oesophagectomy is required, a section of bowel may be used to reconstruct the oesophagus. This is termed a colonic graft or interposition.

The transthoracic approach

This approach involves only a thoracotomy. For oesophageal tumours of the lower third of the oesophagus, a thoracotomy is performed on the left side between the seventh and eighth ribs. For tumours located in the middle third of the oesophagus the thoracotomy is on the right side at the level of the sixth rib.

The transhiatal approach

In this procedure the thorax is not directly entered. This is a one-stage procedure carried out entirely through a laparotomy and an incision in the left side of the neck. The oesophageal tumour is mobilised blind and the anastomosis is formed in the neck.

Other procedures

Occasionally a laryngo-pharyngo-oesophagectomy is required for patients with extensive tumour spread. This surgical procedure involves removal of the larynx, pharynx and oesophagus. The stomach is raised to join the remaining oesophagus and the surgeon will also perform a tracheostomy.

Post-operative management and care

All patients should initially recover in the intensive care unit prior to returning to the surgical ward. Oesophagectomy is a long operation lasting between 6 and 8 hours and for a proportion of that time (2–2$\frac{1}{2}$ hours) the patient will be ventilated on a single lung due to right lung decompression during the thoracic stage of the surgery. This will give rise to an increased risk of intra-operative hypoxia and post-operative atelectasis in the left lung. The patient will therefore need ventilation for a short time post-operatively. This also reduces the risk of aspiration. The patient should be nursed at an angle of greater than 45 degrees to reduce the incidence of aspiration pneumonia. The fact that the stomach has been lifted into the thoracic cavity increases the likelihood of gastric contents 'leaking' into the lungs. In general the patient will require humidified oxygen therapy and epidural analgesia to allow for adequate mobilisation.

Post-operative nutritional management

The patient will be nil-by-mouth post-operatively until the anastomosis has healed. Intravenous fluids and total parenteral nutrition are provided to maintain an adequate fluid balance and the necessary nutrients to allow healing to occur. Provision of approximately 2.5 litres of fluid and avoidance of weight loss are two of the mainstays of post-operative management following an oesophagectomy. A nasogastric tube will be inserted to prevent any abdominal distension and alleviate any nausea and vomiting that the patient may experience.

Care of thoracic drainage

The patient will have had a thoracotomy. This is the surgical opening of the chest cavity and is usually performed to inspect or operate on the heart or lungs. When combined with a general anaesthetic and analgesia the patient is exposed to the possibility of developing atelectasis, pulmonary infection and sputum retention. The patient will have two thoracic drains in situ post-operatively – one basal to drain fluid and one apical to drain air (see Figure 8.8). The drainage must be recorded daily, as removal of the drains will depend on the amount of drainage. The apical drain will usually be removed after 48 hours if the patient does not have a pneumothorax. The basal drain will be removed when the daily total drainage is less than 100 mL. Box 8.4 summarises the principles of care of thoracic drainage in post-oesophagectomy patients.

Swallow assessment

A swallow assessment will need to be performed post-operatively to establish whether the anastomosis has healed. This is performed prior to the patient being recommenced on any oral fluids,

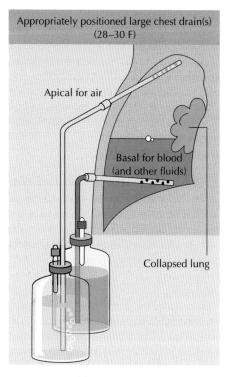

Appropriately positioned large chest drain(s) (28–30 F)

Apical for air

Basal for blood (and other fluids)

Collapsed lung

Figure 8.8   Position of thoracic drains following thoracotomy.

usually around the sixth or seventh post-operative day. This will be a contrast barium swallow.

Post-operative complications

Oesophageal leak

The most urgent post-operative complication is an intrathoracic anastomosis breakdown leading to an oesophageal leak and mediastinitis, inflammation of the midline partition of the thoracic cavity. This breakdown could be due to a tear or secondary to an infection and carries a 50% mortality rate. Often mediastinitis leads to fibrosis, which may cause compression of neighbouring structures within the chest, particularly the bronchial tree and superior vena cava. This is obviously detrimental to respiratory and cardiac function. This complication most commonly occurs in an Ivor Lewis oesophagectomy due to the anastomosis being created so far away from the blood supply. Treatment includes keeping the patient nil-by-mouth, administering intravenous antibiotics and intercostal drainage. The patient will require surgical exploration and repair. Box 8.5 lists the signs of an oesophageal leak.

Box 8.4   Care of thoracic drainage in post-oesophagectomy patients.

- Explanation and reassurance are vital whilst the drain is in situ
- Routine vital sign monitoring (BP, HR, RR, O_2 saturations) before and after insertion of the thoracic drain is necessary for comparison as well as monitoring whilst in situ
- The British Thoracic Society stipulate that the patient must have analgesia whilst the drain remains in situ – not just on insertion (BTS, 2003)
- Patients should remain sitting up and mobilise to increase the use of the lungs whilst the drain is in situ
- The patient should be encouraged to perform deep breathing and coughing exercises
- Regular physiotherapy should be provided
- Drains should **never** be clamped (unless changing bottles or following accidental disconnection), as this may result in a tension pneumothorax
- Observe for 'bubbling' in the apical drain – should only be seen when the patient exhales or coughs and demonstrates the evacuation of air from the pleural space

- Observe for 'swinging' in the basal drain – any swinging movement reflects pressure changes in the pleural cavity with respiration – this movement should lessen as the lung expands
- Accurate recording of thoracic drainage is vital for diagnosis
- Observe for signs of tension pneumothorax or surgical emphysema
- Ensure there are no kinks or loops within the tubing – this may impede drainage
- Consider removing drains when drainage and fluid fluctuations have stopped, breath sounds return to normal and chest X-ray shows no air or fluid in the pleural space
- Patients must be advised to increase intrathoracic pressure on removal by inhaling and then attempting to exhale without letting any air escape – this will prevent air entering the pleural cavity as the drainage tube is removed and the wound covered with 'sleek' tape or the purse-string suture tightened

Box 8.5   Signs of an oesophageal leak.

- Pyrexia
- Tachycardia
- Surgical emphysema
- Shock
- Increased chest drainage
- Chest pain
- Widening mediastinum on a contrast chest X-ray
- Evidence of leak on barium swallow

Gastric disorders

Applied pathophysiology

Peptic ulcers

A peptic ulcer is an erosion in the wall of the gastrointestinal tract that has been exposed to gastric secretions (Walsh, 2002). The erosion is caused by the digestive action of hydrochloric acid and pepsin and although peptic ulcers can occur anywhere in the gastrointestinal tract, the most common sites are the stomach and the duodenum. The majority of peptic ulcers are caused by the presence of the *Helicobacter pylori* (*H. pylori*) bacterium within the stomach. *H. pylori* is able to penetrate the mucosal layer of the stomach and some strains produce cytotoxins that attack and weaken the membranes (Ellis *et al.*, 2002). This, along with inflammation, results in an impaired gastric mucosal barrier and damage by gastric acid. Peptic ulceration can result in a primary malignancy, perforation or haemorrhage

Gastric cancer

Gastric carcinomas are common and are the fifth biggest cancer killer in the UK, secondary only to lung, colorectal, breast and prostate tumours (Ellis *et al.*, 2002). The risk factors include predisposing conditions, such as chronic peptic ulceration or pernicious anaemia; environmental factors, such as *H. pylori* infection; and genetic factors, such as blood group A. According to McCance & Huether (2002), gastric cancer begins in the glands of the stomach mucosa and therefore all carcinomas are adenocarcinomas. Atrophic gastritis has been closely linked to the development of gastric cancer as insufficient acid secretion creates an alkaline environment, which allows bacteria to multiply (McCance & Huether, 2002). These bacteria act on nitrates to form nitrosamines which damage deoxyribonucleic acid (DNA) promoting neoplasia.

Investigations and diagnosis

An oesophago-gastroscopy is the most sensitive way of determining whether a gastric tumour is present or not. It is possible to take biopsies during this endoscopic procedure and the location of the tumour can also be pinpointed. Double-contrast barium meals may also be used. In order to highlight any distant metastases the patient will require a CT scan. The use of endoscopic ultrasound is increasing and provides the surgeon with information regarding the invasiveness of the tumour. Almost 50% of patients with gastric carcinoma are anaemic and therefore, if there is no other apparent cause for the anaemia, a haemoglobin test should be performed to indicate the need for further investigation. A staging laparoscopy is sometimes used to determine the resectability of the tumour.

Pre-operative assessment, monitoring and preparation for gastrectomy

Nutritional status

Patients with a gastric carcinoma are at risk of malnutrition and many will be anorexic at the time of diagnosis. Many patients will receive pre-operative total parenteral nutrition if it is confirmed that they are at risk of malnutrition. It has been found that the primary advantage of this is the reduction in postoperative infections (Henry & Thompson, 2005).

Tumour staging

Gastric cancers are staged using the tumour–nodes–metastases (TNM) system (see Table 8.2).

Surgical procedures – partial and total gastrectomy

Only approximately 30–40% of patients are suitable for curative resection of their gastric tumour,

Table 8.2 TNM staging system for gastric cancer.

Primary tumour (T)

TX	Primary tumour cannot be assessed
T0	No evidence of primary tumour
Tis	Tumour in situ
T1	Tumour invades lamina propria or submucosa
T2a	Tumour invades beyond lamina propria
T2b	Tumour invades subserosa
T3	Tumour invades serosa (no surrounding organ involvement)
T4	Tumour invades adjacent structures and blood vessels

Regional lymph nodes (N)

NX	Regional lymph nodes cannot be assessed
N0	No regional lymph node metastasis
N1	1–6 lymphatic nodes affected
N2	7–15 lymphatic nodes affected
N3	More than 15 lymphatic nodes affected

Distant metastasis (M)

M0	No distant metastasis
M1	Distant metastasis

Stage grouping

Stage	T	N	M
0	Tis	N0	M0
IA	1	0	0
IB	1	1	0
	2a/b	0	0
II	1	2	0
	2a/b	1	0
	3	0	0
IIB	1	1	0
	2	1	0
IIIA	2a/b	2	0
	3	1	0
	4	0	0
IIIB	3	2	0
IV	4	1–3	0
	Any	3	0
	Any	Any	1

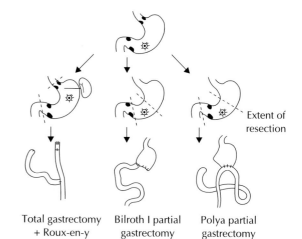

Total gastrectomy + Roux-en-y oesophago-jejunostomy | Bilroth I partial gastrectomy | Polya partial gastrectomy | Extent of resection

Figure 8.9 Types of gastric resection.

mortality and morbidity associated with radical resections (Henry & Thompson, 2005). A gastro-enterostomy is performed following a partial gas-trectomy and here the remaining stomach is joined to the duodenum or small intestine. The most common is a gastroduodenostomy. Figure 8.9 shows the different types of gastric resection.

Post-operative management and care

Post-operative nutritional management

The patient is likely to return from theatre with a nasogastric tube in situ to allow for drainage of the stomach during the anastomotic healing process. This drainage should be accurately monitored and regular aspiration should be undertaken. Peristalsis will have ceased, and to avoid abdominal disten-sion, all oral food and fluids will be withheld. The patient will have intravenous fluids to correct any dehydration caused by the surgery and nasogastric drainage. Some surgeons may allow small amounts of water post-operatively; some will wait until the return of bowel sounds. When the signs of peri-stalsis are evident, the patient will be allowed to gradually increase their oral intake of fluids and eventually receive a soft diet after approximately seven days. Continuous observation takes place for signs of abdominal distension, regurgitation and vomiting, as these will indicate paralytic ileus, or

although around 70% of tumours are considered resectable (Henry & Thompson, 2005). This is due to the fact that gastric cancer develops and meta-stasises rapidly, often spreading to adjacent struc-tures such as the oesophagus or duodenum (Walsh, 2002). The choice of whether to remove all or part of the stomach mostly depends on tumour size and location. However, there appear to be international variations in practice. In Japan, total gastrectomies are performed most frequently, but in the west partial gastrectomies are preferred due to the high

further loss of peristaltic action. Once food is re-introduced, the patient should be advised to have small, bland meals and drinks.

Post-operative complications

Anaemia

Following a gastric resection, the absorption of vitamins will be affected and the patient will need vitamin B_{12} supplements. The absorption of vitamin B_{12} is dependent on the production of intrinsic factor in the stomach and following gastric resection, the patient has an increased risk of developing pernicious anaemia. There is also an increased risk of developing iron deficiency anaemia as normal absorption of iron is facilitated by gastric hydrochloric acid (Walsh, 2002), the volume of which is reduced post-gastrectomy.

Dumping syndrome

Dumping syndrome is a post-operative complication of gastric surgery that occurs after eating (Alexander et al., 2000). Patients may complain of a consistent feeling of fullness and discomfort, sweating, an increase in peristalsis and sometimes diarrhoea. The symptoms are caused by the sudden emptying of fluid into the small bowel resulting in rapid distension of the jejunal loop anastomosed to the stomach. This, in conjunction with a large volume of water leaving the vascular system within the jejunum to dilute the high concentration of electrolytes and sugars, leads to the patient also complaining of a feeling of faintness. Patients must be advised to eat small, frequent meals, reduce carbohydrate intake and avoid drinking fluids during a meal.

Gallbladder disorders

Applied pathophysiology

Gallstones

Gallstones are round or oval-shaped solids found within the biliary tract. They contain cholesterol, calcium carbonate, calcium bilirubinate or a mixture of these elements. Bile is a complex solution of cholesterol, bile pigments, bile salts, calcium and water. Under certain situations, the lining of the gallbladder becomes diseased and the solution becomes unstable leading to crystal formation. Eventually the crystals will form stones. Ninety per cent of gallstones are likely to be asymptomatic, however, occasionally they pass through the biliary system and may cause biliary colic or pancreatitis. Cholelithiasis is the term used when gallstones are formed within the gallbladder.

Cholecystitis

Cholecystitis is inflammation of the gallbladder and is usually caused by the presence of gallstones. This is an acute condition in which the gallbladder becomes inflamed and swollen because flow of bile into the duodenum is blocked by gallstones. This results in biliary colic – intense pain in the upper right abdomen or between the shoulders. The patient will usually complain of severe pain and indigestion, especially after fatty food. Nausea, with or without vomiting, may ensue and if left untreated, the condition can lead to jaundice and occasionally, if the gallbladder ruptures, to peritonitis.

Investigations and diagnosis

Various substances present in bile, including calcium and cholesterol, may contain solid particles, which cause few symptoms while they remain in the gallbladder; in fact, many gallstones are discovered during routine scans or X-rays. An abdominal ultrasound is the main investigative procedure for patients suspected of gallbladder disorders. The scan will reveal any gallstones, thickening of the gallbladder wall or dilatation in the ducts. The scan is non-invasive, quick and relatively inexpensive, causing minimum discomfort to the patient.

If a patient is suspected of having biliary disease they may undergo an endoscopic retrograde cholangio-pancreatogram (ERCP) or percutaneous transhepatic cholangiography (PTC). ERCP will be discussed later. A PTC is a method of outlining the bile ducts and pancreatic ducts with radio-opaque dyes. A needle is inserted into the liver until it reaches a dilated duct where contrast medium is injected.

Pre-operative assessment, monitoring and preparation for cholecystectomy

Dietary factors

The gallbladder stores and concentrates bile, which is produced by the liver and helps to digest dietary fat. There is no particular evidence to demonstrate that any particular dietary substance influences the development of gallstones. However, many patients complain of increased severity of pain following a 'fatty' meal. To assist the digestion of fats, the gallbladder contracts to release bile and this contraction may cause the abdominal discomfort felt by patients with gallstones or gallbladder disease.

Endoscopic retrograde cholangio-pancreatography (ERCP)

Sometimes the surgeon will request an ERCP prior to surgery (see Box 8.6). This provides detailed X-rays of the bile duct and/or pancreas enabling diagnosis and treatment of gallstones, inflammatory strictures, leaks and cancer. If the examination shows gallstones in the bile duct, the ampulla of Vater can be cut using diathermy. This is known

---

Box 8.6   Endoscopic retrograde cholangio-pancreatography (ERCP).

- To allow for a clear view the patient must be nil-by-mouth for at least 6 hours pre-ERCP
- The ERCP can take anything from 30 minutes to 2 hours
- Standard pre-operative monitoring and preparation including removal of dentures and contact lenses, jewellery and other metal objects (see Chapter 2)
- The patient lies on their left-hand side at the start of the procedure
- Following administration of an intravenous sedative and anaesthetic spray to numb the patient's throat, an endoscope is passed through the mouth, oesophagus, stomach and duodenum until it reaches the junction where the biliary tree and pancreas empty into the duodenum
- The patient is then turned into a prone position
- Radio-opaque dye is injected down the endoscope and a series of X-rays are taken following which the endoscope is removed

---

as a sphincterotomy and for this the patient's pre-operative International Normalised Ratio (INR) should be below 1.0, due to the high risk of haemorrhage. The INR is a standard measurement of prothrombin ratio that is usually recorded to monitor the effect of warfarin. The higher the INR, the less likely the blood is to clot and thus the patient is at higher risk of haemorrhage. The stones can then either be extracted via a wire basket passed through the endoscope or left to drain into the duodenum. Possible complications of an ERCP include pancreatitis, infection, bleeding and perforation of the duodenum.

Surgical procedures – laparoscopic and open cholecystectomy

An attack of acute pancreatitis, cholangitis or obstructive jaundice is usually an indication for prophylactic cholecystectomy. Cholecystectomy is commonly performed as a laparoscopic procedure and carries a very low mortality rate. There are several advantages to the patient: a reduced stay in hospital, early mobilisation and therefore reduced risk of post-operative complications and a speedy return to normal life. The patient is anaesthetised and the surgeon passes a laparoscope into the abdomen at the level of the umbilicus. The abdomen is then insufflated with carbon dioxide to allow the gallbladder to be clearly visualised. Following three more incisions in the abdomen, an intra-operative cholangiogram is performed to highlight any gallstones which, if present, can be removed. The gallbladder is then resected and extracted through the incision near the umbilicus. All wounds are closed with subcutaneous sutures.

If it is thought too dangerous to perform laparoscopic surgery, the surgeon may opt for a traditional open cholecystectomy. This is the removal of the gallbladder and occasionally a small portion of the liver and all the lymph nodes surrounding the gallbladder will also be removed – termed an extended cholecystectomy (Cancer Help UK, 2002). This would also be performed for a patient with a diagnosis of cancer of the gallbladder. A difficult laparoscopic cholecystectomy can be converted to open cholecystectomy – often consent will be obtained for both procedures, just in case. An open cholecystectomy involves a cut of about six inches long to the right upper abdomen just below the ribcage. The gallbladder is then resected from its bed and removed prior to the wound being sutured or stapled. This surgery is more extensive than the laparoscopic option and therefore patients will be more acutely ill. Often they need to stay in hospital for a longer time and will not be able to resume work for at least six weeks. After the operation in both types of surgery, the patients will notice that the symptoms have disappeared and that they do not need to avoid fatty foods.

Post-operative management and care

Care of T-tube

A T-tube is a T-shaped tube inserted into the common bile duct. When the patient has a cholecystectomy, the duct becomes inflamed and oedematous. This has the potential to obstruct the flow of bile into the duodenum. The purpose of the T-tube is to keep the duct open to allow drainage of the bile. It is important that a record is kept of the amount of bile drained through the tube, as this will indicate the patency of the duct. It is possible to dislodge the T-tube accidentally due to the weight that can

be placed on it, therefore the drainage bag must be regularly emptied and the contents measured. Should bile leak around the tube, there is a local risk to the integrity of the skin and staff should maintain regular checks and cleansing if required.

Before removal of the T-tube, a cholangiogram will be performed to check the patency of the bile duct and the flow of the bile into the duodenum. This is usually carried out approximately 8–10 days post-operatively. If the duct is patent then the tube will be removed, however, if there are any stones left then the tube will remain in situ until either the stones pass spontaneously into the duodenum or they are physically removed.

Acute pancreatitis

Applied pathophysiology

Acute pancreatitis is an inflammatory disorder of the pancreas (Figure 8.10) that results in self-destruction of the pancreas through auto-digestion. This is a very serious condition, which can be life threatening. There are two types of acute pancreatitis: interstitial, which involves inflammation and oedema of the interstitium; and haemorrhagic,

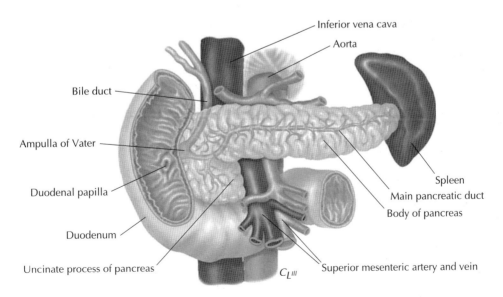

Figure 8.10 The pancreas.
(Reprinted from *Clinical Surgery*, p. 350, Henry & Thompson (2005), with permission from Elsevier)

> **Box 8.7** Physiological consequences of pancreatic auto-digestion.
>
> Pancreatic auto-digestion will result in carrying degrees of:
>
> - Oedema
> - Haemorrhage
> - Necrosis
> - Abscess or cyst formation
>
> in and around the pancreas.

which entails severe inflammation, haemorrhage and necrosis of the pancreatic tissue. Following an attack, the pancreas returns to normal. If there are residual structural changes, the patient would be classified as having chronic pancreatitis. There are numerous causes of acute pancreatitis but the most common are the presence of gallstones and the excessive consumption of alcohol.

Within the pancreas the acinar cells produce digestive enzymes. These enzymes are in an inactive state. One of these enzymes, trypsinogen, is secreted from the pancreas, is activated by intestinal juices and converted to trypsin which acts as a catalyst for activating other enzymes. This activation of enzymes usually occurs in the duodenum where the digestion of food continues. It is thought that alcohol or obstruction by a gallstone causes spasm in the sphincter of Oddi. This sphincter normally controls the release of bile and pancreatic juice into the duodenum but the spasm causes reflux. Intestinal juice is carried into the pancreatic duct and digestive enzymes are prematurely activated causing auto-digestion (see Box 8.7).

Digestive enzymes, in their activated state, also increase capillary permeability, resulting in large volumes of fluid escaping from the vascular system into the peritoneal and retroperitoneal cavities. The patient develops hypovolaemic shock and could eventually develop acute renal failure due to the severe loss of circulating blood volume.

Investigations and diagnosis

Accurate diagnosis should be made within 48 hours of admission. Clinical examination of a patient with suspected pancreatitis will reveal a history of upper abdominal pain and vomiting, with diffuse epigastric tenderness. These symptoms could be attributed to a number of acute abdominal conditions and clinical examination alone is often not used as a reliable source of data for diagnosis. Biochemical analysis is used to aid in the diagnosis of pancreatitis. Diagnosis of acute pancreatitis is made by serum amylase activity four times above normal according to the British Society of Gastroenterology (BSG) (1998) guidelines for the management of acute pancreatitis. Normal values range from 100–300 iu/L and a value > 1000 iu/L strongly suggests pancreatitis within the previous 48 hours. Amylase is an enzyme found in pancreatic juice which is activated by trypsin and therefore levels rise in a patient with pancreatitis. Serum amylase values need to be considered with caution as any increase is transient and a normal value does not necessarily rule out pancreatitis. Also, only approximately 40% of normal serum amylase is pancreatic in origin, the remainder is primarily salivary, and therefore prolonged high levels do not necessarily signify continued inflammation of the gland.

A chest X-ray will exclude air under the diaphragm (indicating gastrointestinal perforation rather than pancreatitis) and also highlight whether the patient has a left-sided pleural effusion, which is a frequent pulmonary complication of pancreatitis (Hughes, 2004). A particular complication of severe acute pancreatitis is also acute respiratory distress syndrome (ARDS) and this can also be diagnosed from a chest X-ray. An abdominal ultrasound scan will highlight any gallstones that are present, however it is sometimes difficult to see the pancreas if the patient is obese or has a lot of bowel gas, therefore these sometimes produce inconclusive results. Should the clinical and biochemical results be inconclusive, a CT scan will demonstrate if the pancreas is enlarged and swollen, if any peripancreatic fluid collections are present, or the presence of any pseudocysts or tumours. Any necrosis of the gland will also be seen on a CT scan. An endoscopic retrograde cholangio-pancreatogram (ERCP) can be performed to outline the biliary and pancreatic ducts but only usually if surgery is indicated. In the early diagnosis of pancreatitis this is not recommended, as an ERCP may aggravate the already inflamed gland.

(see Chapter 13)

Box 8.8   Ranson Criteria.

- Age > 55 years
- Decrease in Hb > 10%
- WCC > 16 000
- Urea > 16 mmol/L
- Glucose > 10 mmol/L
- Ca++ < 2 mmol/L
- Fluid loss > 6L

Severe disease is present if three or more factors detected

Box 8.9   Glasgow Criteria.

- Age > 55 years
- WCC > 15 000
- Urea > 16 mmol/L
- Glucose > 10 mmol/L
- Ca++ < 2 mmol/L
- Albumin < 32 g/L

Severe disease is present if three or more factors detected

Assessment and monitoring

Severity rating – Ranson and Glasgow Criteria

Modified early warning system (MEWS) charts can be used to determine the deterioration or improvement of a patient's condition and are an effective method of haemodynamic monitoring (Hughes, 2004) (see Chapter 13). Early identification of deterioration is vital in pancreatitis so that patients can receive appropriate high-dependency care. Severity stratification should be made at presentation or within 48 hours (BSG, 1998). For the purpose of objective measurement two sets of criteria have been designed – the Ranson Criteria and the Glasgow Criteria (Boxes 8.8 and 8.9).

APACHE II score

The acute physiology and chronic health evaluation (APACHE II) scoring system is used to identify 12 physiological variables, the patient's age, any history of severe organ or system dysfunction, or if the patient is immunocompromised. If the patient gains a score of 9 or higher on the APACHE II

system they are considered to have severe pancreatitis (BSG, 1998). The disadvantage of this system is that is takes a long time to complete and is therefore rarely used.

Management and care

All cases of severe acute pancreatitis should be managed in a high-dependency or intensive care unit setting with full monitoring and systems support (BSG, 1998). However, many patients with less fulminant disease are managed in the general surgical ward environment.

Pain control

Adequate pain management is one of the priorities in the management of a patient with pancreatitis. Ideally any analgesia will not stimulate spasms in the sphincter of Oddi or exacerbate pancreatic inflammation. Patients are managed with regular intramuscular pethidine or, if this is inadequate, patient-controlled analgesia can be used (Hughes, 2004). Morphine can cause spasm in the sphincter of Oddi and is therefore generally avoided. Non-pharmacological measures sometimes ease the pain and patients can be assisted into a sitting position where they can lean forward over a table.

Suppression of pancreatic function

The patient will require absolute rest of the gastrointestinal system and must remain nil-by-mouth until the acute episode has resolved. Anything taken by mouth will stimulate the release of pancreatic enzymes and increase the pain and damage to the patient. Patients will often have a nasogastric tube in situ to further reduce the risk of stimulation of the pancreas by preventing gastric secretions from entering the duodenum. The nasogastric tube will require regular aspiration to relieve vomiting and abdominal distension. The colour, consistency and amount of drainage must be recorded to enable accurate fluid balance management.

Correction of shock

Depending on the severity of the pancreatitis, the patient may be suffering from hypovolaemic shock, particularly if haemorrhagic pancreatitis has been diagnosed. Observation of the patient's vital signs is paramount. These should be monitored at least hourly, along with haemodynamic status and urinary output. Correction of this shock will include the provision of intravenous fluids and oxygen therapy. Refer to Chapter 13 for further information on the management of shock.

Monitoring blood glucose levels

All patients should have regular blood glucose monitoring during their admission, as the patient is at risk of developing diabetes as a result of the reduced endocrine function of the pancreas.

Controlling infection risk

The risk of infection in patients with severe acute pancreatitis is high and usually attributed to the disease process, the treatment received or the nutritional and immunological status of the patient on admission. The administration of a broad-spectrum antibiotic is recommended as it has been seen to provide some prophylaxis (BSG, 1998) and the majority of patients will receive intravenous therapy.

Complications – haemorrhage, cardiac and renal failure, acute respiratory distress syndrome

Whether the patient is diagnosed with haemorrhagic pancreatitis or there is ulceration due to the premature activation of digestive enzymes, the patient is at risk of haemorrhaging. This will lead to cardiovascular collapse and massive exudation of fluid into the retroperitoneal tissues. The patient will be predisposed to cardiac and renal failure due to their hypovolaemic state. Occasionally, depending on the severity, the patient may require dialysis for their renal failure (Walsh, 2002). A patient with acute pancreatitis may develop acute respiratory distress syndrome due to acid–base abnormalities and the inability to fully expand the lungs caused by abdominal distension. These patients should be cared for in an intensive care environment. Treatment for sepsis and careful monitoring of fluid balance is important, as any overhydration will exacerbate the problem. Figure 8.11 summarises the complications associated with acute pancreatitis.

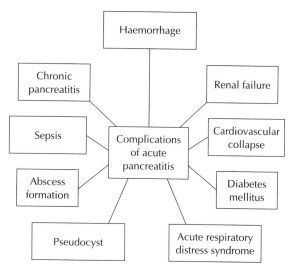

Figure 8.11   Complications associated with acute pancreatitis.

Pancreatic cancer

Applied pathophysiology

Most pancreatic tumours are ductal adenocarcinomas and arise from the ductal epithelium (O'Rourke & D'Ath, 1998). Tumours can be located in the head, body or tail of the pancreas with the head being the most common (Figure 8.12). These tumours spread to the duodenum, obstruct the bile duct, invade backwards into the retroperitoneal space and forwards into the peritoneal cavity. Patients are generally asymptomatic until the tumour invades surrounding tissues or obstructs the duct. Often patients will complain of back pain, and jaundice is a frequent symptom. Due to the impaired enzyme secretion and flow to the duodenum as a result of pancreatic cancer the patient will frequently display signs of fat and protein malabsorption (McCance & Huether, 2002), for example, steatorrhoea. This results in weight loss.

Pre-operative assessment, monitoring and preparation

Obstructive jaundice

Jaundice is the yellow discoloration of the skin and sclera caused by an excess amount of the bile

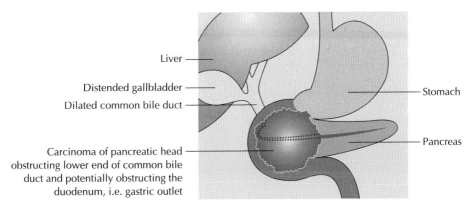

Figure 8.12   Carcinoma of the head of the pancreas.
(Reprinted from *Essential Surgery*, 3rd edn, Fig. 17.3a, Burkitt & Quick (2001) with permission from Elsevier)

pigment bilirubin in the body. If a patient presents with obstructive jaundice – that is, anything that blocks the release of bilirubin from the liver cells or prevents its secretion into the duodenum – the cause could be pancreatic carcinoma.

Diabetes

All patients should have regular blood glucose monitoring during their admission as there is a risk of developing diabetes: a pancreatic neoplasm may reduce the endocrine function of the pancreas.

Endoscopic retrograde cholangio-pancreatography (ERCP)

The patient may undergo an ERCP (see above) prior to surgery to outline the biliary tract and high-light any abnormalities and the potential resect-ability of the pancreatic tumour.

Surgical procedures

Pancreatico-duodenectomy (Whipple's procedure)

As with many other malignant tumours, surgical resection offers the only chance of cure, but for cancer of the pancreas only between 10 and 20% of patients will be suitable candidates (O'Rourke & D'Ath, 1998). This is due to fact that patients often present when their tumour has infiltrated

the surrounding area or there are distant meta-stases present. During this procedure the patient's distal stomach, gallbladder, common bile duct, head of pancreas, duodenum and upper jejunum are resected (Figure 8.13). Survival following sur-gery is limited to two years on average.

Palliative surgical bypass

If the tumour is thought to be localised, the patient will be taken for laparotomy and resection. If, however, the tumour turns out to be unresectable the surgeon may opt to perform a diversionary procedure. An alternative passage between the common bile duct and duodenum is created that relieves obstructive jaundice. The use of diversion-ary surgery needs to be considered carefully in light of the long-term outlook for the patient and the potential for post-operative complications (Fitzsimmons, 2003) and is in fact rarely performed these days. The majority of surgeons prefer to opt for endoscopic stent insertion. Occasionally the sphincter of Oddi requires sphincterotomy prior to placement of a self-retaining plastic stent, either percutaneously or endoscopically.

Post-operative management and care

Replacement of pancreatic function

Following pancreatic resection, the patient is left unable to maintain adequate digestive function.

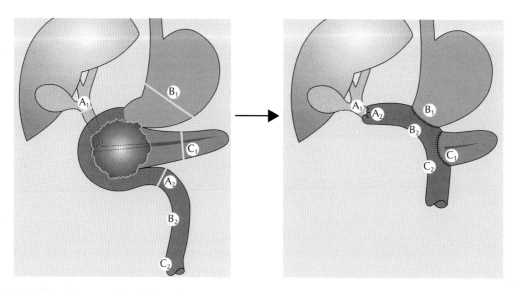

Figure 8.13   Whipple's pancreatico-duodenectomy.
(Reprinted from *Essential Surgery*, 3rd edition, Fig. 17.5, Burkitt & Quick (2001) with permission from Elsevier)

The disruption to the endocrine and exocrine functions of the pancreas leads to diabetes and the inability to break down certain food types. The patient may well require insulin and a pancreatin preparation to replace the lost function. This will be in combination with dietary modifications for the rest of the patient's life.

Self-test questions

1. Describe oesophageal varices and list the three treatment options.
2. List three factors that lead to the development of oesophageal carcinoma.
3. If a patient complains of dysphagia what are the two investigations that they should definitely have?
4. What investigations are undertaken to fully stage an oesophageal carcinoma?
5. What is a thoracotomy?
6. List the risk factors for carcinoma of the stomach.
7. What are the common routes of spread of gastric carcinoma?
8. List the important factors for T-tube management.
9. What are the physiological consequences of pancreatic auto-digestion?
10. List the five key areas of management for a patient with acute pancreatitis.

Reference list and further reading

Alexander MF, Fawcett JN & Runciman PJ (2000) *Nursing Practice Hospital and Home: the Adult* (2nd edn). Edinburgh: Churchill Livingstone

American Joint Committee for Cancer (AJCC) (1997) *Cancer Staging Manual* (5th edn). Philadephia: Lippincott-Raven

British Society of Gastroenterology (BSG) (1998) *United Kingdom guidelines for the management of acute pancreatitis* (online). www.bsg.org.uk/pdf_word_docs/pancreatic.pdf (Accessed 04.01.07)

British Society of Gastroenterology (BSG) (2002) *Guidelines for the management of oesophageal and gastric cancer* (online). www.bsg.org.uk/pdf_word_docs/ogcancer.pdf (Accessed 04.01.07)

British Thoracic Society (BTS) (2003) *Guidelines for the Management of Spontaneous Pneumothorax* (online). www.brit-thoracic.org.uk/public_content.php?pageid=7andcatid=36andsubcatid=187 (Accessed 04.01.07)

Burkitt HG & Quick CRG (2001) *Essential Surgery*. Edinburgh: Churchill Livingstone

Cancer Help UK (2002) *Glossary* (online). www.cancerhelp.org.uk/glossary.asp?search=e (Accessed 04.01.07)

Cuschieri A, Grace PA, Darzi A, Borley N & Rowley DI (2003) *Clinical Surgery*. Oxford: Blackwell Publishing

Ellis H, Calne R & Watson C (2002) *General Surgery* (10th edn). Oxford: Blackwell Publishing

Fitzsimmons D (2003) 'Pancreatic cancer: optimising the patient experience' *Cancer Nursing Practice* 2(10): 21–25

Grace PA & Borley NR (2002) *Surgery at a Glance* (2nd edn). Oxford: Blackwell Publishing

Henry MM & Thompson JN (eds) (2005) *Clinical Surgery* (2nd edn). Edinburgh: Elsevier Saunders

Hughes E (2004) 'Understanding the care of patients with acute pancreatitis' *Nursing Standard* 18(18): 45–52

Lattimer CR, Wilson NM & Lagattolla NRF (2002) *Key Topics in General Surgery* (2nd edn). Oxford: Bios

McCance KL & Huether SE (2002) *Pathophysiology: The Biologic Basis for Disease in Adults and Children* (4th edn). St Louis: Mosby

O'Rourke K & D'Ath S (1998) 'Clinical update: pancreatic cancer' *Primary Health Care* 8(8): 17–21

Pudner R (ed.) (2000) *Nursing the Surgical Patient*. Edinburgh: Baillière Tindall

Walsh M (ed.) (2002) *Watson's Clinical Nursing and Related Sciences* (6th edn). Edinburgh: Baillière Tindall

9 Surgery of the Lower Gastrointestinal Tract

Ian Felstead

Introduction

The large bowel, or colorectal region of the gastrointestinal tract, starts at the ileo-caecal junction where the ileum joins the caecum. Attached to the caecum is the appendix. The large bowel continues from the caecum with the ascending colon. This section of the colon bears left at the hepatic flexure into the transverse colon, which turns downwards at the splenic flexure into the descending colon. This leads into the sigmoid colon that eventually becomes the rectum and the anus. Figure 9.1 shows the overall structure of the large bowel.

The aims of this chapter are to provide information for nurses working on acute surgical wards that care for patients who have undergone colorectal surgery. Information will firstly be presented on the common pathophysiological conditions detailing the investigations used to aid diagnosis. The major surgical procedures will then be addressed to include detail on the specific pre-operative assessment, monitoring and preparation required, the operative procedure and the specific post-operative management and care (see Box 9.1).

Chapter 1 has discussed the general principles of pre-operative assessment and preparation of the patient for surgery. Patients who are to undergo colorectal surgical procedures require some additional specific assessment and preparation, as detailed within this chapter. They also require the

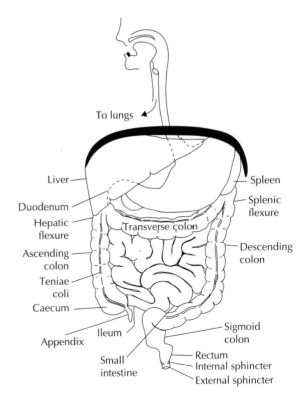

Figure 9.1   The gastrointestinal tract.

Box 9.1 Aims of the chapter.

- To introduce the reader to the most common pathophysiological conditions in the colorectal region
- To discuss the common investigations and diagnostic tests performed on patients with the common conditions
- To discuss the major surgical procedures undertaken on the large bowel with regards to specific pre-operative assessment, monitoring and preparation; the surgical procedure and post-operative care and management

same general post-operative care as those patients undergoing other major surgical procedures. The overall principles of post-operative management have been discussed in Chapter 3 and these should be considered alongside the information presented here.

Applied pathophysiology of colorectal disorders

Diverticulitis

This is inflammation of a diverticulum (a small pouch or pocket in the lining of the intestine) (see Figure 9.2).

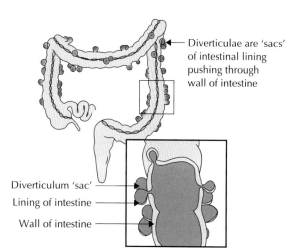

Diverticulae are 'sacs' of intestinal lining pushing through wall of intestine

Diverticulum 'sac'

Lining of intestine

Wall of intestine

Figure 9.2 Diverticulum.
(Reproduced courtesy of the Canadian Digestive Health Foundation)

This inflammation causes bacteria to collect in the pouches resulting in varying degrees of infection, inflammation, fever and abscess formation, which eventually will enlarge to a stage where they can cause obstruction of the bowel lumen. Ellis *et al.* (2002) state that an inflamed diverticulum will either perforate, produce chronic infection or haemorrhage. A patient with chronic diverticular disease may display the same symptoms as a patient with carcinoma of the colon, including altered bowel habit, large bowel obstruction and passage of blood and mucus from the rectum.

Colorectal cancer

Colorectal cancer is believed to develop through a process known as the adenoma–carcinoma sequence. Initially cells in the luminal part of the colonic crypt begin to proliferate due to a mutation in the adenomatous polyposis coli (APC) gene found on chromosome 5 (Snoo, 2003). These rapidly growing cells create an outgrowth, or polyp, which is described as an adenoma. Further mutation to various oncogenes produces a larger adenoma. This adenoma increases in size and mutates until eventually an invasive carcinoma is formed with the ability to metastasise.

The causes of colorectal cancer are unknown but it is thought that diet, genetic factors and pre-existing disease are all risk factors (see Box 9.2). Diets that are low in fibre and high in fats are thought to reduce the transit time within the large bowel putting the mucosa in contact with potential carcinogens for an increased length of time. The main types of inherited colorectal cancer are familial adenomatous polyposis (FAP) and hereditary non-polyposis colorectal cancer (HNPCC). These

Box 9.2 Risk factors for colorectal cancer.

- Diet high in fat and low in fibre
- Genetic predisposition – hereditary non-polyposis colorectal cancer and familial adenomatous polyposis
- Smoking
- Inflammatory bowel disorders – Crohn's disease, ulcerative colitis
- Lack of exercise

account for approximately 1% and 6% respectively (Snoo, 2003). Patients with inflammatory bowel disease, particularly ulcerative colitis, are at higher risk of developing colorectal cancer.

Gastrointestinal obstruction

Normal functioning of the small and large bowel is dependent on an open lumen for movement of intestinal contents as well as adequate innervation and circulation to sustain peristalsis. Anything that interferes with any of these factors may lead to a bowel obstruction. Obstruction can either be classified as mechanical or non-mechanical.

Mechanical obstruction means that the intestinal lumen has been affected and can be caused by adhesions, hernias, a volvulus, tumours, diverticulitis or faecal impaction. Non-mechanical obstruction can be caused by paralytic ileus, rib, spinal or pelvic trauma, or drugs, and relates to the peristaltic action of the bowel. These conditions cause nerve or muscle dysfunction and are sometimes known as functional or neurogenic obstruction. The lumen of the bowel remains patent. Box 9.3 summarises the causes of mechanical and non-mechanical obstruction.

The obstruction triggers a series of events whose clinical manifestations depend on the location of the obstruction and degree of circulatory compromise. When the obstruction occurs there is an accumulation of intestinal contents such as swallowed air, intestinal gas and digestive secretions, proximal to the obstruction (Shelton, 1999). As a result of the loss of tone and distension of the proximal section, the distal bowel collapses. Intestinal secretions are stimulated and the absorption of fluids is reduced, leading to further increase of fluid and air proximal to the obstruction. The raised pressure in the bowel lumen causes increased capillary permeability and extravasation of fluid and electrolytes from the plasma to the peritoneal cavity (see Box 9.4).

The proximal sequestration of fluid and resultant increase in pressure also leads to necrosis from impaired blood supply and possible rupture of the bowel wall. The bowel becomes increasingly permeable to bacteria, leading to peritonitis. The movement of fluid from the plasma and reduced absorption also leads to dehydration and in severe cases hypovolaemic shock. (See Chapter 13 for further discussion of shock.)

Normal homeostatic functioning requires a stable pH (7.35–7.45) – the measure of the concentration

---

Box 9.3   Mechanical and non-mechanical causes of obstruction.

Mechanical
- Adhesions
- Hernia
- Volvulus
- Tumour
- Diverticulitis
- Impaction
- Intussusception
- Stenosis

Non-mechanical
- Paralytic ileus
- Electrolyte imbalance
- Rib, spine or pelvic trauma
- Drugs that reduce bowel motility, e.g. opioids

Box 9.4   Pathophysiology of gastrointestinal obstruction.

Fluid, gas and intestinal contents accumulate proximal to the point of obstruction
↓
The distal bowel may collapse
↓
Distension and oedema of the bowel wall reduces the absorption of fluids and stimulates intestinal secretions
↓
Increased fluid leads to increased pressure in the bowel lumen
↓
Increased pressure leads to increased capillary permeability and extravasation of fluid and electrolytes into the peritoneal cavity
↓
This leads to oedema, congestion and necrosis from impaired blood supply and possible rupture of the bowel
↓
Increased bacteria (anaerobes) lead to increased endotoxins and sepsis
↓
Retention of fluid in the intestine and peritoneal cavity leads to hypotension and hypovolaemic shock

of hydrogen ions in a solution and therefore its acidity or alkalinity. Metabolic alkalosis is a pH imbalance in which the body has either accumulated too much of an alkaline substance, such as bicarbonate, or has lost an acidic substance, such as hydrogen. There is insufficient acid to return the extracellular pH to neutrality (pH 7.4). The body becomes more alkaline: it has a higher pH. High gastrointestinal obstructions cause vomiting of the acidic gastric contents and loss of hydrogen ions leading to metabolic alkalosis and dehydration (through water loss). As a result, muscular weakness and cramps may develop.

Metabolic acidosis is the reverse where the body cannot excrete enough of an acidic substance or suffers a sudden increase in an acidic substance, for example in sepsis. The pH becomes lower. Patients with a low obstruction may develop metabolic acidosis due to an increased loss of bicarbonate from bile that cannot be reabsorbed. Symptoms include headache, lack of energy, drowsiness, rapid and shallow respirations, nausea and vomiting. The increase in intestinal secretions also leads to abdominal distension, reverse peristalsis and eventual vomiting of faeculent matter.

Clinical manifestations of intestinal obstruction

The signs and symptoms of intestinal obstruction can be attributed to either a primary cause (the obstruction itself) or secondary (arising due to the obstructive process) (Shelton, 1999). Primary manifestations will include altered bowel sounds, abdominal discomfort and distension, whereas secondary manifestations can include nausea and vomiting, malnutrition, hypotension and fever. These signs and symptoms will vary according to whether the obstruction is located in the small or large bowel (see Table 9.1) (Shelton, 1999).

Investigations and diagnosis of colorectal disorders

An understanding of the investigations commonly undertaken may be helpful for health professionals dealing with patients' queries. Intestinal obstruction has a range of causes and the ideal diagnostic test should distinguish between functional or mechanical obstruction and partial or complete obstruction (Shelton, 1999). Some obstruction is caused by malignant disease, so investigations

Table 9.1 The signs and symptoms of intestinal obstruction.

Characteristics	Location of tumour		
	Duodenum/jejunum	Late jejunum/ileum	Colorectal region
Abdominal pain	Epigastric region, increasing and decreasing in 4–5-minute intervals	Right upper quadrant, similar to cramp, intermittent in 15–20-minute intervals	Lower quadrants (suprapubic), intermittent
Pain timing in relation to eating	Immediately after eating	Approximately 1 hour after eating	Several hours after eating
Bowel sounds	Hyperactive in left upper quadrant, low or absent elsewhere	Hyperactive in left and right upper quadrants, low or absent in lower quadrants	Hyperactive in upper quadrants and proximal to obstruction, low or absent in lower quadrants
Abdominal distension	Not prominent	Prominent in upper abdomen – epigastric region	Lower abdominal and pelvic region
Vomiting	Clear fluid from stomach or green from duodenum	Green from jejunum, bile if from below bile duct, faeculent if from caecum	Usually no vomiting
Stool	Watery diarrhoea	No stool output following distal tract evacuation	Thin ribbon-like stool with partial obstruction, watery fluid otherwise (overflow)

(Adapted from Shelton, 1999)

Box 9.5   Factors to include in an abdominal assessment.

- Changes in contours of the abdomen
- Abnormal veins
- Scars on the abdominal wall
- Striae gravidarum (stretch marks)
- Changes at the umbilicus
- Visible peristalsis
- **Remember** to include palpation, auscultation and percussion

(Gray & Toghill, 2001)

Box 9.6   Clinical manifestations of bowel perforation and contrast leak.

- Abdominal pain
- Nausea and vomiting
- Pyrexia
- Signs of shock

Box 9.7   Sigmoidoscopy and colonoscopy.

- Both of these investigations are endoscopic procedures.
- Endoscopy refers to the visualisation of the interior of the body cavities and hollow organs by means of a flexible fibre-optic instrument (Alexander *et al.*, 2000).
- A sigmoidoscopy is an examination of the rectum and sigmoid colon with a sigmoidoscope (inserted through the anus). This will either be a rigid instrument of approximately 25 cm in length or a flexible tube approximately 60 cm in length.
- A colonoscopy is an internal examination of the entire colon and rectum, introduced through the anus and guided by way of visual and X-ray control.
- Both of these procedures also enable the collection of specimens for histological examination.

may be undertaken to establish whether a tumour is present. Some tests are undertaken to identify any metastatic spread from colorectal cancer, for example a liver ultrasound may be used to detect hepatic metastases, and a chest X-ray may indicate the presence of pulmonary metastases. Explanations might sometimes need to be brief, to avoid unnecessary distress to a patient who is subsequently found to be free of malignant disease.

History and physical examination

A history of the patient's normal bowel habit will help to identify any potential obstruction or other bowel disorder. Physical examination may indicate a mass palpable in either the abdomen or rectum. Jaundice or ascites may indicate tumour spread (see Box 9.5).

Abdominal X-ray

A plain abdominal film will enable differentiation between functional and mechanical impairment of the bowel. It may help to establish whether the bowel is being compressed by any external force that is causing the obstruction. An abdominal X-ray may also show bowel distension, volvulus and adhesions.

Barium studies – swallow or enema

A barium enema may demonstrate diverticula as globular outpouchings and also there may be evidence of a stricture. This investigation should not be performed in the acute phase of disease, however, as it may cause perforation of an inflamed and friable bowel. Barium studies will be effective in demonstrating the presence of a tumour. Enemas must not be performed if there is specific risk or evidence of bowel perforation as the contrast used could leak into the peritoneal cavity leading to peritonitis (Box 9.6).

Sigmoidoscopy/colonoscopy

These diagnostic procedures are very useful in demonstrating any neoplasms (see Box 9.7). A colonoscopy may enable colonic diverticula to be seen, although it is difficult for the endoscopist to pass the scope through the rigid and narrow sigmoid that may occur in this condition.

Box 9.8   Endoanal ultrasound.

Endoanal ultrasound is a variation of endorectal ultrasound, where the balloon, which surrounds the transducer, has been replaced with a plastic cone. The shape and the dimensions of this cone facilitate its painless insertion in the anal canal while the acoustic contact is optimal with minimal deformation of the anal canal walls. With ultrasonic examination, a depth of 5 cm is visualised.

   This examination is very useful in the assessment and investigation of perianal fistulas, faecal incontinence and rectal neoplasms.

Box 9.9   Faecal occult blood test.

The faecal occult blood test (FOB test) detects small amounts of blood in the patient's faeces that are not normally visible to the naked eye.

   A small sample of faeces is smeared onto a piece of card using a small scraper to scrape some faeces off toilet tissue that has just been used following a bowel motion.

   A chemical is added to the sample on the card and if there is a change in colour after adding the chemical, it indicates that some blood is present.

   The FOB test only informs that the patient is bleeding from somewhere in the lower GI tract – not where. For this reason if the test is positive then further tests will be scheduled, for example, sigmoidoscopy.

Computed tomography scan/magnetic resonance imaging

A computed tomography (CT) scan helps to identify the specific cause and location of mechanical obstruction (Shelton, 1999). CT scans are also very useful in determining the extent of a primary colorectal tumour and whether any metastatic spread has occurred. Magnetic resonance imaging (MRI) scans are predominantly used in rectal cancer to determine whether there is any invasion or metastatic spread beyond the rectum.

Endoanal ultrasound

This diagnostic test (see Box 9.8) is sometimes performed to outline the layers of the rectal wall and detect any lymph node involvement in colorectal cancer.

Biochemical testing

A full blood count may show a raised white cell count due to an inflammatory process. If dehydration is present, a high haemoglobin concentration may be present due to reduced plasma volume and urea and electrolyte examination may demonstrate a raised sodium and potassium level.

Faecal occult blood testing (FOBT)

General observation of the stool will not necessarily show any blood, therefore a FOBT (see Box 9.9) will be needed to test for its presence or absence.

Conservative management of GI obstruction

Patients presenting with gastrointestinal obstruction may be treated conservatively if there is no immediate threat to bowel viability. This conservative management will incorporate proximal decompression and fluid/electrolyte replacement.

   There are many priorities associated with the management of gastrointestinal obstruction. Pain is often a common clinical manifestation requiring assessment and management. The pattern and severity of the pain may help to establish a diagnosis, for example, the timing of abdominal pain in relation to eating helps diagnosis of the level of obstruction. If a patient complains of cramping, intermittent pain in the right upper quadrant, occurring at intervals of approximately 15–20 minutes, the obstruction may be located in the lower jejunum or ileum (Shelton, 1999). If the patient is hypovolaemic, intramuscular analgesia may be relatively ineffective, because muscle perfusion and absorption of the medication into the bloodstream is reduced. Intravenous medication may be needed instead.

   The presence or absence of nausea and vomiting may help to establish the level of obstruction. If the vomitus is faeculent, this suggests an obstruction in the lower intestinal tract (Shelton, 1999). Nasogastric intubation helps to decompress and empty the stomach, reducing the risk of vomiting and aspiration and making the patient more comfortable. If the patient is receiving opiate analgesia, the use of anti-emetics is particularly important due to the nauseating effect of these drugs on the chemo-receptor trigger zone in the emetic centre of the brain.

Correction of dehydration and electrolyte imbalance via the administration of intravenous fluids is often regulated according to the patient's urine output and biochemical analysis. Monitoring of fluid balance is extremely important considering the patient may have sequestration of fluid into the peritoneal cavity causing hypovolaemia. This is often achieved through the measurement of naso-gastric tube output, catheter output (usually hourly measurements) and central venous pressure (CVP) measurement.

Finally, observation and monitoring of the patient's vital signs (pulse and blood pressure, temperature, respiratory rate and oxygen saturation) as well as bowel function and abdominal distension are important when caring for patients with GI obstruction.

If this conservative treatment fails to resolve the obstruction, the patient will require surgery. Surgery is also essential if there is established or suspected strangulation or complete large bowel obstruction. In such cases, the patient may experience tenderness in the right iliac fossa.

Pre-operative assessment, monitoring and preparation for bowel surgery

Staging and classification – TNM and Dukes

Clinical and pathological staging are used to assess the prognosis and plan treatment. Colorectal cancer is staged using the tumour–nodes–metastases (TNM) and Dukes classification systems (Table 9.2, Box 9.10, Figure 9.3).

Table 9.2 TNM staging system for colorectal cancer.

Primary tumour (T)

TX	Primary tumour cannot be assessed
T0	No evidence of primary tumour
Tis	Carcinoma in situ – intraepithelial or invasion of lamina propria
T1	Tumour invades submucosa
T2	Tumour invades muscularis propria
T3	Tumour invades through muscularis propria into subserosa or into non-peritonealised pericolic or perirectal tissues
T4	Tumour directly invades other organs of structures and/or perforates visceral peritoneum

Regional lymph nodes (N)

NX	Regional lymph nodes cannot be assessed
N0	No metastases in regional lymph node
N1	Metastases in one to three regional lymph nodes
N2	Metastases in four or more regional lymph nodes

Distant metastasis (M)

MX	Distant metastases cannot be assessed
M0	No evidence of distant metastases
M1	Distant metastases

TNM in relation to Dukes classification:

Dukes A	T1	N0	M0
Dukes B	T3	N0	M0
Dukes C	Any T	N1	M0
Dukes D	Any T	Any N	M1

Box 9.10 Dukes classification for colorectal cancer.

DUKES A	Tumour confined to the muscle coat, lymph node free of tumour
DUKES B	Tumour reaching serosa; lymph nodes free of tumour
DUKES C	Any cancer with lymph node involvement by tumour C1 – if apical node not involved by tumour C2 – if apical node involved by tumour
DUKES D	Distant metastases

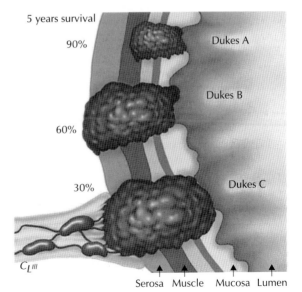

Figure 9.3 Dukes classification of colorectal cancer. (Reprinted from *Clinical Surgery*, p. 405, Henry & Thompson (2005), with permission from Elsevier)

> **Box 9.11**   Types of bowel preparation.
>
> - Suppositories
> - Phosphate enema
> - Oral laxatives
>   - Picolax
>   - Kleen prep

Bowel preparation

In elective procedures the patient may require bowel preparation. This will usually be at the discretion of the surgeon and may differ from unit to unit. The overall aim of bowel preparation is, however, the same: to improve visibility during the operation, to prevent any faecal soiling of the anastomosis or operative site and to prevent any faecal impaction post-operatively. Bowel preparation usually takes the form of colonic lavage or bowel washouts and laxatives (Box 9.11). It is normal for patients to lose a significant amount of fluid when receiving laxative bowel preparation: this could lead to dehydration and is compounded in older people who may already be in a negative fluid balance. It is therefore common for patients to be given intravenous fluids to ensure fluid homeostasis in the pre-operative period.

Stoma siting

In elective surgery, the stoma nurse specialist is usually responsible for the correct siting of the stoma; however, in an emergency this is undertaken by the surgeon. There are several considerations necessary when siting a stoma (see Box 9.12).

These factors, incorporated with an assessment of the patient's eyesight, manual dexterity, mental state and cultural needs, should help to create a stoma that the patient is able to cope with successfully (Hyde, 2000). The allocated site must be marked pre-operatively with an indelible marker pen and in some cases it is advisable for the patient to wear an appliance before the actual surgery to enable some psychological preparation for the stoma's presence post-operatively. Siting of the stoma is one of the most important pre-operative tasks to be carried out in this type of surgery, as it

> **Box 9.12**   Sites to avoid when positioning a stoma.
>
> - Old scars
> - Bony prominences
> - The umbilicus
> - Groin creases
> - Pubic areas
> - The waistline
> - Fatty bulges or creases (lying, sitting and standing)
> - Underneath large breasts
> - Areas affected by skin disorders
> - The site of the proposed surgical incision
> - A site which cannot be seen by the patient
>
> www.coloplast.co.uk 'An Introduction to Stoma Care'

> **Box 9.13**   Types of colostomy.
>
> **Loop colostomy**
> A loop colostomy is usually formed to divert faeces and protect an anastomosis. A loop of the colon is brought to the surface of the body through a small incision and is supported by a 'bridge' until the stoma has healed and is fixed in position. A loop colostomy is usually temporary and can be closed after 6 to 8 weeks. More commonly a loop ileostomy is formed, as there is a better blood supply to facilitate bowel closure (Ellis *et al.*, 2002).
>
> **End (or permanent) colostomy**
> An end colostomy is usually formed in the treatment of rectal or anal carcinoma. If the rectum is involved in the disease process it will need to be removed. The remaining colon is then mobilised and the cut end brought up to the abdominal surface and usually sited in the left iliac fossa.

will minimise any future difficulties due to interference by clothing, or skin problems caused by a leaky appliance. Box 9.13 shows different types of colostomies.

Major surgical procedures

The patient's post-operative notes will detail the procedures that have been undertaken. An explanation of the surgery is given here to heighten understanding of the patient's post-operative condition.

Hemicolectomy

A right hemicolectomy is performed to remove tumours of the caecum, ascending colon and hepatic flexure. Following laparotomy the terminal ileum, ascending colon and hepatic flexure are mobilised, the tumour and surrounding bowel resected and an anastomosis formed between the ileum and the transverse colon.

A left hemicolectomy is usually performed for the removal of a tumour of the splenic flexure or descending colon that is not obstructing the bowel lumen. The left side of the colon is mobilised and the growth is resected. The two ends are joined in an end-to-end anastomosis. A radical left hemicolectomy involves the resection of the regional lymph nodes followed by anastomosis of the transverse colon to the recto-sigmoid colon. If this is performed as an emergency, the patient may be left with a temporary colostomy. If a tumour is present in the sigmoid colon, the patient may have a sigmoid colectomy. Figure 9.4 shows the segments of bowel removed in these procedures, whilst Figure 9.5 illustrates a total colectomy.

Transverse colectomy

A transverse colectomy is performed to remove a non-obstructive tumour of the transverse colon. Following full mobilisation of the transverse section of the colon it is resected and an end-to-end anastomosis formed between the right and left colon. If the operation is being performed for malignant disease, the omentum is usually included in the resection.

Hartmann's procedure and formation of colostomy

If a patient suffers a perforated diverticulum or any other left-sided colonic emergency, they may require a Hartmann's resection. This is an emergency procedure and therefore an end-to-end anastomosis is not usually performed, as there has been insufficient time to cleanse the bowel. This increases the risk of infection and contamination, which could cause the anastomosis to break down. A Hartmann's procedure involves a resection and

a. Right hemicolectomy

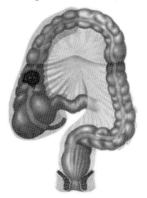

b. Left hemicolectomy

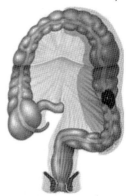

c. Sigmoid colectomy

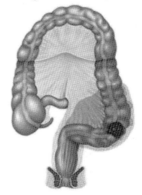

(Shaded areas show resected section)

Figure 9.4   Types of colectomy.
(Reprinted from *Clinical Surgery*, p. 407, Henry & Thompson (2005), with permission from Elsevier)

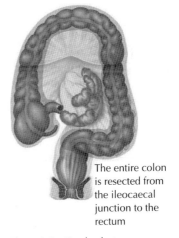

The entire colon is resected from the ileocaecal junction to the rectum

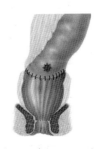

Ileorectal anastomosis

Figure 9.5   Total colectomy.
(Reprinted from *Clinical Surgery*, p. 400, Henry & Thompson (2005), with permission from Elsevier)

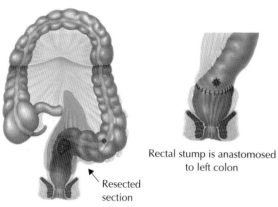

Rectal stump is anastomosed
to left colon

Resected
section

Figure 9.6   Anterior resection.
(Reprinted from *Clinical Surgery*, p. 409, Henry & Thompson
(2005), with permission from Elsevier)

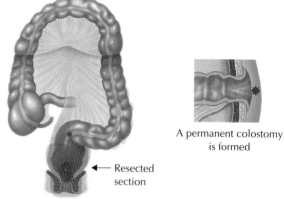

A permanent colostomy
is formed

Resected
section

Figure 9.7   Abdomino-perineal resection.
(Reprinted from *Clinical Surgery*, p. 409, Henry & Thompson
(2005), with permission from Elsevier)

formation of a colostomy at the proximal end of the colon in the left iliac fossa. The remaining rectal stump is sutured or stapled and left in situ to allow for stoma reversal at a later date when the bowel has sufficiently healed.

Anterior resection

An anterior resection is performed to excise rectal carcinomas that are more than 10 cm from the anal verge but below the recto-sigmoid junction (Figure 9.6). The operation is usually performed through a vertical incision extending from above the umbilicus to the pubis. The rectum is mobilised and the tumour excised with a distal margin of usually 5 cm. An anastomosis is formed between the rectal stump and the left colon. Generally a transverse loop colostomy is carried out as a protective measure.

Abdomino-perineal resection and formation of colostomy

An abdomino-perineal resection is performed to remove rectal carcinomas when the tumour is less than 10 cm from the anal verge (Figure 9.7). The operation is usually performed through a vertical incision from above the umbilicus to the pubis and with an incision around the anus. It is not possible to clear the cancer without removing the anus and therefore the patient will be left with a permanent

colostomy. The rectum is mobilised and the lower rectum and anus are excised leaving the area to be sutured. The sutured area is a major source of post-operative pain for patients so good analgesic management is needed.

Post-operative management and care

Stoma care

Post-operatively the patient with a stoma requires specific care and management (Box 9.14). In theatre a skin-protective wafer will probably have been applied around the stoma and a drainable, transparent appliance placed over the top. This appliance must be transparent to allow for observation

---

Box 9.14   Principles of post-operative ostomy care.

- Use only transparent appliances to allow visualisation of the stoma
- Observe for:
  - Stoma colour
  - Stoma size
  - Stoma output
  - Signs of oedema or necrosis
- Leave initial appliance in situ for at least 48 hours
- Empty bag regularly
- Accurately record output – haemoserous fluid, liquid stool, gas

of stoma colour (a pink and healthy appearance indicates a good blood supply), size and output. It will take several days for a new stoma to act (Dougherty & Lister, 2004). This initial appliance will usually remain in situ for at least 48 hours. The bag must be emptied regularly as, if it becomes too full, the weight could result in a leak. Any liquid stool or gas must be noted, as this is an indication of the return of peristalsis. It must be remembered that all stomas produce haemoserous fluid for one to three days post-operatively before any faecal matter is passed (Collett, 2002).

The stoma must be observed for signs of oedema and necrosis. These are immediate complications and usually occur within 24 hours of surgery (Collett, 2002). All stomas are swollen following surgery due to handling of the bowel but this should decrease over the following days. Necrosis of the stoma is due to an insufficient blood supply to the section of the bowel used to form the stoma. The new stoma will become a dusky purple colour and the bowel may become necrotic and odorous (Collett, 2002). Usually the necrotic tissue will slough off when the stoma is cleaned, however, if it extends deeper than 2 cm surgical excision may be necessary.

Post-operative psychological care

Post-operatively, a patient with a new stoma may grieve the loss of normal function. Careful consideration must be given to the patient's psychosocial needs, including addressing any issues of altered body image. Information and reassurance is needed to enable the patient to feel supported. Involvement of the patient's family may also help to address social and sexual relationship issues that may be affected by the presence of a stoma. A key member of the interprofessional team is the stoma care nurse specialist, whose knowledge can help the patient to come to terms with their 'new' body function and who should be involved from the pre-operative period right through into the community following discharge of the patient. It may also be appropriate to introduce the patient to other ostomy patients who have learnt to adjust successfully following stoma surgery. (See Chapter 5 for further discussion of body image and sexuality issues.)

Physiological changes in the post-operative period

Following bowel surgery, whether a stoma or an anastomosis has been formed, the patient's body needs to adjust physiologically to the loss of part of the bowel. The body can compensate to some extent for the loss of the colon. Transit time can be increased within the small intestine and the absorptive area can be increased. However, if the bowel surgery is higher in the gastrointestinal tract and the patient has an ileostomy formed, for example, there is a risk of dehydration and electrolyte imbalance. These patients tend to lose almost 500 mL of fluid every day and can suffer from large losses of sodium, magnesium, calcium and water. Accurate monitoring and recording of fluid balance is vital, as well as observation for signs of hypovolaemic shock (see Chapter 13).

Post-operative complications

Paralytic ileus

Paralytic ileus is the term used to describe stasis within the bowel. When the bowel is operated on, the nerve pathways are interrupted, and this can result in the temporary loss of peristalsis. This condition means that patients are unable to consume anything orally due to their inability to pass any matter through the bowel. The time period until peristalsis returns is an individual phenomenon and cannot be generalised between patients, therefore the surgical team will listen for bowel sounds on a daily basis and usually commence the patient on small amounts of water gradually building up to free fluids and full diet over a number of days.

Haemorrhage

Post-operative haemorrhage can be relatively unnoticeable even with the presence of wound drains. Vigilant observation for the classic signs of shock is vital if extensive complications are to be avoided. The majority of patients who suffer post-operative haemorrhage will require a substantial blood transfusion and admission to the intensive care unit following further surgery (Anderson, 2003).

Box 9.15   Clinical manifestations of an anastomotic leak.

- Bowel contents in wound drain
- High fever
- Generalised peritonitis
- Generalised sepsis
- Less obvious symptoms
  ○ Unexplained pyrexia
  ○ Elevated white blood cell count
  ○ Prolonged ileus
  ○ Chest infection developing at a later stage
- Longer term complications
  ○ Localised abscess
  ○ Fistulae

Anastomotic breakdown

Resting the bowel post-operatively should enable the anastomosis to heal prior to coming into contact with bowel matter. There is a risk of breakdown or leak from the joined ends of the bowel and this could lead to varying degrees of peritonitis and haemorrhage. The actual risk of anastomotic leakage is reasonably high. Between 5 and 15% of all colonic anastomoses are susceptible to breakdown (Anderson, 2003). Should the patient suffer an anastomotic leak, the only course of action is to return them to theatre for a second operation, often involving the formation of an ileostomy. The clinical manifestations of an anastomotic leak are outlined in Box 9.15; however, leakage should be considered whenever there is unexplained post-operative deterioration (Anderson, 2003).

Damage to bladder function and sexual dysfunction

One potential complication that must be explained to patients pre-operatively is that despite how careful the surgeon is there is the risk of damage to the nerves in the pelvic region. This will not only affect bladder function but also could affect sexual function. The bulkier and lower the tumour is in the bowel, the higher the risk that the surgery could result in permanent bladder and/or sexual dysfunction.

Self-test questions

1. List the different parts of the large bowel in order, starting at the ileo-caecal junction.

2. List four mechanical and non-mechanical causes of gastrointestinal obstruction.
3. What is diverticulitis?
4. What are the risk factors for colorectal cancer?
5. How would you recognise if barium contrast had leaked into the patient's peritoneum?
6. Which aspect of nursing care is vital when patients are receiving bowel preparation?
7. List the factors that need to be considered when siting a stoma.
8. Name the emergency procedure that a patient is likely to undergo if they suffer a perforated diverticulum.
9. What are the principles of post-operative stoma management?
10. How would you recognise an anastomotic leak in a patient following gastrointestinal surgery?

References and further reading

Alexander MF, Fawcett JN & Runciman PJ (2000) *Nursing Practice Hospital and Home: The Adult* (2nd edn). Edinburgh: Churchill Livingstone

Anderson ID (ed.) (2003) *Care of the Critically Ill Surgical Patient* (2nd edn). London: Hodder Arnold

Canadian Digestive Health Foundation (2005) (online). www.cdhf.ca (Accessed 04.01.07)

Collett K (2002) 'Practical aspects of stoma management' *Nursing Standard* 17(8): 45–52, 54–55

Cuschieri A, Grace PA, Darzi A, Borley N & Rowley DI (2003) *Clinical Surgery*. Oxford: Blackwell Publishing

Dougherty L & Lister S (eds) (2004) *The Royal Marsden Hospital Manual of Clinical Nursing Procedures* (6th edn). Oxford: Blackwell Science

Ellis H, Calne R & Watson C (2002) *Lecture Notes on General Surgery* (10th edn). Oxford: Blackwell Science

Forbes CD & Jackson WF (2002) *Color Atlas and Text of Clinical Medicine* (3th edn). St Louis: Mosby

Gray D & Toghill P (2001) *An Introduction to the Symptoms and Signs of Clinical Medicine*. London: Arnold

Henry MM & Thompson JN (eds) (2005) *Clinical Surgery* (2nd edn). Edinburgh: Elsevier Saunders

Hyde C (2000) 'Diverticular disease' *Nursing Standard* 14(51): 38–43

Knowles G (2002) 'The management of colorectal cancer' *Nursing Standard* 16(17): 47–52, 54–55

Shelton B (1999) 'Intestinal obstruction' *Advanced Practice in Acute Critical Care* 10(4): 478–491

Snoo L (2003) 'Colorectal cancer' *Primary Health Care* 13(1): 43–49

10 Urological Surgery

Ian Felstead and Jane McLean

Introduction

Urology as a speciality is now commonplace in most general hospitals, although in many areas urological patients are located on general acute surgical wards. The urinary system comprises the kidneys, ureters, bladder and urethra. In the male patient the genito-urinary system also includes the accessory male reproductive organs, namely the prostate gland, penis and testes. The aims of this chapter (see Box 10.1) are to provide information for nurses working on acute surgical wards that care for patients who have undergone urological surgery. Information will be presented on the common pathophysiological conditions detailing the

---

investigations used to aid diagnosis. The major surgical procedures will be addressed including detail on the specific pre-operative assessment, monitoring and preparation required; the operative procedure; and the specific post-operative management and care. Urinary stone, prostate and bladder surgery will be discussed.

Chapter 1 has discussed the general principles of pre-operative assessment and preparation of the patient for surgery. Patients who are to undergo urological surgical procedures also require some specific assessment and preparation, as detailed within this chapter. Patients undergoing urological surgery will require the same general post-operative care as those patients undergoing other major surgical procedures. The overall principles of post-operative management have been discussed in Chapter 3 and these should be considered alongside the information presented within this section.

Urological investigations and diagnosis

Urinalysis/midstream specimen of urine (MSU)/catheter sample of urine (CSU)

Routine urinalysis should be performed in all patients on admission as it provides important information regarding systemic as well as urological disease. Sensory inspection of a urine sample is

---

Box 10.1   Aims of the chapter.

- To provide an understanding of the investigations and tests that are used to aid diagnosis within the urological setting
- To discuss the pathophysiology in relation to a number of common urological conditions including urinary stone disease, bladder and prostatic carcinoma
- To provide an understanding of the pre-, intra- and post-operative care of patients undergoing a number of common urological surgical procedures
- To enable the reader to recognise potential complications of urological surgery

also an important diagnostic procedure and should include colour, consistency and smell. It is important to test urine whilst fresh, as at room temperature bacteria will grow rapidly in a sample and make results invalid (Fillingham & Douglas, 2004). Other important urine sample collections for culture and sensitivity are MSU and CSU. Box 10.2 lists urological investigations and diagnostic tests.

Digital rectal examination

Digital rectal examination (DRE) is routinely performed when patients are suspected of having prostate enlargement. With the patient in a left lateral position, a trained practitioner inserts a finger into the rectum and palpates the prostate gland. An experienced practitioner will be able to estimate the size of the gland and also feel the texture. A healthy prostate should feel smooth and slightly soft whereas a suspicious gland can feel hard and nodular (Jones, 2003).

Prostate-specific antigen

The prostate-specific antigen test (or PSA test) is a diagnostic blood test used when prostate cancer is suspected. PSA is an enzyme that prevents semen from solidifying. High levels of prostate-specific

antigen enzyme in the bloodstream have been linked to cancer, but they have also been linked to other disorders of the prostate and therefore the test in isolation lacks specificity. In practice a digital rectal examination is used in conjunction with a PSA to increase its predictive value (Jones, 2003). The American Urologic Association (AUA, 2003) recommends PSA screening for men over the age of 50; however, in the UK it is believed that the test is unnecessary for asymptomatic men. Advocates, however, consider that PSA enzyme screening detects early stage carcinomas 80% of the time, and that deaths from prostate cancer have dropped since the procedure was approved. Opponents are unconvinced that screening has reduced cancer deaths, and argue that PSA screening yields 'false positive' results in 20% of cases, suggesting malignant growth where none exists. For this reason a policy has been developed in the UK that stipulates that only patients who request PSA testing will be offered the assay, rather than general practitioners broaching the subject. A common site for spread of a carcinoma of the prostate is the liver and therefore liver function tests (LFTs) will also be performed if this diagnosis is suspected.

Urodynamic investigation

Urodynamic studies (Box 10.3) are used to assess the neuromuscular function of the lower urinary tract, that is, the urethra, bladder and sphincters. The pressure, volume and flow relationships in the lower urinary tract are studied.

Uroflowmetry

Uroflowmetry is a simple diagnostic procedure used to calculate the flow rate of urine over a period of time. It is also used to assess the bladder and bladder sphincter function. An array of techniques has been used to measure urine flow rate, two of which are discussed here. The gravimetric method involves urine being passed into a container which is continuously weighed. This technique suffers from the amount of processing that is required to eliminate artefacts from vibration or movement. The other most common method is using the rotating disc mictiometer. Here the urine is directed onto a spinning disc whose rotational velocity is kept constant by a tachometer and feedback circuit. As fluid hits the disc, more electrical energy is required to maintain the constant angular velocity, and measurement of the extra current can be used to give flow rate. Patients have to be warned not to move the stream when voiding as this can produce artefacts.

Uroflowmetry is used to assist in the evaluation of the function of the lower urinary tract or to determine if there is an obstruction to normal urine outflow. During urination, the initial stream starts slowly, but almost immediately speeds up until the bladder is nearly empty. With urinary tract obstruction, the pattern of flow is altered, with increases and decreases that are more gradual (Figure 10.1). The uroflowmetry graphs this information, taking into account the patient's age and gender. It has to be remembered, though, that flow rates vary from day to day and a poor flow rate

> **Box 10.4**   Medical conditions that can alter normal flow rate.
>
> - Benign prostatic hypertrophy (BPH) – a benign enlargement of the prostate that usually occurs in men over the age of 50 years. Enlargement of the prostate interferes with normal passage of urine and can obstruct the bladder altogether if left untreated
> - Cancer of the prostate or bladder tumour
> - Urinary incontinence
> - Urinary blockage – obstruction of the urinary tract can occur for many reasons along any part of the urinary tract form the kidneys to the urethra. Urinary obstruction can lead to backflow of urine causing infection, scarring, or kidney failure if left untreated
> - Neurogenic bladder dysfunction – improper function of the bladder due to an alteration in the nervous system such as spinal cord lesion or injury
> - Frequent urinary tract infections (UTIs)

may not necessarily mean obstruction (Blandy, 1998) (Box 10.4). Nevertheless, an impaired flow rate is significant in diagnosing prostate or bladder outflow problems.

In females the normal flow rate is 20–40 mL/s and in males it is 15–30 mL/s. Accurate measurement of flow rate is facilitated by a voided volume greater than 150 mL. Patients are therefore encouraged to have a full bladder when attending for this test (Box 10.5). Uroflowmetry may be performed in conjunction with other diagnostic procedures such as cystometry.

Cystometry

Cystometry is a test of bladder function in which pressure and volume of fluid in the bladder is measured during filling, storage and voiding. A cystometry study is performed to diagnose problems with voiding, including incontinence, urinary retention and recurrent urinary tract infections (UTIs). Urinary difficulties may occur because of a weak or hyperactive bladder sphincter or detrusor, or a poor co-ordination of their two activities. Infection of the bladder or urethra may cause incontinence, as can obstruction of the urethra from scar tissue, prostate enlargement, and other benign or cancerous growths. A loss of sensation due to nerve damage can lead to chronic overfilling of the

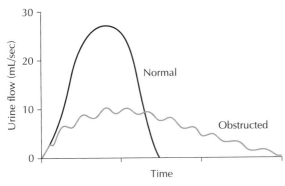

Figure 10.1   Urine flow rate graph.
(Reprinted from *Clinical Surgery*, p. 617, Henry & Thompson (2005), with permission from Elsevier)

Box 10.5   Uroflowmetry procedure.

The procedure must be explained to the patient, allowing time for any questions and to gain informed consent. No specific preparation is required prior to the procedure. The patient is asked to drink about four to five glasses of water several hours before the test is performed to ensure a full bladder. This process may be started at home or when the patient attends a special outpatient clinic (flow clinic). If the process is started at home, the patient is requested not to empty his or her bladder before arriving at the clinic for the procedure.

If the patient is pregnant, she needs to advise medical staff. The patient should also advise a health professional if any current medications, either prescription, over the counter and any herbal supplements, are being taken.

The patient advises the staff when they have a feeling of bladder fullness and the need to void. They are then instructed on how to use the flowmeter device. When ready to void, the patient presses the flowmeter start button and then counts 5 seconds before voiding into a funnel device that is attached to a commode. The flowmeter will record information as the patient is voiding. When finished, the patient waits a further 5 seconds then presses the flowmeter button again. They are asked not to put toilet paper into the funnel device.

Post-procedure
When the patient has emptied his/her bladder a bladder scan can be undertaken to assess residual volume.

Box 10.6   Cystometrogram procedure.

The patient should arrive for the CMG with a full bladder, the procedure is explained and informed consent gained. The patient is asked to void urine into the flow rate machine, and the time required to begin voiding and the size, force and continuity of the urinary system is recorded. The amount of urine, how long voiding took and the presence of straining, hesitancy and dribbling are also recorded.

The patient is asked to lie down and a double-lumen catheter is inserted with one lumen for pressure measurement and the other for filling the bladder. The pressure lumen is filled with water and connected to a pressure transducer wired to a recorder. The filling lumen is connected to room temperature normal saline via an administration set.

The bladder pressure line records the intravesical pressure. A rectal line is inserted to exclude a pressure

rise due to an extravesical component due to straining or coughing. This line can record the intra-abdominal pressure separately, which is later subtracted from the intravesical pressure, giving the detrusor pressure. Once both the catheter and the rectal lines are in situ and flushed with water, the patient is asked to cough to raise the abdominal pressure and therefore the total bladder pressure. The detrusor pressure should not rise.

The patient is asked to identify when the first sensation of bladder filling is felt and the volume is noted. The filling continues and the patient is then asked to advise staff when he feels a strong urge to void and the instilled volume is recorded.

The patient may be required to jog on the spot or the taps turned on to induce leakage, whereupon the cystometer will record the pressure at the point when the leakage occurred.

---

bladder. A pressure flow study with imaging is known as a cystometrogram (CMG).

Cystometrogram (CMG)

Cystometrogram provides information regarding the normal bladder function, and about obstruction either of the nerves supplying the bladder or the bladder muscle. The procedure measures changes in the bladder as it fills, the total bladder capacity and the presence of any residual urine after the bladder has contracted. Box 10.6 explains the cystometrogram procedure.

Cystometrogram might indicate a cause for UTIs, diminished bladder capacity, multiple sclerosis,

cerebrovascular accident, spinal cord injury, bladder outlet obstruction or an overactive bladder. If the patient has a current UTI, there is an increase in the possibility of a false result. The test itself may increase the possibility of spreading infection and may cause some haematuria.

Urological imaging

Kidney–ureter–bladder (KUB)

This plain radiographic image is useful for examining the position of the structures and identifying calculi (stones), the majority of which are

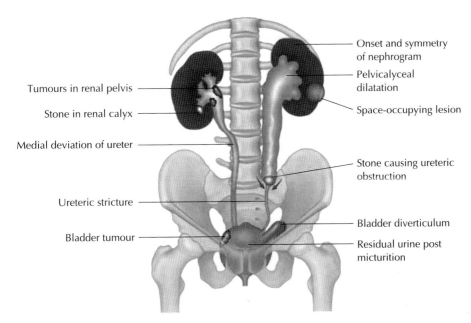

Tumours in renal pelvis

Stone in renal calyx

Medial deviation of ureter

Ureteric stricture

Bladder tumour

Onset and symmetry of nephrogram

Pelvicalyceal dilatation

Space-occupying lesion

Stone causing ureteric obstruction

Bladder diverticulum

Residual urine post micturition

Figure 10.2   Guide to intravenous urogram interpretation.
(Reprinted from *Clinical Surgery*, p. 593, Henry & Thompson (2005), with permission from Elsevier)

radio-opaque. Generally two images are taken from the anterior and posterior aspects, each with the patient in a standing position. This film is often used prior to an intravenous urogram (IVU).

Intravenous urogram (IVU)

An intravenous urogram (IVU) is used to obtain a more detailed anatomical assessment of the urinary tract. Following an initial film, a radio-opaque contrast medium is given intravenously and then a series of X-rays are taken at timed intervals following injection. This allows visualisation of the kidneys, ureters and bladder and is useful in identifying any kidney or bladder masses. Figure 10.2 presents a guide to the interpretation of an intravenous urogram.

Urethrogram

A urethrogram is an X-ray in which X-ray contrast dye is instilled up the urethra and the area is viewed on the X-ray screen to check anatomical integrity. This is potentially a very uncomfortable procedure for the patient, as the usual process is for the patient to have a catheter inserted part-way and the balloon inflated inside the urethra. This blocks

the urethra and prevents any contrast dye from escaping, thus enabling X-rays to be taken of the ascending urethra. It is likely that the patient will suffer localised trauma and may pass some blood post-procedure.

Cystogram

Cystography uses X-rays and contrast dyes to study the bladder, enabling the urologist to check the structure of the bladder while identifying disorders such as tumours, infections and stones. A catheter is inserted through the patient's urethra and the dye is injected through the catheter into the bladder. A series of X-rays are taken, usually at various stages of filling and from various angles to enable full visualisation of the bladder. Additional films are taken after drainage of the dye (known as a voiding cystourethrography). The procedure takes about an hour and a half.

Computed tomography (CT scan)

CT scans are widely used to provide a detailed image of any masses or calcification within the body. The scan provides information regarding the density of various tissues at different levels within the body. Very effective in helping to stage cancer, the scan is used in the identification and evaluation of renal, ureteric and bladder tumours. They are not, however, very effective in the identification of prostate carcinoma. CT scanning is also used to provide images of the abdomen, chest and lymph nodes to indicate any metastatic spread (Fillingham & Douglas, 2004).

Magnetic resonance imaging (MRI scan)

For a more detailed scan of the prostate gland, including effective assessment and staging of a tumour, the urologist may opt for an MRI rather than a CT scan. The indications for an MRI are the same as for CT scanning and may be chosen over CT scanning as there is no requirement for the use of contrast media.

Bone scan

One of the primary sites for metastatic disease in prostate cancer is bone, and therefore the patient is likely to undergo a plain abdominal X-ray and an isotopic bone scan. For the bone scan the patient is intravenously injected with an isotopic agent and then, approximately three hours later, scans of the entire skeletal structure are taken. A bone scan will demonstrate increased blood supply in areas of malignancy, as tumour development depends on a good blood supply. This must be viewed with caution, though, as many elderly men suffer from arthritis and may have suffered fractured ribs in the past (Blandy, 1998), which can cause a false positive result due to the altered vasculature.

Transrectal ultrasonography (TRUS) and biopsy

Ultrasonography is cheap, painless and uses no dangerous contrast media. Transrectal ultrasonography (TRUS) is an effective way of gaining accurate information regarding the amount of growth and density of the prostate. This is an extremely useful aid in the staging of prostatic carcinoma as the size, shape and infiltration of the prostate gland can be assessed. Urologists also use TRUS to obtain samples of the prostate gland core for histological analysis. An ultrasound probe is inserted into the rectum to enable accurate guidance of a biopsy needle where six to ten biopsies are taken depending on the size and volume of the gland. Post-procedure

rectal bleeding is a risk and the patient must be closely monitored for this.

Cystoscopy

Cystoscopy allows direct visualisation of the urethra and internal surface of the bladder and is a very common investigative procedure in urological services. If a flexible cystoscope is used, the patient does not require an anaesthetic. However, a rigid cystoscopy is carried out under general anaesthetic and sometimes forms the first part of any prostate or bladder surgery. Once the cystoscope has traversed the urethra into the bladder, biopsies can be taken for histological analysis. It is also possible to obtain an internal view of the ureters and renal pelvis through the use of a ureteroscope, a smaller and thinner version of a cystoscope. This procedure also allows tissue samples to be taken and fine catheters can be passed into the ureters to allow medical imaging – a retrograde ureterogram.

Urinary stone disease

Applied pathophysiology

The incidence of urinary stones in the United Kingdom is approximately 2–3% of the population and more common in males than in females by a ratio of 3:1 (Alexander *et al.*, 2000). A surgical stone is defined as a stone that is symptomatic: either causing obstruction or with the potential to cause obstruction, or is a source of infection (Tolley & Segura, 2002).

Stone formation is a complex process that involves the combination of crystals and other miscellaneous material, and is usually of an unknown cause. Most commonly patients with a stone-forming tendency have abnormal crystallisation in the urine (Fillingham & Douglas, 2004). This tendency to crystallisation is enhanced by diseases that lead to increased concentrations of solutes in the urine, such as calcium, oxalate, amino acids (for example, cystine) and urates. This leads to five major types of stones (see Box 10.7). Other potential causes are the presence of another fragment of stone or of a foreign body such as a urinary catheter.

The increased concentration of solutes leads to precipitation in the urine and formation of a nucleus or matrix. This promotes further precipitation and enlargement of the stone (Walsh, 2002). Renal colic, typically characterised by the sudden onset of severe pain radiating from the flank to the groin, is most commonly caused by the passage of calculi through the urinary tract. The pain of renal colic is due to obstruction of urinary flow, with subsequent increasing wall tension in the urinary tract. Rising pressure in the renal pelvis stimulates the local synthesis and release of prostaglandins and subsequent vasodilation induces a diuresis, which further increases intrarenal pressure. Prostaglandins also work directly on the ureter to induce spasm of the smooth muscle.

Pre-operative assessment, monitoring and preparation

Most renal calculi pass spontaneously and so management should focus on rapid pain relief, confirmation of the diagnosis and recognition of complications requiring immediate intervention.

Both non-steroidal anti-inflammatory drugs (NSAIDs) and opioids provide pain relief in acute renal colic, both alone and in combination. Other pre-operative nursing priorities include monitoring urine output for volume, haematuria and passage of stones. Urine should be sieved from a plastic bottle or bedpan as it is possible that any excreted stones could 'stick' to the cardboard versions.

Surgical procedures

Insertion of nephrostomy tube

A nephrostomy is a surgical procedure by which a tube, stent or catheter is inserted through the skin and into the kidney and is undertaken to relieve obstruction and subsequent renal damage. Firstly, the patient is given an anaesthetic to numb the area where the tube will be inserted. A needle is then inserted into the kidney. The needle is guided to the correct place either under ultrasound or CT guidance. A guide wire is inserted following the needle and then the tube follows the guide wire to its proper location. The tube is secured by tying a suture located at the distal end (outside the body). When this suture is tightened the end of the tube in the kidney curls up and for this reason the tube is often called a 'pig-tail' drain. A bag is connected to the end of the drain that collects the urine. The procedure usually takes one to two hours.

Retrograde stent insertion

Ureteric double-J stents are frequently used in urological practice. This includes patients with a stricture at the vesico-ureteric junction due to a blockage of urine from the kidney, or scarring from the presence of a stone narrowing the ureter. The stent tube drains urine from the kidney to the bladder. Symptoms may include tiredness, nausea and anorexia due to the build-up of salts in the bloodstream that the kidneys would normally have filtered out. Permanent kidney damage may occur if the condition is ignored.

The ureteric stent is a specially designed hollow plastic tube, which is flexible enough to be placed into the urinary system (bladder or ureter). It can be left in situ for 6–8 months and can then either be removed or replaced. The stent is inserted under general anaesthetic via a cystoscope. It is placed into the ureter and kidney via the opening of the ureter in the bladder. If a nephrostomy tube is already in situ, the stent may be inserted from the kidney to the bladder.

Ureteroscopic removal

Following a general anaesthetic, a camera is inserted through the urethra into the bladder and then moved up into the ureter until it reaches the stone. A basket-type attachment is inserted alongside the camera and passed along to the stone where the basket is opened, put around the stone and closed. The basket is then removed from the ureters, bladder and urethra, with the stone inside. This is normally a straightforward procedure and is useful for small stones that are not too far up the ureters.

> **Box 10.8**   Complications of lithotripsy.
>
> - Bleeding
> - Infection
> - Anaesthetic risks
> - Temporary decreased kidney function
> - Incomplete breakup of stone, requiring further procedures

Extracorporeal shock wave lithotripsy (ESWL)

Lithotripsy is used to break up renal stones with sound waves. The fragments of stone are then passed in the urine. The process uses a device called a lithotripter. One type makes sound waves, whilst the other makes ultrasound waves. These travel easily through soft tissues of the body without causing damage. The stones absorb the energy from these waves and break up. Stone fragments are then passed with the urine. The procedure is done under X-ray or ultrasound guidance to localise the stone during the procedure. The treatment itself is not painful, but passing the stone fragments can be. Certain types of stones will respond to this treatment better than others. Box 10.8 lists the complications of lithotripsy.

Post-operative management and care

Care of nephrostomy tube

If a nephrostomy tube is inserted as an outpatient the patient is expected to stay in hospital for up to 12 hours after the procedure to make sure the tube is functioning properly. Inpatients may stay in the hospital several days. Soreness at the insertion site is not unusual for up to one week post-insertion.

As the nephrostomy tube is located in the patient's back, it is usual for them to require assistance with its care. The nephrostomy tube should be kept dry and protected from water when taking showers. The skin around it should be kept clean, and the dressing over the area changed frequently. Strict aseptic technique is vital when dealing with the nephrostomy tube and changing the surrounding dressing as the tube provides a direct entry for bacteria to the kidney and patients are very susceptible to infection.

Care of double-J stent

Following insertion of a double-J stent, an X-ray may be taken to ensure that it is in the correct position. The various complications of the procedure include possible increase in frequency of micturition, an irritation similar to a urinary infection, a mild increase in the need to void urine with urgency, a sensation of incomplete emptying of the bladder, haematuria and a small risk of a stone forming around the site of the stent.

These complications may be reduced by maintaining a good fluid intake of between 1.5 to 2 litres of fluid daily. The patient may experience pain and discomfort in the pelvis and kidney area, which may be worse at the end of their stream.

Prostate obstruction

Applied pathophysiology

Benign prostatic hyperplasia

Benign prostatic hyperplasia (BPH) is an enlargement of the prostate gland that over time causes varying degrees of irritative and/or obstructive symptoms (see Box 10.9). Hyperplasia is the term used to describe an increased production and growth of normal cells and in BPH nodules form and grow in the inner portion of the gland. This, in conjunction with atrophy of the smooth muscle segments, leads to hypertrophy of the gland (Gutierrez & Peterson, 2002). Hypertrophy refers to the increase in size of an organ or gland brought about by the enlargement of its cells rather than by cell multiplication and sometimes BPH is described as benign prostatic hypertrophy (see Figure 10.3).

The cause of BPH is unknown but the condition is thought to develop due to fluctuating levels of

> **Box 10.9**   Symptoms of BPH/prostate carcinoma.
>
> | **Irritative** | **Obstructive** |
> | --- | --- |
> | - Urgency | - Slow urinary flow |
> | - Frequency | - Incomplete emptying |
> | - Nocturia | - Hesitancy |
> | - Haematuria | - Post-micturition |
> | (carcinoma) | dribble |
> | - Urinary infection | - Dysuria |

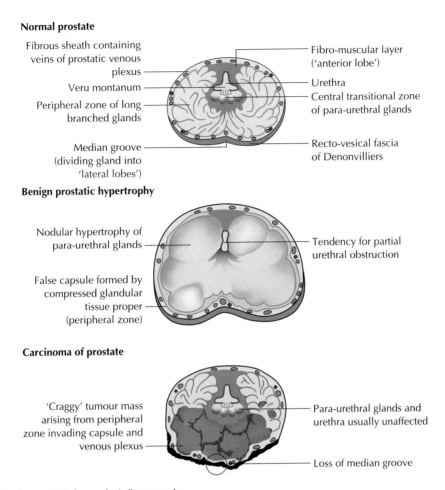

Normal prostate

Fibrous sheath containing veins of prostatic venous plexus

Fibro-muscular layer ('anterior lobe')

Veru montanum

Urethra

Peripheral zone of long branched glands

Central transitional zone of para-urethral glands

Median groove (dividing gland into 'lateral lobes')

Recto-vesical fascia of Denonvilliers

Benign prostatic hypertrophy

Nodular hypertrophy of para-urethral glands

Tendency for partial urethral obstruction

False capsule formed by compressed glandular tissue proper (peripheral zone)

Carcinoma of prostate

'Craggy' tumour mass arising from peripheral zone invading capsule and venous plexus

Para-urethral glands and urethra usually unaffected

Loss of median groove

Figure 10.3 Benign prostatic hyperplasia/hypertrophy.
(Reprinted from *Essential Surgery*, 'Chapter 29, Diseases of the Prostate', Figure 10.1, Burkitt & Quick (2001), with permission from Elsevier)

androgen and oestrogen (Henry & Thompson, 2005). Testosterone, primarily produced by the testes, is converted in the prostate by the enzyme 5-alpha-reductase to dihydrotestosterone (DHT) (Figure 10.4). This is the most active androgen in the prostate and is a steroid hormone responsible for the development of the male sex organs and male secondary sexual characteristics. Increased levels of testosterone possibly lead to increased levels of DHT and, although this is necessary for normal prostate growth, its role in the development of BPH remains unclear (Gutierrez & Peterson, 2002).

Carcinoma of the prostate

Most prostatic carcinomas are adenocarcinomas that, in contrast to BPH, begin at the periphery of the prostate gland (Gutierrez & Peterson, 2002). The tumours are usually slow growing and confined to the prostatic capsule (see Figure 10.5). As with BPH, the cause of prostate cancer is unknown; however, it is thought that there could be a hormonal influence in the transformation of normal cells into cancerous ones (Alexander *et al.*, 2000). Prostate cancer has the potential to spread either locally, in the periprostatic and perirectal soft

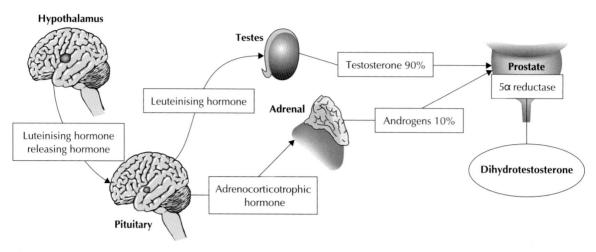

Figure 10.4   Hormonal control of prostate gland.
(Reprinted from *Clinical Surgery*, p. 630, Henry & Thompson (2005), with permission from Elsevier)

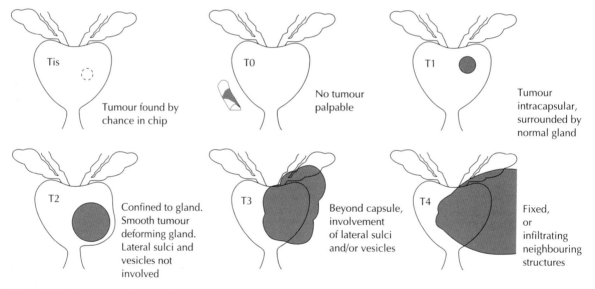

Figure 10.5   Carcinoma of the prostate.
(Reprinted from *Lecture Notes on Urology*, p. 208, Blandy (1998), with permission from Blackwell)

tissues, via the lymphatic system to the iliac and para-aortic nodes, or via the blood, primarily to the bone (Henry & Thompson, 2005).

Diagnosis of the disease is difficult, as the patient is often asymptomatic and symptoms only develop when the disease is advanced. At this stage the patient is likely to exhibit haematuria plus symptoms similar to those shown in patients with BPH. In advanced disease the patient may also exhibit the symptoms of metastatic disease – bone pain and

leg swelling from lymphatic obstruction (Henry & Thompson, 2005).

Carcinoma of the bladder

Applied pathophysiology

Tumours of the bladder occur more commonly in men than in women (4:1 ratio) (Alexander *et al.*,

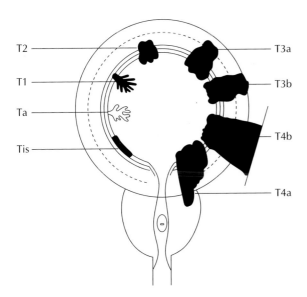

T2

T1

Ta

Tis

T3a

T3b

T4b

T4a

Figure 10.6 Carcinoma of the bladder.
(Reprinted from *Lecture Notes on Urology*, p. 164, Blandy
(1998), with permission from Blackwell)

2000). Approximately 95% of all tumours are malignant and the remaining 5% have a tendency to recur following what appears to be successful treatment. Several histological types of tumour can arise in the bladder but transitional cell carcinoma (TCC) accounts for almost 90% (Bailey & Sarosdy, 1999) (Figure 10.6). These tumours arise from the epithelial lining and can be categorised into papillary and superficial (70–75%) or solid and invasive (20–25%). Another type, carcinoma in situ (CIS), will occur in approximately 10% of cases (Bailey & Sarosdy, 1999). This is a flat intraepithelial malignant tumour that either occurs as an isolated lesion (primary CIS) or in association with either papillary or solid tumours (secondary CIS).

The first symptom that a patient will exhibit is usually intermittent painless haematuria, or cystitis. Other symptoms such as dysuria and frequency may present but unfortunately many men opt not to report these symptoms to their GP due the embarrassment. If the tumour is low in the bladder, it may partially obstruct the urethral orifice and cause hesitancy and a weakened urinary stream. If the tumour obstructs the ureteral orifice eventually the patient may complain of pain associated with hydronephrosis. Box 10.10 lists bladder cancer symptoms related to the location of the tumour.

Box 10.10   Bladder cancer symptoms and location of tumour.

- Intermittent painless haematuria
- Cystitis
- Dysuria
- Urinary frequency

If the tumour is low in the bladder:

- Partial obstruction of urethra causing hesitancy and weakened stream

If the tumour is higher and obstructs the ureteral orifice:

- Pain associated with hydronephrosis

Pre-operative assessment, monitoring and preparation for patients undergoing prostate and bladder surgery

Chapter 1 has discussed the general principles of pre-operative assessment and preparation of the patient for surgery. Patients who are to undergo prostate or bladder surgical procedures also require some specific assessment and preparation, as detailed within this section.

International Prostate Symptom Score (IPSS)

Although several scoring systems have been developed, the IPSS is the most commonly used tool, although many practitioners find this tool too cumbersome and difficult for the patient to understand (see Table 10.1). This scoring system enables practitioners to evaluate the symptoms experienced by the patient in order to determine how severe the problem is and how much of an impact it is posing on the patient's quality of life.

Grading and staging

Once the diagnosis of either prostate or bladder cancer has been confirmed, assessment of the extent of the tumour is necessary to indicate the patient's prognosis and decide on the best treatment plan (Jones, 2003; Templeman, 2003). Prostate and bladder cancers are staged using the tumour–nodes–metastases (TNM) system. The grading systems vary. For prostate tumours the Gleason method, which is based on the glandular pattern of

Table 10.1   International Prostate Symptom Score (IPSS)

	Not at all	Less than 1 time in 5	Less than half the time	About half the time	More than half the time	Almost always	Your score
Incomplete emptying Over the past month, how often have you had a sensation of not emptying your bladder completely after you have finished urinating?	0	1	2	3	4	5	
Frequency Over the past month, how often have you had to urinate again less than two hours after you had finished urinating?	0	1	2	3	4	5	
Intermittency Over the past month, how often have you found you stopped and started again several times when you urinated?	0	1	2	3	4	5	
Urgency Over the last month, how difficult have you found it to postpone urination?	0	1	2	3	4	5	
Weak stream Over the past month, how often have you had a weak urinary stream?	0	1	2	3	4	5	
Straining Over the past month, how often have you had to push or strain to begin urination?	0	1	2	3	4	5	

	None	1 time	2 times	3 times	4 times	5 times or more	Your score
Nocturia Over the past month, how many times did you most typically get up to urinate from the time you went to bed until the time you got up in the morning?	0	1	2	3	4	5	

Total IPSS score	

Interpretation of symptoms according to total score: 0–7 mild
8–19 moderate
20–35 severe

Quality of life due to urinary symptoms	Delighted	Pleased	Mostly satisfied	Mixed – about equally satisfied and dissatisfied	Mostly dissatisfied	Unhappy	Terrible
If you were to spend the rest of your life with your urinary condition the way it is now, how would you feel about that?	0	1	2	3	4	5	6

the tumour and the expected rate of growth, is used (Templeman, 2003). For bladder tumours there is a three-grade system that has been adopted by the majority of pathologists that scores the degree of cell differentiation (Bailey & Sarosdy, 1999).

Catheterisation

Many patients will require the insertion of a catheter pre-operatively, particularly if they have been admitted with urinary retention. Often these patients will be discharged home with the catheter in situ to await surgery. If the emergency patient is catheterised and is passing haematuria they will require catheterisation with a three-way catheter to allow for bladder irrigation. Once the urine is clear the catheter will be changed to a long-term one and the patient will be discharged to await surgery if this is required.

General issues

Due to the high risk of haemorrhage following prostate and bladder surgery, it is important that patients who are on anticoagulation therapy, warfarin for example, are identified. Often these patients are admitted to the ward several days before their surgery so that they can stop taking their medication and be treated with a low molecular weight anticoagulant. Pre-operative coagulation screening is an important aspect of pre-operative preparation for patients undergoing prostate or bladder surgery and ideally the patient should have an International Normalised Ratio (INR) of less than 1.0 prior to going into theatre (see Box 10.11).

Box 10.11 International Normalised Ratio.

Prothrombin time (PT) is the time taken for blood clotting to occur in a sample of blood to which calcium and thromboplastin have been added. This is standardised with the International Normalised Ratio (INR), allowing for uniform measurement of the anticoagulation status for patients.

It is generally accepted that an INR of at least 2.0 is required for effective anticoagulation.

The risk of bleeding increases with an increasing INR, and may increase dramatically above an INR of 4.5–5.0; therefore patients undergoing surgery are usually required to have an INR of below 1.0.

Should the patient suffer extensive blood loss following surgery it is likely that they will require a blood transfusion to prevent them becoming haemodynamically unstable. To prevent post-operative anaemia the patient must have an adequate haemoglobin level pre-operatively and correction of any pre-operative anaemia is imperative.

Surgical procedures

There are various surgical procedures for benign prostatic hyperplasia, prostate carcinoma and carcinoma of the bladder. This section considers the most common procedures and provides an explanation of the surgery.

Rigid cystoscopy

A rigid cystoscopy is a telescopic examination of the bladder and the urethra and is performed immediately prior to prostate and bladder surgery. The patient is placed in the lithotomy position (see Chapter 2) and the cystoscope is passed along the urethra into the bladder. A rigid cystoscope has an instrument channel that allows a variety of instruments to be inserted into the bladder (Blandy, 1998). This means that a number of procedures can be performed, including the taking of biopsies and the resection of tumours.

Transurethral resection of the prostate (TURP)

A TURP is performed to 'hollow out' the inside of the prostate and open up the urethral lumen to allow clearer passage for the drainage of urine. Following the insertion of a rigid cystoscope, a resectoscope is passed into the urethra and small sections of the prostate are chipped away. Carried out under general or spinal anaesthetic, depending on the overall physical status of the patient and the presence of concurrent disease, the procedure takes approximately 30 minutes (Basketter, 2002). During the procedure the area is continuously flushed out with irrigation fluid, usually glycine. This is to enable an adequate view of the prostate throughout surgery (Steggall, 1999). Glycine is generally used as it is an isotonic and non-electrolyte solution. This is vital for patient safety as diathermy is used to cauterise the bleeding points during surgery. The principle of diathermy is the production

Table 10.2   The TNM staging system for prostate cancer.

Tumour (T)		Nodes (N)		Metastasis (M)	
TX	Primary tumour cannot be assessed	NX	Regional lymph nodes cannot be assessed	MX	Presence of distant metastasis cannot be assessed
T0	No evidence of primary tumour	N0	No regional lymph node metastasis		
T1	Clinically inapparent tumour not palpable or visible by imaging			M0	No distant metastasis
T1a	Tumour incidental histological finding in 5% or less of tissue resected	N1	Metastasis in a single lymph node, 2 cm or less in greatest dimensions	M1	Distant metastasis
				M1a	Non-regional lymph nodes
T1b	Tumour incidental histological finding in more than 5% of tissue resected	N2	Metastasis in a single lymph node, more than 2 cm but not more than 5 cm in greatest dimension, or multiple lymph nodes, none more than 5 cm in greatest dimension	M1b	Bone
T1c	Tumour identified by needle biopsy			M1c	Other sites
T2	Palpable tumour confined within prostate				
T2a	Tumour involves half of a lobe or less				
T2b	Tumour involves more than half of a lobe, but not both lobes				
T2c	Tumour involves both lobes	N3	Metastasis in a lymph node more than 5 cm in greatest dimension		
T3	Tumour extends through the prostatic capsule				
T3a	*Unilateral* extracapsular extension				
T3b	*Bilateral* extracapsular extension				
T3c	Tumour invades seminal vesicle(s)				
T4	Tumour is fixed or invades adjacent structures other than seminal vesicles				
T4a	Tumour invades external sphincter and/or bladder neck and/or rectum				
T4b	Tumour invades levator muscles and/or is fixed to pelvic wall				

of heat by means of a high-frequency electric current passed between two electrodes. If during resection an electrolyte solution is used, there is a substantial risk to the patient of the electric current being translocated to other parts of the body, potentially causing cardiovascular disruption.

It is estimated that this operation carries an operative risk of less than 1% (Blandy, 1998) and approximately 80% of men will experience symptom improvement (Basketter, 2002). However, it is not without its complications.

Retropubic or open prostatectomy

If the prostate is very large, open prostatectomy may be required. The entire prostate gland is removed via the abdomen. The risks are similar but greater than in TURP (Basketter, 2002).

Radical prostatectomy

If resection of the prostate is required for carcinoma, the patient may undergo a radical pros-

tatectomy. This is a major operation where the entire prostate and surrounding lymph nodes are resected using a retropubic or perineal approach (Blandy, 1998; Jones, 2003).

Laser treatment

In many district general hospitals TURP is now rarely performed due to the development of alternative treatments and minimally invasive procedures. TURP is usually only carried out when other treatments have proven ineffective or are contraindicated. In particular the use of laser surgery has 'overtaken' TURP as the surgery of choice as it has been found to reduce the risk of post-operative bleeding and other complications associated with a more invasive procedure or TURP. Dysuria and urinary tract infections are risks post-procedure. Patients undergoing laser treatment via the urethra tend to have the procedure performed in a day surgery setting as opposed to an inpatient stay thus reducing costs and trauma to the patient.

Table 10.3   The TNM staging system for bladder cancer.

Tumour (T)		Nodes (N)		Distant metastasis (M)			
TX	Primary tumour can not be assessed	NX	Regional lymph nodes can not be assessed	MX	Distant metastasis cannot be assessed		
T0	No evidence of primary tumour			M0	No distant metastasis		
Ta	Non-invasive papillary carcinoma	N0	No regional lymph node metastasis	M1	Distant metastasis		
Tis	Carcinoma in situ 'flat tumour'						
T1	Tumour invades sub-epithelial connective tissue	N1	Metastasis in a single lymph node 2 cm or less in greatest dimension	Stage 0	Ta or Tis	N0	M0
				Stage I	T1	N0	M0
T2	Tumour invades muscle			Stage II	T2a or T2b	N0	M0
T2a	Tumour invades superficial muscle (inner half)	N2	Metastasis in a single lymph node 2 cm to 5 cm or multiple lymph nodes	Stage III	T3a or T3ba or T4a	N0	M0
T2b	Tumour invades deep muscle (outer half)		not more than 5 cm in greatest dimensions	Stage IV	T4b	N0	M0
T3	Tumour invades prevesical fat				Any T	N1 to N3	M0
T3a	Microscopically	N3	Metastasis in a lymph node more than 5 cm in greatest dimension		Any T	Any N	M1
T3b	Macroscopically (extravesical lesion)						
T4	Tumour invades any of the following; prostate, uterus, vagina, pelvic wall, or abdominal wall						
T4a	Tumor invades prostate, uterus or vagina						
T4b	Tumor invades pelvic wall or abdominal wall						

Transurethral resection of a bladder tumour (TURBT)

A TURBT is the mainstay of treatment, particularly for patients with limited disease. If the tumour is small, solid and muscle-invasive, complete resection is possible and often patients do not require further treatment other than regular cystoscopic surveillance (Bailey & Sarosdy, 1999).

The procedure follows the same process as a TURP. The patient will have a general or spinal anaesthetic followed by insertion of a rigid cystoscope and resectoscope and the tumour is cut away from the bladder wall. Again, there are a number of complications with this procedure, which will be discussed in the next section.

Cystectomy and formation of ileal conduit

A patient with invasive bladder carcinoma may require a total cystectomy and urinary diversion, the most common of which is the formation of an ileal conduit (Alexander *et al.*, 2000). This procedure involves the excision of the lower ureters, bladder, prostate, seminal vesicles and urethra in men and also the uterus, ovaries, fallopian tubes and vaginal vault in women. Patients must be made

aware that sexual function is usually lost in both sexes following this radical resection.

To form an ileal conduit, the surgeon removes a segment of the ileum with an intact blood supply, and creates an anastomosis between the open ends of the ileum to restore intestinal continuity (Walsh, 2002). One end of the resected ileal portion is closed and the other is brought through the abdominal wall to create a stoma. The detached ends of the ureters are then anastomosed to the isolated section of the ileum and a stoma bag is placed over the exposed stoma (Figure 10.7).

In some cases it is possible to perform reconstructive surgery and use bladder substitutes in place of urinary diversion (Alexander *et al.*, 2000). This would involve part of the intestine being directly anastomosed to the urethra to provide a reservoir for the urine.

Post-operative management and care

Patients undergoing prostate and bladder surgery will require general post-operative care. There are, however, several issues that are specific to the post-operative management and care of patients undergoing prostate and bladder surgery and these

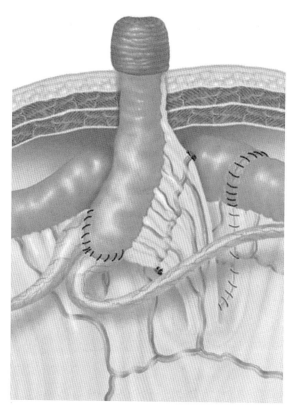

Figure 10.7 Ileal conduit.
(Reprinted from *Clinical Surgery*, p. 615, Henry & Thompson (2005), with permission from Elsevier)

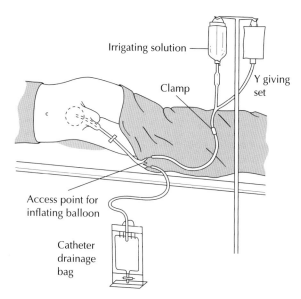

Figure 10.8 Bladder irrigation.
(Reprinted from *Marsden Manual of Clinical Nursing Procedures*, p. 125, Mallet & Dougherty (2000), with permission from Blackwell)

are considered here. The overall principles of post-operative management have been discussed in Chapter 3 and these should be considered alongside the information presented here.

Bladder irrigation

There is a risk following prostate or bladder surgery that patients could develop clot retention leading to obstruction of the urethra, or, if catheterised, the catheter lumen. To prevent this relatively common post-operative complication, bladder irrigation is used (Scholtes, 2002).

A sterile fluid is continuously instilled into the bladder through a three-way catheter. This is a large indwelling catheter that has three separate channels – one for the instillation of the irrigation fluid, one for the drainage of the urine and one to enable the inflation of the retaining balloon (Scholtes, 2002). The catheter allows the simultan-

eous entry and drainage of fluid out of the bladder (Figure 10.8).

The rate of administration of the irrigation fluid is dependent on the colour of the urine. The darker the urine, often referred to as claret-coloured (Scholtes, 2002), the more heavily blood-stained it is and the faster the irrigation needs to be delivered. As the urine begins to lighten, the bleeding is slowing and the irrigation rate can be reduced. This titration continues until the urine is only slightly blood-stained. The patient is advised to drink plenty of fluids following the surgery and particularly following discontinuation of the irrigation.

The recommended irrigation fluid is normally 0.9% sodium chloride; it is the mechanical action of the fluid that removes and dislodges any clots rather than the properties of the sodium chloride (Steggall, 1999). Water is not recommended due to the risk that it could be absorbed via the severed prostatic veins and the patient could develop transurethral resection (TUR) syndrome (see later).

Bladder lavage

Occasionally during bladder irrigation, a small blood clot becomes trapped in the eye of the

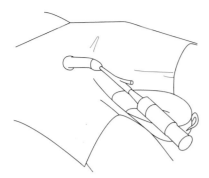

Figure 10.9   Bladder lavage.
(Reprinted from *Lecture Notes on Urology*, p. 203, Blandy (1998), with permission from Blackwell)

catheter preventing the bladder from draining. This will lead to the patient displaying the clinical manifestations of urinary retention. The instillation of the irrigation fluid is immediately stopped until the blockage has been cleared. It is possible to dislodge the clot by increasing the pressure within the lumen of the catheter by either squeezing the catheter tube or 'milking' it using milking tongs (Lowthian, 1991, cited in Scholtes, 2002). If this is unsuccessful, bladder lavage will be necessary.

Bladder lavage, or a bladder washout, is the instillation of fluid via a syringe or prepacked solution into the bladder to flush away any debris or dissolve any encrustation (Rew, 1999) (Figure 10.9). In this case water is generally used as the fluid will drain from the bladder immediately after instillation and therefore there is limited time for any absorption of the lavage fluid. If the fluid fails to drain from the bladder, gentle suction can be applied to the syringe. However, care needs to be taken not to suck the urothelium into the eye of the catheter causing pain, trauma and possibly infection (Baxter, 2000).

Intravesical therapy

Intravesical chemotherapy may be used after transurethral resection of a bladder tumour to prevent local recurrence of disease. The chemotherapeutic agent is instilled into the bladder via a catheter and the patient is requested to retain the solution for at least an hour (Bailey & Sarosdy, 1999). Usually the catheter is left in situ and a 'gate' clamp is used to prevent the bladder from draining. During the hour the patient must move around to ensure that all inner surfaces of the bladder are coated. The solution is then voided normally. Care needs to be taken when removing commode pans or emptying catheter bags following the administration of the solution due to its toxic nature. This type of therapy is effective when administered following TURBT and then at weekly intervals; however, clinical trials have found that the administration of BCG immunotherapy is superior (Bailey & Sarosdy, 1999).

BCG (Bacillus Calmette-Guérin) is commonly known as a vaccine that is given to protect people from tuberculosis, but it can also be used as an immunotherapeutic agent (Cumisky, 2000). BCG is instilled into the bladder and stimulates local activation of the immune system. This promotes an inflammatory response and results in the elimination or reduction in the number of superficial cancerous cells.

Due to the implications for health and safety and risk of cross-infection, intravesical therapy should only be administered by suitably qualified practitioners – usually the urology nurse practitioner or clinical nurse specialist.

Specific urological post-operative complications

Acute complications following prostate or bladder surgery are primarily concerned with loss of blood. The risk of haemorrhage is high, particularly following prostatic surgery, due to the highly vascular nature of the prostate and the fact that during surgery the prostatic veins are severed. Careful monitoring of the patient's vital signs and urine colour is necessary to identify the early signs of haemorrhage.

Blood loss could lead to the patient becoming anaemic and requiring a blood transfusion. The majority of patients will be cross-matched for at least two units of leucocyte-depleted red blood cells (LDRBC) pre-operatively.

One particular complication specific to transurethral resection of the prostate is that of transurethral resection syndrome (TUR syndrome). The syndrome has a 7% incidence and 1% mortality rate (Gnahem & Ward, 1990, cited in Steggall, 1999). It is believed that this syndrome develops as a result of irrigation fluid, usually glycine, being absorbed into the severed prostatic veins during the procedure, causing haemodilution (Steggall,

Box 10.12 Clinical manifestations of TUR syndrome.

- Cardiovascular effects
  - ○ Chest pain
  - ○ Hyper- and hypotension
  - ○ Bradycardia
- Electrocardiographic (ECG) changes
- Central nervous system effects
  - ○ Generalised seizures
  - ○ Restlessness
  - ○ Confusion
  - ○ Nausea
  - ○ Vomiting
  - ○ Headache
- Visual disturbances

Box 10.13 Potential complications of prostate and bladder surgery.

- Anxiety
- Pain
- Perforation of the bladder wall
- Urinary tract infection
- Urethral stricture
- Urinary retention
- Urinary incontinence
- Impotence
- Retrograde ejaculation

1999). This is known as intravascular absorption and leads to hyponatraemia. There is also the possibility of extravascular absorption whereby the irrigation fluid accumulates in the retroperitoneal spaces. This syndrome can result in a variety of clinical manifestations (Box 10.12).

Vigilance of the staff caring for the patient post-operatively is vital if the clinical manifestations of this syndrome are to be recognised, particularly as it can take up to 10 hours for the development of any symptoms if the cause is extravascular absorption. Treatment of the syndrome is centred on returning the sodium level in the blood plasma to the 'normal' range, through administration of saline solution and restriction of oral fluids (Steggall, 1999).

There are other complications from prostate and bladder surgery, some of which can be long-term (see Box 10.13). The patient must be made aware of these risks prior to consenting to any procedure.

Renal cancer

Pathophysiology

Cancer of the kidney can arise from the urothelium or from the tissue of the kidney itself. Tumours of the urothelium account for approximately 9% of all urothelial tumours (Fillingham & Douglas, 2004). The most common renal tumours in adults are adenocarcinomas; they are more likely to occur in men (2:1) and have a peak incidence of between 65 and 75 years of age. It is rare for patients to develop bilateral adenocarcinomas – approximately 3%. Renal tumours are staged using the TNM system and graded according to their level of differentiation.

Patients with renal tumours may present with haematuria, loin pain, an abdominal mass, recurrent fever, weight loss, hypertension and oedema. These signs and symptoms could be due to a number of conditions and therefore investigation and diagnosis is vital. The first-line investigation for patients with an abdominal mass or loin pain should be an ultrasound. With an ultrasound it is possible to distinguish between a cyst and a solid renal tumour. A CT scan will be required should a renal mass be diagnosed to look for evidence of spread. This will enable accurate staging. Biopsy of a renal tumour is not recommended due to the risk of seeding the biopsy tract (Reynard et al., 2006). Surgical management is by way of a partial or total nephrectomy.

Partial or total nephrectomy

In a partial nephrectomy only the diseased portion of the kidney is removed. In a radical nephrectomy the whole kidney is removed, along with a portion of the ureter, the adrenal gland and the fatty tissue surrounding the kidney. The patient has a general anaesthetic and the incision is made on the side or the front of the abdomen. Many urological surgeons perform laparoscopic nephrectomy where surgical instruments are manoeuvred through four small incisions and the excised kidney is removed through a larger incision in the front of the abdominal wall. This allows for a faster recovery time, shorter hospital stays and a reduction in post-operative pain. Pre-operative preparation of the nephrectomy patient will include taking a blood sample to cross-match as the patient may require a blood transfusion. The patient will also have a catheter inserted into the bladder. It is also important through pre-operative investigation to establish that the patient has two kidneys and that the kidney that will remain is healthy. Renal function tests, urinalysis, cytology, culture and sensitivity will normally be performed.

Post-operative management

One of the most important aspects of post-operative management for the nephrectomy patient is pain control. Patients often express severe pain at the site of the incision. This can be reasonably well controlled with the use of a patient-controlled analgesia system (Fillingham & Douglas, 2004). The proximity of the incision to the diaphragm may make deep breathing exercises difficult and uncomfortable and increase the patient's susceptibility to chest infections. This can often be reduced by appropriate positioning of the patient. The patient should either be in a semi-recumbent position supported by pillows or lying on their unaffected side (opposite to incision). Side lying will encourage maximum chest expansion on the side of the incision (Fillingham & Douglas, 2004).

After the excision of a kidney, it is vital that the patient's urine output is closely monitored to ensure the adequate function of the kidney that is left. Accurate maintenance of fluid input and output is imperative as well as hourly urine measurements.

Psychologically, patients need reassurance that it is perfectly possible to live with only one kidney provided that it is healthy.

Self-test questions

1. Name the structures within the urinary system, including the accessory male reproductive organs.
2. Urodynamic procedures could include measurement of four aspects – list the four aspects.
3. What do KUB and IVU stand for?
4. What are the three main focuses of renal calculi management?
5. List three aspects of nephrostomy tube care.
6. List the irritative and obstructive symptoms of benign prostatic hypertrophy.
7. What fluid is used for bladder irrigation during urological surgery and why?
8. How would you recognise if a patient had transurethral syndrome?
9. What are the potential complications of prostate and bladder surgery?
10. Briefly explain hormonal control of the prostate gland and its relation to benign prostatic hyperplasia.

Reference list and further reading

Alexander MF, Fawcett JN & Runciman PJ (2000) *Nursing Practice Hospital and Home: The Adult* (2nd edn). Edinburgh: Churchill Livingstone

American Urological Association (2003) *Prostate Cancer Screening* (online). www.urologyhealth.org/adult/index.cfm?cat=09andtopic=250 (Accessed 08.01.07)

Bailey M & Sarosdy M (1999) *Fast Facts: Bladder Cancer.* Oxford: Health Press

Basketter V (2002) Benign prostate disease. *Nursing Times Plus* 98(28): 53–54

Baxter A (2000) 'Bladder lavage and irrigation' *in*: Mallett J & Dougherty L (eds) *The Royal Marsden Hospital Manual of Clinical Procedures* (5th edn). London: Blackwell Science

Blandy J (1998) *Lecture Notes on Urology* (5th edn). London: Blackwell Publishing

Bristol Urology Associates (2004) *The International Prostate Symptom Score (IPSS)* (online). www.bristolurology.co.uk/documents/ipss.pdf (Accessed 08.01.07)

Burkitt HG & Quick CRG (2001) *Essential Surgery.* Edinburgh: Churchill Livingstone

Chambers A (2002) 'Transurethral resection syndrome – it does not have to be a mystery' *AORN* 75(1): 155–176

Cumisky S (2000) 'BCG immunotherapy for carcinoma of the urinary bladder' *Nursing Standard* 14(37): 45–47

Cuschieri A, Grace PA, Darzi A, Borley N & Rowley DI (2003) *Clinical Surgery.* Oxford: Blackwell Publishing

Fillingham S & Douglas J (2004) *Urological Nursing* (3rd edn). Edinburgh: Baillière Tindall

Gnahem AN & Ward JP (1990) 'Osmotic and metabolic sequelae of volumetric overload in relation to the TURP syndrome' *British Journal of Urology* 66(1): 71–78

Gutierrez KJ & Peterson PG (2002) *Pathophysiology.* Philadelphia: WB Saunders Company

Henry MM & Thompson JN (eds) (2005) *Clinical Surgery* (2nd edn). Edinburgh: Elsevier Saunders

Jones A (2003) 'Prostate cancer – an overview' *Cancer Nursing Practice* 2(1): 31–38

Lowthian P (1991) 'Using bladder syringes sparingly' *Nursing Times 87*: 10

Mallet J & Dougherty L (eds) (2000) *Marsden Manual of Clinical Nursing Procedures* (5th edn). Oxford: Blackwell

National Institute of Diabetes and Digestive and Kidney Diseases (online). www.kidney.niddk.nih.gov (Accessed 08.01.07)

Rew M (1999) 'Use of catheter maintenance solutions for long-term catheters' *British Journal of Nursing 8*: 11

Reynard J, Brewster S & Biers S (2006) *Oxford Handbook of Urology*. Oxford: Oxford University Press

Scholtes S (2002) 'Management of clot retention following urological surgery' *Nursing Times Plus 98*(28): 48–50

Steggall MJ (1999) 'TUR syndrome: a risk after prostatic surgery' *Professional Nurse 14*(5): 323–326

Templeman H (2003) 'The management of prostate cancer' *Nursing Standard 17*(21): 45–53

Tolley DA & Segura JW (2002) *Fast Facts: Urinary Stones*. Oxford: Health Press

Walsh M (ed.) (2002) *Watson's Clinical Nursing and Related Sciences* (6th edn). Edinburgh: Baillière Tindall

11 Women's Health

Fiona J McArthur-Rouse

Introduction

Advances in surgical and anaesthetic techniques over recent years mean that many gynaecological surgical procedures are carried out as day cases or require only a few days of inpatient care. The remit of gynaecological wards has thus evolved in many district general hospitals to include the provision of emergency services and early pregnancy assessment clinics (EPACs), colposcopy services and surgical pre-assessment clinics. In some NHS trusts they have developed into women's health centres that also provide care to women undergoing breast surgery. The main *major* surgical procedures seen in such wards include abdominal hysterectomy, salpingo-oophorectomy, ovarian cystectomy, salpingectomy, vaginal hysterectomy, anterior or posterior repairs and breast surgery. These are carried out for a variety of reasons such as malignant or benign tumours, endometriosis, urinary symptoms and ectopic pregnancy. The majority of procedures are undertaken as elective admissions; however some patients, such as those suffering from an ectopic pregnancy or ruptured ovarian cyst, may require emergency surgery. Box 11.1 identifies the aims of this chapter. Readers may find it useful to revise their knowledge of the normal structure and function of the female reproductive system at this point.

Box 11.1 Aims of the chapter.

- To explain the underlying pathophysiology of common disorders that may lead women to require major surgical intervention
- To discuss the investigations, diagnosis and surgical management of these women and their disorders
- To discuss the specific care requirements of women undergoing major surgical interventions

---

Endometriosis

Endometriosis is a common benign disease in which deposits of endometrial tissue (the lining of the uterus) are found outside of the uterine cavity. The cause is unclear but one theory proposes that during menstruation some blood flows out of the fallopian tubes into the pelvic cavity. This is known as retrograde menstruation (Barron, 2001). The displaced endometrial tissue is responsive to cyclical hormones in the same way as that in the uterine cavity and therefore bleeds at regular intervals. Ultimately, the area of bleeding may heal by the formation of scar tissue (McKay Hart & Norman, 2000) and frequently adhesions are formed to surrounding structures. Symptoms include pain, dyspareunia, menstrual disturbance and infertility.

Although the pain is not necessarily proportionate to the severity of the disease, it is often underestimated and may be severe, particularly before and during menstruation.

Diagnosis of endometriosis is usually achieved by laparoscopy and treatment will depend on the severity of the disease and the patient's desire to maintain or enhance fertility. Initially medical treatments may be offered which aim to prevent bleeding either by direct action on the endometrium or by preventing oestrogen production (Barron, 2001); however these tend to have unpleasant side-effects and the treatment can only be maintained for limited periods of time.

Patients with endometriosis may be admitted to the gynaecological ward for surgical treatment. This may be a laparoscopic procedure using a diathermy laser to eradicate lesions, or in severe cases a laparotomy, total abdominal hysterectomy, bilateral salpingo-oophorectomy, division of adhesions and possibly bowel surgery may be required. If it is suspected that the disease involves the bowel, bowel preparation may be administered pre-operatively (see Chapter 9). The pre- and post-operative management of patients undergoing total abdominal hysterectomy is discussed later in this chapter.

Uterine fibroids (fibromyomata, leiomyomas)

Uterine fibroids (fibromyomata or leiomyomas) are benign tumours that arise from the muscular wall of the uterus and sometimes the cervix. They are the most common tumours of the female genital tract, affecting 20% of women over the age of 35 and having a peak incidence between the ages of 35 and 45 (Gangar, 2001). They occur more frequently in black women and may be single or multiple.

Uterine fibroids are thought to be oestrogen-dependent, although the cause is not clearly understood. They usually grow slowly – however, pregnancy can result in increased growth whilst after the menopause growth tends to cease and they may atrophy. Malignant change can occur, but fortunately this is rare. Most fibroids occur in the body of the uterus and the location describes the type (see Figure 11.1).

a. Subserous fibroids lie beneath the serous lining of the uterus. May project from peritoneal surface and become pedunculated

b. Submucous fibroids lie beneath the endometrial lining and protrude into uterine cavity. May become polypoid

c. Intramural fibroids occur in the myometrium (muscle layer of uterus)

d. Cervical fibroids occur in the cervix

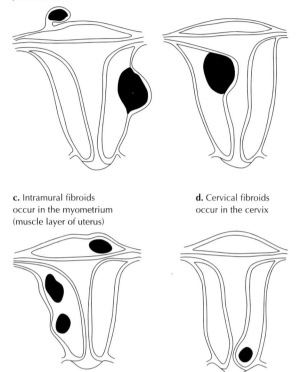

Figure 11.1   Types of uterine fibroid.

Clinical manifestations of uterine fibroids

Many women are asymptomatic even with quite large fibroids. However, depending on the location, urinary frequency and constipation can occur. Submucosal fibroids are often a cause of menorrhagia and if they become polypoid may cause dysmenorrhoea as the uterus attempts to expel them. Pain is generally associated with complications such as torsion of a polypoid fibroid, degeneration, infection or sarcomatous (malignant) change.

Investigations and diagnosis

Because they are often asymptomatic, fibroids are sometimes diagnosed during routine examination. Large fibroids may be palpable on bimanual examination and the uterus often has an irregular shape. An ultrasound scan is usually performed but does not always give a clear idea of size, number or location of the fibroid and an examination under anaesthetic may be required.

Treatment

Treatment options for uterine fibroids include medical management, embolisation procedures, surgical removal of the fibroids (myomectomy) or hysterectomy (see Box 11.2). The choice of treatment depends upon the patient's age and desire to conserve the uterus.

Total abdominal hysterectomy and bilateral salpingo-oophorectomy

Pre-operative assessment and preparation

The usual pre-operative assessment and preparation is undertaken as described in Chapter 1, including prophylactic antibiotics and antithrombotic therapy. A full blood count is taken to assess haemoglobin levels pre-operatively as these may be low due to menorrhagia. An iron supplement may be prescribed for several weeks before surgery or, if the haemoglobin level is particularly low, a blood transfusion may be required. Blood will also be taken for routine cross-matching as it may be needed during surgery. The patient should be counselled pre-operatively regarding the procedure as some patients experience great sadness at the finality of hysterectomy and the loss of fertility. Psychosocial aspects of surgery are discussed further in Chapter 5.

Post-operative considerations

The patient will usually return to the ward following surgery with an intravenous infusion (IVI) in situ, a Redivac drain, a urinary catheter and a patient-controlled analgesia pump (PCA). The usual post-operative monitoring is undertaken (see Chapter 3) with the addition of observation of vaginal blood loss, a small amount of which is normal. Early mobilisation is encouraged and the patient will usually be able to sit out of bed with assistance on the first post-operative day. Oral fluids and diet are gradually introduced and the patient must be able to tolerate adequate oral fluids

---

Box 11.2   Treatment options for uterine fibroids.

Medical management – Gonadotrophin-releasing hormone (GnRH) analogues suppress the secretion of luteinising hormone and follicle-stimulating hormone, thus causing the ovaries to reduce their production of oestrogen. Menopausal side-effects can occur and patients may require 'add-back' HRT to reduce these. Once treatment ceases the fibroids may grow back. It is sometimes used pre-operatively to shrink the fibroids before surgery.
Embolisation of uterine artery – This procedure is carried out under local anaesthesia and sedation. It involves the introduction of micro-particles into the uterine arteries to impair the blood supply to the fibroids and cause them to shrink. The procedure usually involves an overnight stay in hospital. The technique is relatively new and long-term effectiveness is still being evaluated.
Myomectomy – This is the surgical removal of the fibroids, which are 'shelled out'. It is usually performed under general anaesthetic via a transverse incision in the abdomen, although some subserosal or pedunculated fibroids may be managed laparoscopically. Following treatment the fibroids may recur. This procedure is normally used for younger women who have not completed their families, and post-operative management is the same as that for a total abdominal hysterectomy.
Total abdominal hysterectomy (TAH) – This is the most common procedure for uterine fibroids in women who have completed their families. It involves removal of the uterus and cervix and is usually performed under general anaesthesia via a transverse or *pfannenstiel* incision unless the fibroids are very large, in which case a midline incision may be required. In women who are menopausal the ovaries may also be removed (bilateral salpingo-oophorectomy).
Laparoscopic assisted vaginal hysterectomy (LAVH) – This procedure is sometimes used following shrinkage of the fibroids with GnRH. It avoids the need for an abdominal incision and thus reduces recovery time. It is performed under general anaesthetic and the procedure may take longer than an abdominal approach. The uterine vessels are ligated via the laparoscope and then the uterus is removed vaginally.

before discontinuing the IVI. Gynaecological patients are at increased risk of post-operative nausea and vomiting (PONV) and prophylactic anti-emetics should be administered regularly. Bowel preparation (if it has been administered) and long periods of pre-operative fasting followed by excessive PONV can lead to severe dehydration in these patients. Therefore, it is important to closely monitor fluid balance and ensure that intravenous infusion regimens are reviewed if necessary.

The drains, infusions and catheter are usually removed by the second day and urinary voiding patterns should be observed following removal of the catheter to ensure that the patient is not retaining urine. Early mobilisation should be encouraged to avoid post-operative complications and the use of antiembolic prophylaxis should continue until the patient is fully mobile. Patients often suffer 'post-op blues' and become very tearful around the third post-operative day. The reason for this is not clear but patients should be reassured that it is common. If there are no complications the patient is usually discharged home on the fourth or fifth post-operative day. Arrangements will need to be made for removal of staples if she is discharged with them still in situ. If the ovaries have been removed, hormone replacement therapy (HRT) may be prescribed.

Box 11.3   Types of genital prolapse and their symptoms.

Cystocele – The bladder and upper part of the anterior wall of the vagina prolapse, causing herniation between the bladder and the vagina. Symptoms include stress incontinence, dysuria, urgency and frequency of micturition.
Urethrocele – There is descent of the lower anterior vaginal wall and herniation between the urethra and vagina. It often occurs with cystocele.
Rectocele – The anterior wall of the rectum protrudes into the posterior wall of the vagina. Symptoms include difficulty emptying the rectum and feelings of rectal pressure.
Enterocele – The upper part of the vaginal wall prolapses with herniation of the pouch of Douglas. Small bowel or omentum may descend. Enterocele is often associated with uterine prolapse.
Uterine prolapse – The uterus descends below its normal level and there is inversion of the vaginal vault. The patient may feel a dragging sensation. There are three degrees of uterine prolapse:

- 1st degree – The uterus becomes retroverted and descends into the vagina but the cervix does not reach the introitus
- 2nd degree – The cervix is visible at the introitus and may appear ulcerated
- 3rd degree – The uterus descends completely and comes to lie outside of the vulva. This is sometimes referred to as procidentia.

Genital prolapse

Pathophysiology and clinical manifestations

Genital prolapse is common and tends to result from damage to the supporting structures during childbirth. The onset may be gradual or quite sudden and often occurs after the menopause when the tissues of the genital tract begin to atrophy. Box 11.3 explains the types of prolapse and their symptoms. The different types of prolapse may coexist.

Investigations and diagnosis

Diagnosis of a prolapse is usually made following vaginal examination. A Sims' speculum is sometimes used with the patient in the left lateral position.

Pre-operative assessment and preparation

If admitted as an emergency with a procidentia, it may be necessary to treat the prolapsed uterus with saline-soaked gauze. Sometimes a prolapsed uterus can be gently reduced and kept in place with a ring pessary. This is a palliative procedure that may be used if the patient is unfit for surgery or to keep her comfortable before the operation.

Patients are usually assessed in the pre-assessment clinic and prepared for surgery as discussed in Chapter 1. Because of their age special consideration needs to be given to co-morbidity, however, most older women tolerate vaginal surgery well. Following vaginal surgery for genital prolapse there is often some shortening of the vagina and the vaginal wall is tightened. Therefore, pre-operatively the surgeon ascertains whether or

---

Box 11.4 Surgical procedures undertaken for genital prolapse.

Anterior colporrhaphy – This procedure is undertaken for a cystocele and is sometimes referred to as an anterior repair. The anterior vaginal wall is opened up and the fascial layer between the cystocele and the vaginal wall is tightened with sutures. Redundant vaginal wall tissue is removed.

Posterior colpoperineorrhaphy – This is carried out for a rectocele and is often referred to as a posterior repair. It is a similar procedure to that described above; however, the posterior wall of the vagina is repaired and the procedure includes repair of the perineal muscles.

Vaginal hysterectomy – This is usually carried out for uterine prolapse and may be combined with an anterior and/or posterior repair. The uterine ligaments are stretched and divided and the uterus is removed.

---

not the patient is sexually active. This is to ensure that a functional vagina is maintained if necessary.

Treatment

Surgical procedures for genital prolapse depend on the type of prolapse and include anterior colporrhaphy, posterior colpoperineorrhaphy and vaginal hysterectomy. Box 11.4 explains these procedures, which can be carried out individually or in combination. Usually they are performed under general anesthesia but if the patient's condition precludes this, they are sometimes conducted under epidural or spinal anaesthesia (see Chapter 4).

Vaginal hysterectomy and anterior–posterior repair

Post-operative considerations

The patient normally returns to the ward post-operatively with an intravenous infusion in progress, a urinary catheter, a vaginal pack in situ and possibly a patient-controlled analgesia (PCA) pump. The usual post-operative monitoring is undertaken with the addition of observation of loss via the vaginal pack. This is a length of cream-soaked gauze that is inserted into the vagina at the end of surgery to act as a pressure dressing on the vaginal sutures. The pressure can give a sensation of bladder and bowel fullness and this should be explained to the patient, who may feel that she needs the toilet. The pack and catheter are usually removed on the first post-operative day, as are the intravenous infusion and PCA. Following their removal it is important to continue to monitor vaginal loss and ensure that the patient is able to void urine effectively. Patients who have had vaginal surgery usually recover more quickly than those who have had abdominal hysterectomies because there is no abdominal incision. They are usually able to tolerate diet and fluids more quickly too. It is not uncommon for those with good home support to be discharged on the second or third day post-operatively.

Genuine stress incontinence

Genuine stress incontinence (GSI) is the involuntary leakage of urine that occurs when the intravesical pressure (pressure within the bladder) exceeds the maximum urethral closure pressure in the absence of detrusor (bladder muscle) contraction (Rosevear, 2002). A number of surgical procedures have been developed to treat genuine stress incontinence and most aim to elevate and support the bladder neck. Burch colposuspension was the procedure of choice, but in recent years this has been superseded by the tension-free vaginal tape (TVT), which is showing comparable results and is less invasive. Box 11.5 outlines the priorities of care for patients suffering from GSI and undergoing TVT procedures.

Ectopic pregnancy

The term ectopic pregnancy refers to a pregnancy that occurs outside of the uterus. Whilst the majority (approximately 95%) occur in one or other of the fallopian tubes, usually near the ampullary

---

Box 11.5   Priorities of care for patients suffering from GSI and undergoing TVT procedures.

- Signs and symptoms of GSI can be embarrassing for the patient leading to delay in seeking help:
  - ○ Leakage of urine during coughing, sneezing, exercise, laughing
  - ○ Frequency of micturition
  - ○ Urgency and urge incontinence
- The investigations for GSI need to distinguish between genuine stress incontinence and detrusor instability (a condition in which the bladder contracts involuntarily during filling) and involve:
  - ○ Detailed history, frequency volume chart, urinalysis and midstream urine sample (MSU)
  - ○ Simple urodynamic investigation such as cystometry (see Chapter 10)

Tension-free vaginal tape (TVT) procedure – This procedure is performed under sedation and local or spinal anaesthetic via a small vaginal incision, a Prolene mesh tape is inserted as a tension-free sling on either side of the urethra and drawn through two small incisions just above the pubic bone. The tape is adjusted during a series of coughs by the patient.

Post-operative considerations
- The patient usually returns to the ward with a urinary catheter in situ and an intravenous infusion (IVI) in progress. The IVI is usually removed on return to the ward and the patient can eat and drink immediately
- If a spinal anaesthetic has been used it is necessary to wait for normal sensation to return in the lower limbs before mobilising
- The catheter is usually removed on the night of the surgery and following removal the amount of urine voided and the residual urine are measured on two or three occasions to ensure adequate voiding
- Residual urine is measured using a bladder scanner and if this is less than a third of the amount passed, this is usually considered satisfactory
- The patient is usually discharged on the day following surgery and is followed up by the urogynaecological specialist nurse

---

end, the fertilised ovum can embed in any tissue with an adequate blood supply including the ovary, cervix and peritoneal cavity (see Figure 11.2). Whilst the incidence of ectopic pregnancy is difficult to measure (Whitton *et al.*, 2001) the rate is thought to be increasing and appears to be related to the prevalence of salpingitis. Salpingitis is inflammation of the fallopian tubes that causes damage to the ciliated epithelium and produces adhesions between folds of the tube. It is usually attributed to sexually transmitted disease such as *Chlamydia trachomatis*. However, any condition that affects the patency of the fallopian tubes and slows the passage of the fertilised ovum towards the uterus will increase the likelihood of an ectopic pregnancy occurring. Box 11.6 summarises the risk factors associated with ectopic pregnancy.

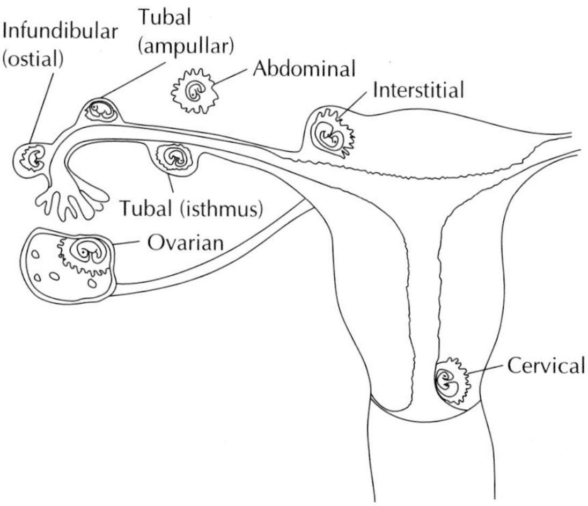

Figure 11.2   Sites of ectopic pregnancy. (Adapted from Smeltzer & Bare, 2000)

Box 11.6   Risk factors associated with ectopic pregnancy.

- Salpingitis/pelvic inflammatory disease
- Intra-uterine contraceptive devices (IUCD)
- Previous tubal surgery, including sterilisation
- Post-partum or post-abortion infection
- Endometriosis
- Migration of the ovum across the pelvis to the opposite tube
- Infertility treatments
- Past history of ectopic pregnancy

Pathophysiology

The uterus has a thick layer of decidua in which the fertilised ovum is able to embed. However, when it attempts to implant in a fallopian tube there is only a thin layer of connective tissue separating the epithelium from the muscle. Thus it is easy for the trophoblast to erode into the muscle layer of the tube where it may rupture a large blood vessel. Blood can burst into the tube or into the peritoneal cavity. Occasionally an abdominal pregnancy occurs where the developing embryo perforates the tube without causing severe haemorrhage, survives and attaches to abdominal contents. It is possible for such a pregnancy to continue to term (Clayton et al., 2000).

Clinical manifestations of ectopic pregnancy

Patients suffering from an ectopic pregnancy usually present as an emergency with abdominal pain, either via their general practitioner (GP) or the early pregnancy assessment clinic (EPAC). At this stage they may not even be aware that they are pregnant. Table 11.1 identifies the common symptoms of ectopic pregnancy.

Investigations and diagnosis

Diagnosis of ectopic pregnancy can be difficult as symptoms are similar to those of an early miscarriage, torsion or rupture of an ovarian cyst or even appendicitis. A detailed history is taken, including menstrual history, particularly any recent deviations from the patient's normal cycle. Examination may reveal a tender swelling in one lateral fornix and a slightly enlarged uterus. The patient is asked to provide a urine specimen so that a pregnancy test can be undertaken. However, if the urine is very dilute this may not be reliable. Measuring the serum levels of beta human chorionic gonadotrophin hormone (hCG) provides a more accurate assessment, however, in itself this is not definitive. In a normally progressing pregnancy the serum beta hCG levels double every 48 hours during the first six weeks of pregnancy. Levels that are lower than normal, plateau or take longer than 48 hours to double, are suggestive of ectopic pregnancy or a failing intrauterine pregnancy. The absence of beta hCG almost completely excludes a diagnosis of ectopic pregnancy.

An ultrasound scan is usually undertaken in order to locate the suspected ectopic pregnancy. Transvaginal scans are thought to provide clearer detail than abdominal scans but even these are frequently inconclusive. Colour Doppler sonography is sometimes used to identify increased blood flow to the tubal arteries, which may be indicative of an ectopic pregnancy.

Laparoscopy is the most useful method of diagnosis of ectopic pregnancy enabling the visualisation of the peritoneal cavity, uterus and fallopian tubes. However, it requires a general anaesthetic and is an invasive procedure that is best avoided if there is some chance that the pregnancy is intrauterine. For this reason monitoring of hCG levels and repeat scans may be ordered. Patients often find the delay in a definitive diagnosis anxiety-provoking and require detailed explanations about the process.

Pre-operative assessment and preparation

If a diagnostic laparoscopy is ordered, or an ectopic pregnancy is confirmed, the patient is prepared for theatre as described in Chapter 1. She will usually consent to a laparoscopy and proceed to laparotomy and possible salpingectomy. This is often undertaken as an emergency procedure, particularly if the ectopic has ruptured. The patient requires close monitoring of vital signs as she is at risk of hypovolaemic shock due to internal haemorrhage (see Chapter 13). An intravenous infusion is commenced and sometimes a blood transfusion

Table 11.1   Common symptoms of ectopic pregnancy.

Unruptured ectopic	Ruptured ectopic
• Pain in lower abdomen, usually unilateral, intermittent, vague and cramping	• Sudden severe pain, sometimes referred to the shoulder tip
	• Distended abdomen
• Vaginal bleeding occurs usually after the death of the ovum. Blood is usually dark brown and scanty	• Bleeding, pallor, fainting and signs of shock

or colloids are required. The patient will also require analgesia and usually an intramuscular opioid injection is given with an anti-emetic. These events can cause great anxiety for the patient, who may be in fear of her life and distraught at the loss of her baby. The patient's partner also requires support at this time.

Treatment

Surgical management

The aim of treatment is to control bleeding and remove the cause of the problem. The embryo cannot be salvaged so the focus is on restoring the woman to health and, if possible, conserving fertility. A laparoscopy is usually performed in the first instance to assess the damage to the tube and the subsequent surgery is often carried out laparoscopically. The extent of the surgery undertaken will depend upon the site of the pregnancy and the degree of tubal damage. If the tube has not ruptured and the pregnancy is at the fimbrial end, it can sometimes be 'milked' out, conserving the tube. An unruptured ectopic pregnancy in the isthmus is often removed via a small incision in the tube, which is then either closed carefully (salpingotomy) or left open to heal (salpingostomy) (Whitton *et al.*, 2001). If the tube is irreparable or there is uncontrollable bleeding it is necessary to remove the tube completely (salpingectomy) and occasionally the ovary has to be removed as well (salpingo-oophorectomy). Sometimes only part of a damaged tube is removed (partial salpingectomy). If there are adhesions in the pelvis or if visibility is obscured by excessive bleeding, it is necessary to perform a laparotomy in order to undertake these procedures. A 'mini-laparotomy' is usually performed via a small *pfannenstiel* incision.

Conservative management

Although surgery is generally the treatment of choice for ectopic pregnancy, in some cases a tubal mole (where haemorrhage occurs around the embryo causing its death) will resolve spontaneously either by resorption or tubal abortion. Thus expectant management may be indicated if the patient is asymptomatic and the beta hCG

levels are falling. However, this type of management requires regular follow-up measurement of the beta hCG levels and there is the possibility that the tube will remain blocked.

Medical management of ectopic pregnancy has been introduced as an alternative to surgery in some areas and can be successful in patients who are diagnosed early whilst the tube is intact, the ectopic pregnancy still small and the beta hCG levels low (Whitton *et al.*, 2001). The treatment involves systemic or local administration (under ultrasound guidance) of drugs such as methotrexate, prostaglandins or hyperosmolar glucose. Whilst these have the advantage of reducing the need for tubal surgery, the side-effects can be unpleasant and regular follow-up monitoring is required. (See Whitton *et al.* (2001) for further details of medical management.)

Post-operative considerations

When the patient returns to the ward, she will require the usual post-operative monitoring and observation of wound site(s) and vaginal blood loss. She will have an intravenous infusion in progress and possibly a blood transfusion. If a mini-laparotomy has been performed, she may have a Redivac drain in situ and possibly a urinary catheter and patient-controlled analgesia pump. These are all normally removed on the first or second day post-operatively and if all is well she will be discharged from hospital on the third or fourth day. If the procedure has been undertaken laparoscopically the recovery process is much quicker and depending on the time of surgery the patient may be treated as a day case or overnight stay.

Of particular importance for patients who have suffered an ectopic pregnancy is the post-operative counselling. These women will often say things like 'I'm being silly' and 'it was not a real baby' when they become upset post-operatively. It is important that the woman and her partner are allowed to grieve the loss of their pregnancy and need to be reassured that their feelings are legitimate. The feelings of loss may be compounded by the loss of or damage to a fallopian tube and the effects on fertility. For women who already have one damaged or missing tube due to previous surgery or ectopic pregnancy the effects can be devastating. Issues of loss in relation to surgery are discussed in Chapter 5.

Gynaecological malignancies

Gynaecological cancers are a diverse group of diseases, the most common being cervical, ovarian and endometrial. However, compared to other cancers such as breast, lung and bowel cancer they are relatively rare. For this reason it has become necessary to centralise expertise in some areas of the UK to ensure that patients receive appropriate treatment from clinicians who deal regularly with these cancers (NHS Executive, 1999). Most patients with early stage cervical and endometrial cancers are treated in cancer units in district general hospitals, whereas patients with advanced disease or ovarian, vaginal or vulval cancers tend to be referred to cancer centres where they are treated by specialist multiprofessional gynaecological oncology teams.

This section considers the pathophysiology, risk factors, clinical manifestations, investigation and treatment of invasive cervical cancer, benign and malignant tumours of the ovary and endometrial cancer. Specific post-operative considerations relating to all of these are then discussed.

Invasive carcinoma of the uterine cervix

The incidence of invasive carcinoma of the uterine cervix has declined in the UK in recent years and this has been attributed to the cervical screening programme. Pre-invasive disease usually affects young women up to 30 years of age, whereas invasive cancer occurs mostly in women aged between 35 and 50. Fortunately the cervical screening programme means that the majority of lesions are diagnosed and treated at the pre-invasive stage, usually in the colposcopy clinic. Invasive carcinoma of the cervix is defined as a tumour that invades at least some way into the underlying connective tissue.

Pathophysiology

The cervix is the lower portion of the uterus that projects into the vaginal vault and is sometimes

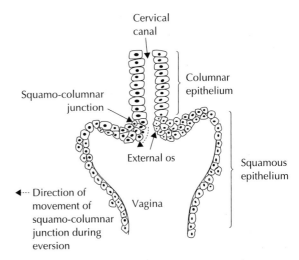

Figure 11.3   Diagram to illustrate squamous metaplasia. At puberty and in pregnancy, the cervix changes shape, and columnar epithelium appears below the external os (eversion). The everted columnar epithelium changes over time to squamous epithelium. This is termed metaplastic change. The area of metaplastic squamous epithelium is termed the **transformation zone**.

referred to as the neck of the womb. The vagina and outer part of the cervix (the ectocervix) are lined with stratified squamous epithelium whereas the inner cervix (endocervix) is lined with columnar epithelium (Figure 11.3). The point at which these cell types meet is called the squamo-columnar junction. At puberty this junction lies at the external os, but hormonal changes during puberty and pregnancy cause the cervix to change shape and the lower part of the endocervical canal becomes everted. The exposed columnar epithelium gradually changes to squamous epithelium, a process referred to as benign squamous metaplasia. This area of metaplastic cells is called the transformation zone and occasionally it gives rise to abnormal (dysplastic) changes and cervical neoplasms. In post-menopausal women, the size of the cervix is reduced and the squamo-columnar junction and part of the transformation zone come to lie in the endocervix.

The majority (80–90%) of cervical cancers are squamous cell in origin arising from the transformation zone whilst 10–20% are adenocarcinomas, most of which arise from the endocervical glandular cells. The location of these lesions within the endocervical canal can make them more difficult to detect and delay diagnosis (Figure 11.4). The

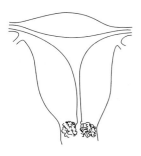 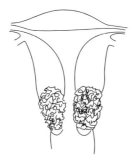

a. Squamous cell carcinoma

b. Adenocarcinoma. Typical bulky lesions creating a barrel-shaped abnormality of the cervix. Spread similar to squamous cell carcinoma

Figure 11.4   Diagram to illustrate the different growth pattern of ecto- and endocervical lesions.

> **Box 11.7**   Risk factors associated with squamous cell carcinoma of the cervix.
>
> - History of infection with sexually transmitted viruses, particularly human papillomavirus (HPV types 16 and 18)
> - Immunosuppression, either due to medication or disease (HIV)
> - Early onset of sexual activity
> - History of multiple sexual partners
> - Smoking
> - Belonging to low socioeconomic groups
> - Multiparity
> - Use of the oral contraceptive pill

> **Box 11.8**   Symptoms of cervical cancer.
>
> - Abnormal vaginal bleeding (post-coital, intermenstrual, menorrhagia)
> - Dyspareunia
> - Watery or blood-tinged discharge
> - Offensive discharge
> - Anaemia (due to persistent bleeding)
> - Haemorrhage
> - Pain in the pelvis, back and legs
> - Oedema in lower legs and feet
> - Dysuria, haematuria, rectal bleeding, constipation, tenesmus
> - Fistula formation (between vagina and bowel or vagina and bladder)

> **Box 11.9**   Investigations undertaken in the clinical staging of cervical cancer.
>
> - Examination under anaesthetic (EUA)
> - Chest X-ray
> - Renal tract imaging
> - Colposcopy and biopsy
> - Cystoscopy
> - Sigmoidoscopy
> - Barium enema

reasons why cervical neoplasms occur are not clear; however, a number of risk factors for the disease have been identified (Box 11.7). The risk factors for adenocarcinomas are different from those cited for squamous cell carcinoma in that sexual behaviour does not appear to be related to the development of the disease (Hughes, 2001).

Clinical manifestations of carcinoma of the cervix

In the early stages carcinoma of the cervix can be asymptomatic. Abnormal vaginal bleeding, particularly post-coital bleeding, and pain on intercourse (dyspareunia) are common presenting symptoms. As the disease progresses and involves adjacent organs, urinary symptoms and bowel problems may be evident (see Box 11.8).

Investigations and diagnosis

History taking and clinical examination are performed and examination under anaesthetic (EUA) is considered essential for accurate staging of the disease. Cervical cancer is staged clinically pre-operatively because if the tumour is advanced the treatment involves radiotherapy rather than surgery. Figure 11.5 illustrates the International Federation of Gynecology and Obstetrics (FIGO) staging according to the extent of spread. Investigations undertaken to clinically stage cervical cancer are listed in Box 11.9.

Each growth is allocated to a stage according to the extent of spread (FIGO, 1995).

Stage 0 CIN III (Carcinoma-in-situ)

Stage Ia Micro-invasive carcinoma not extending more than 5 mm beyond the basement membrane and of a width less than 7 mm

Stage Ib The growth is confined to the cervix

Stage IIa Extension to the vagina not beyond the upper two thirds

Stage IIb Extension into the parametrium but not as far as the pelvic walls

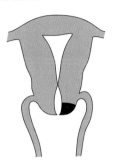 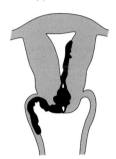 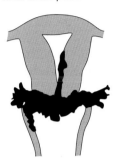

Stage III Extension to lower third of vagina or to pelvic wall

Stage IIIa Carcinoma involving the lower third of the vagina

Stage IIIb Carcinoma extending to the pelvic side wall and/or hydronephrosis due to tumour

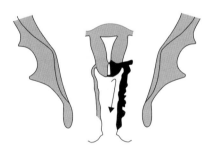 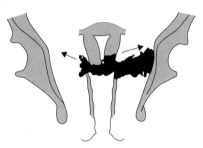

Stage IV Extension through vagina into bladder or outside pelvis

Stage IVa Carcinoma involving bladder, rectum or outside the pelvis

Stage IVb Carcinoma extending to distant organs

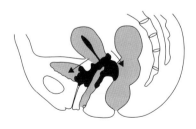 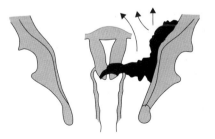

Classification (which is a clinical staging) is made after vaginal and rectal examination followed by cystoscopy and sigmoidoscopy when indicated, and doubtful cases are placed in the less advanced stage.

Figure 11.5   FIGO staging for carcinoma of the cervix.
(Reprinted from *Gynaecology Illustrated* (5th edn), McKay Hart & Norman, 'Diseases of the cervix' pp. 204–205, ©2000, with permission from Elsevier)

Pre-operative assessment and preparation

The usual pre-operative assessment and preparation is undertaken as described in Chapter 1, including prophylactic antibiotics and antithrombotic therapy. Patients who have an objection to receiving blood or blood products will require specific pre-operative counselling as this may result in the tumour being treated with radiotherapy rather than surgery (Hughes, 2001).

Treatment

Treatment for cervical cancer depends on the stage of the disease. Results and survival rates following radiotherapy and surgery for early stage cervical cancer (stage I and IIa) are similar; however, surgery is usually the preferred choice for younger fit patients as it is less likely to impair bowel, bladder and sexual function. Older patients and those who are not medically fit for surgery may be offered radiotherapy as an alternative treatment for early disease. Advanced cancer of the cervix (stage IIb and above) is usually treated with radiotherapy. For further information on radiotherapy see Moore-Higgs *et al.* (2000).

Surgery

A radical hysterectomy is usually undertaken for cancer of the cervix. This involves removal of the whole uterus, the upper third of the vagina, the parametria, the pelvic lymph nodes and sometimes the para-aortic lymph nodes too. The ovaries are usually conserved in younger women, as spread to them is uncommon. Sometimes the ovaries are transposed out of the radiation field in case post-operative radiotherapy is required. The operation is usually undertaken via a midline or transverse incision; however, some surgeons are now able to perform the procedure laparoscopically.

Recent advances in surgical treatment have led to the undertaking of radical trachelectomy for early stage cervical cancer in some hospitals. This involves the removal of the cervix, upper vagina, parametrium and pelvic lymph nodes in an attempt to conserve fertility. However, this procedure is still considered experimental (Hughes, 2001).

Following surgery and full histological examination of the tumour, radiotherapy may be prescribed to prevent recurrence, particularly in those patients whose disease has spread to the lymph nodes.

Ovarian cysts and neoplasms

Ovarian cysts and neoplasms may be benign or malignant. Benign cysts are relatively common and account for a large number of hospital admissions. Larger cysts are often associated with emergency admissions for complications such as torsion or rupture.

Ovarian cancer is the most common gynaecological malignancy with approximately 5000 new cases being diagnosed each year in England and Wales and approximately 4000 deaths (NHS Executive, 1999). It generally affects women aged between 45 and 70 years old and although the causes are unclear, it is thought to be associated with incessant ovulation causing chronic irritation or damage to the ovarian epithelium. Thus nulliparity, early menarche and late menopause are associated with increased risk, whilst pregnancy and use of oral contraception reduce the risk. Box 11.10 identifies the risk factors associated with ovarian carcinoma. Because symptoms are vague, the disease is often in the advanced stages before it is diagnosed. For this reason prognosis and the long-term survival rate for this disease are poor. There is currently no screening programme available and no single screening method that is sensitive and reliable enough to detect ovarian cancer. Hence clinical trials are underway that look at combining tests to improve detection and sensitivity.

Box 11.10   Risk factors for ovarian cancer.

- Hormonal influence:
  - Low or nulliparity
  - Early menses and late menopause
- Genetic/familial factors:
  - Family history of ovarian or breast cancer
  - Lynch II syndrome (associated with ovarian, breast and colon cancer)
  - Blood group A
- Environmental factors:
  - Obesity
  - Use of talcum powder in genital area

Pathophysiology

There are a number of different types of benign and malignant ovarian cysts, the most common of which are described in Box 11.11. They are classified as non-neoplastic (functional) or neoplastic (Gauthier & Carcio, 2000). Non-neoplastic ovarian cysts result from normal ovarian function and are often asymptomatic. They will often regress spontaneously, in which case no treatment is required. Neoplasms of the ovary are diverse and can grow quite large due to the space available in the abdominal cavity. Ovarian neoplasms may arise at any age but are most common between the ages of 30 and 60. They may be benign, malignant or have low malignant potential (borderline malignancy). McKay Hart & Norman (2000, p. 265) suggest their clinical significance to be threefold:

1. They are particularly liable to be or to become malignant.

2. They are asymptomatic and painless in the early stages.
3. They may grow to a large size and undergo mechanical complications such as torsion and perforation.

Clinical manifestations of ovarian tumours

Often ovarian tumours are asymptomatic and the woman may not consult her doctor until the cyst has grown quite large and is causing pressure symptoms such as frequency of micturition, gastrointestinal symptoms and pain. Such vague symptoms (see Box 11.12) are often attributed to irritable bowel syndrome, pre-menstrual or menopausal symptoms. There may be some swelling of the abdomen, but frequently this is attributed to weight gain or even pregnancy. Because of this diagnosis is often delayed, and in the case of malignant tumours this has a detrimental effect on prognosis.

Box 11.11 Common ovarian cysts.

Non-neoplastic cysts

Follicular cysts – These cysts are common and result when normal Graafian follicles exceed the usual 2.0–2.5 cm before rupturing. They rarely reach more than 5 cm in diameter and usually resolve spontaneously, requiring no treatment.

Corpus luteum cysts – These occur when the corpus luteum fails to degenerate normally and becomes distended with blood. They may continue to secrete progesterone, delaying the onset of menstruation. Corpus luteum cysts usually regress spontaneously, but occasionally they rupture and cause symptoms similar to those of an ectopic pregnancy.

Theca-lutein and granulosa lutein cysts – These are caused by the excessive production of gonadotrophin which occurs in association with hydatidiform moles or choriocarcinoma. They may also result from hyperstimulation of the ovary in infertility treatment. These cysts usually regress when the underlying cause is treated.

Endometriotic cysts – These arise due to the condition *endometriosis* in which deposits of endometrial tissue are found outside of the uterine cavity. When this occurs on the surface of the ovary an endometriotic cyst is formed which is responsive to normal hormonal stimulation and bleeding occurs periodically into the cyst. The blood becomes thick and dark and is then referred to as a 'chocolate cyst'.

Neoplastic cysts

Epithelial neoplasms – These are the most common ovarian neoplasms and arise from the layer of epithelial cells that cover the surface of the ovary. There are a number of different types of epithelial neoplasms including serous tumours, mucinous tumours and Brenner tumours. Epithelial neoplasms may be benign or malignant.

Germ cell neoplasms – These arise from the germ cells of the ovary and the most common type is the benign cystic teratoma or dermoid cyst. This type of cyst contains a variety of tissues derived from the primary germ layers and when cut open it is often found to contain cartilage, hair, teeth, skin and sebaceous glands. These cysts are usually benign but malignant changes can occur.

Sex cord stromal tumours – These arise from the main substance of the ovary (the stroma of the cortex) and may contain hormone-secreting cells such as granulosa cells and theca cells (oestrogen producing) or Sertoli cells and Leydig cells (androgen producing). Although rare, these tumours may also become malignant.

Box 11.12   Symptoms of ovarian tumours.

- Frequency of micturition
- Loss of appetite, indigestion and nausea
- Bloating, abdominal swelling, ascites
- Altered bowel habit
- Vague abdominal discomfort
- Dyspareunia
- Dysmenorrhoea
- Bleeding per vagina
- Palpable abdominal mass

Box 11.13   Pre-treatment investigations undertaken for ovarian cancer.

- Abdominal and bimanual pelvic examination
- Pelvic or transvaginal ultrasound scan
- CT scan and MRI
- Barium enema
- Chest X-ray
- Tumour marker – Ca_{125}

Investigations and diagnosis

Although a major concern of diagnosis is to exclude malignancy, it is sometimes impossible to tell, prior to surgery, whether an ovarian tumour is malignant or benign. First, abdominal and bimanual pelvic examinations are undertaken. Also a digital rectal examination may be performed to detect hard deposits in the rectovaginal pouch. On examination a mass may be palpable and either freely movable or adherent to other structures. The presence of ascites is often indicative of advanced malignant disease. The patient may find these examinations intrusive, undignified and unpleasant and the presence of a female chaperone is essential if she is being examined by a male doctor. The chaperone should provide support to the patient as well as assisting the doctor.

In order to exclude an ectopic pregnancy a blood test may be taken to measure the levels of serum beta human chorionic gonadotrophin (hCG) hormone. A pelvic or transvaginal ultrasound scan will also be undertaken. Whilst this cannot confirm the presence of malignancy, it does provide some clues as to the size and nature of the cyst. For example, totally cystic tumours are rarely malignant whilst cysts that are bilateral with irregular borders and solid components are more likely to be malignant. Sometimes, when malignant disease is suspected, computed tomography (CT) scanning or magnetic resonance imaging (MRI) are used for pre-operative evaluation and to monitor response to treatment. A chest X-ray may be requested to detect chest metastases and if bowel involvement is suspected a barium enema may be performed.

Some tumours produce tumour-associated antigens or 'tumour markers' and in cases of suspected ovarian cancer the Ca_{125} marker is measured. However, when minimal disease is present the marker may be undetectable and it may also be raised in non-malignant disease such as endometriosis. A Ca_{125} level of less than 35 U/mL is generally considered normal. The marker is also used post-operatively to assess response to treatment. The pre-treatment investigations undertaken for ovarian tumours are summarised in Box 11.13.

Pre-operative assessment and preparation

In addition to the pre-operative assessment and preparation discussed in Chapter 1, patients undergoing surgery for ovarian tumours should be counselled about the implications of possible findings at surgery. For example, if ovarian cancer is suspected, the patient may need to be prepared for the possible formation of a stoma, and bowel preparation may be required.

Uncertainty about diagnosis and fear of surgery can cause patients to become very anxious and upset. This anxiety is often manifested as withdrawal or aggression, particularly towards their partners and healthcare personnel. Such patients need to be treated with kindness and understanding and their manner should not be taken personally by those caring for them. Partners should be counselled about this too as they may not understand the woman's attitude and may feel alienated and hurt by the rejection. The psychosocial aspects of surgery are covered in more depth in Chapter 5.

Patients admitted with large ovarian tumours or ascites are at risk of malnutrition due to the increased metabolic demands of a fast-growing tumour and the composition of fluid contained in the tumour or ascites. Thus despite apparent weight gain due to girth expansion the patient may appear cachexic. A thorough nutritional assessment is therefore required and the patient may benefit from pre-operative nutritional supplements, particularly protein and carbohydrates. The movement of fluid from the intravascular compartment may also cause dehydration and hypovolaemia and therefore intravenous fluids may be required pre-operatively.

Treatment

If there is no suspicion of malignancy, a patient with a small ovarian cyst may not require any treatment but is reviewed to ensure that the cyst regresses spontaneously. Larger cysts (more than 6–8 cm in diameter) are usually removed via a laparotomy as they present a greater risk of malignancy and complications such as torsion and rupture. When a malignant ovarian tumour is suspected the patient will require urgent treatment as delays may influence long-term prognosis.

Benign ovarian tumours

If the tumour is benign, an ovarian cystectomy is usually performed which involves enucleation of the tumour from its capsule of ovarian tissue (McKay Hart & Norman, 2000). In this procedure the ovary is conserved. However, sometimes it is necessary to remove the ovary as well.

Malignant ovarian tumours

The surgery undertaken for malignant ovarian tumours is based on surgical and pathological findings. The patient will usually consent to an exploratory laparotomy and proceed to a total abdominal hysterectomy, bilateral salpingo-oophorectomy, omentectomy, pelvic and para-aortic lymph node sampling and possible bowel resection. The staging of ovarian cancer is based upon findings at laparotomy and subsequent histological examination (Figure 11.6). A midline incision is made and the surgeon inspects and palpates the intra-abdominal contents, taking biopsies where necessary and specimens of ascitic fluid and peritoneal washings for cytology.

Having staged the disease, the aim of the surgery is to remove as much of the tumour as possible. This is often referred to as 'surgical debulking' or 'cyto-reductive surgery'. In most cases the surgeon will also remove the uterus, fallopian tubes, ovaries, omentum and sometimes the appendix. Partial resection of the bladder and bowel and formation of a stoma may also be required. However, in younger women who have not completed their families and have stage I disease or a tumour with low malignant potential the reproductive organs may be conserved.

The size of the tumour left after debulking is an important prognostic indicator with those with less than 1 cm residual tumour having a better prognosis. Depending on the stage of the disease and the amount of residual tumour, follow-up treatment with chemotherapy and possibly secondary surgery may be required. The reader is directed to Moore-Higg et al. (2000) for further information on this topic.

Complications

Torsion

Torsion is a common complication of ovarian cysts and may occur with any tumour except those with adhesions. The pedicle is usually fairly long and as it twists the veins of the pedicle are occluded first while the arterial blood supply continues. This leads to bleeding into the tumour and sometimes intraperitoneal haemorrhage. If left untreated the tumour will become necrotic.

Torsion of an ovarian tumour is often sudden in onset and the patient will be admitted as an emergency, suffering from severe lower abdominal pain and vomiting. Urgent laparotomy is required to remove the cyst and often it is necessary to remove the affected ovary as well.

Rupture

Spontaneous rupture of an ovarian cyst can sometimes occur or it may follow torsion of a pedicle or bimanual examination. If a small cyst ruptures there may be no symptoms and no treatment required, but if the cyst is large there is usually severe pain and vomiting. Sometimes a blood vessel is torn in the process and large volumes of blood can be lost into the peritoneal cavity causing the patient to suffer associated hypovolaemic shock. Additionally if the ruptured cyst is malignant

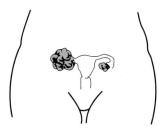

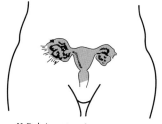

Stage I Growth limited to ovaries
Ia Limited to one ovary. No ascites
Ib Limited to both ovaries. No ascites
Ic Ascites or positive peritoneal washings
    also present or tumour on surface of one
    or both ovaries or capsule ruptured

Treatment: Surgery alone for Ia
and Ib. Add chemotherapy if Ic

Stage II Pelvic extension
IIa Spread to uterus/tubes
IIb Spread to other pelvic tissues
IIc IIb with ascites or positive peritoneal
    washings or tumour on surface of one
    or both ovaries or capsule ruptured

Treatment: Surgery and chemotherapy

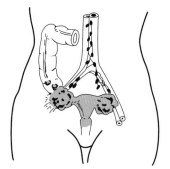

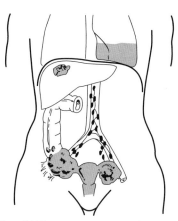

Stage III Extrapelvic intraperitoneal spread
and/or retroperitoneal or inguinal positive
nodes, or superficial liver metastases
IIIa Apparent limitation to true pelvis
    Nodes negative but proven microscopic
    seeding of abdominal peritoneum
IIIb Histologically proven abdominal peritoneal
    superficial implants < 2 cm diameter
IIIc Abdominal implants > 2 cm diameter or
    positive retroperitoneal or inguinal nodes

Treatment: Surgery as extensive as necessary
and possible, followed by chemotherapy

Stage IV Distant metastases or pleural
effusion with positive cytology or
parenchymal liver metastases

Treatment: As much surgical extirpation
as possible, perhaps with colostomy,
followed by chemotherapy. Palliative
radiotherapy may be used here

Figure 11.6   FIGO staging for ovarian cancer.
(Reprinted from *Gynaecology Illustrated* (5th edn), McKay Hart & Norman, 'Diseases of the ovary and fallopian tube', p. 280,
©2000, with permission from Elsevier)

there may be spread of the disease. The patient will usually be admitted as an emergency and need immediate laparotomy. Close observation and monitoring will be required throughout the pre- and post-operative period (see Chapter 13 for further details).

Endometrial cancer

Cancer of the endometrium affects approximately 4200 women in the UK each year and accounts for approximately 800 deaths (Gangar, 2001). It is rare in women under the age of 40 and most commonly

Box 11.14   Risk factors for endometrial cancer.

- Early menarche and late menopause
- History of endometrial hyperplasia
- Use of unopposed oestrogen in HRT
- Obesity
- Nulliparity or low parity
- Polycystic ovary disease
- Oestrogen-secreting tumours of the ovary
- Diabetes and hypertension

Box 11.15   Clinical manifestations of endometrial cancer.

- Intermenstrual bleeding
- Menorrhagia
- Post-menopausal bleeding
- Purulent, blood-tinged discharge
- Pyometria
- Pelvic pressure, lumbosacral or hypogastric pain
- Intestinal obstruction
- Ascites
- Respiratory distress
- Haemorrhage

affects those aged between 50 and 65. If diagnosed and treated early, prognosis is generally good since the tumour is often contained within the uterus.

Pathophysiology

Endometrial cancer is often preceded by endometrial hyperplasia (benign overgrowth of the endometrium). The majority of tumours are endometrioid adenocarcinomas arising from the glandular component of the endometrial mucosa. They may be confined to a single polyp or diffuse growths, commonly involving the upper portion of the uterine cavity. They may be well differentiated (grade 1), moderately differentiated (grade 2) or poorly differentiated (grade 3). Tumours that are moderately or poorly differentiated are associated with a poorer prognosis. The cause of endometrial cancer is not clear but several risk factors have been identified, all of which are associated with excessive exposure of the endometrium to oestrogen (see Box 11.14).

Clinical manifestations of endometrial cancer

The most common manifestation of endometrial cancer is abnormal uterine bleeding, which because of the age of the women most affected tends to present as post-menopausal bleeding (PMB). Pelvic pressure symptoms, pain, ascites and haemorrhage are associated with later disease (see Box 11.15).

Investigations and diagnosis

Patients presenting with PMB are usually seen in a rapid access clinic where a variety of investigations are undertaken. A transvaginal ultrasound scan is usually performed to assess the endometrial thickness and depth of myometrial invasion and endometrial tissue is obtained for pathological examination, often using a Pipelle sampling device. This may be combined with hysteroscopy, either as an outpatient or day case procedure. This involves the passing of a fine hysteroscope through the cervix into the uterus to visualise the uterine cavity, which is expanded by pumping in gas or fluid. Magnetic resonance imaging (MRI) is sometimes used to assist in pre-treatment staging. The tumour grade can be assessed by pathological examination of the biopsy samples and this grading is used alongside ultrasound results to provisionally stage the disease (Figure 11.7).

Pre-operative assessment and preparation

The usual pre-operative assessment and preparation is undertaken as described in Chapter 1 including prophylactic antibiotics and antithrombotic therapy. Because these patients tend to be in the older age group they are more likely to have age-related co-morbidity that requires special consideration.

Treatment

The treatment of choice for endometrial cancer is surgical. A midline incision is made and the procedure involves careful exploration of the intra-abdominal contents, total abdominal hysterectomy

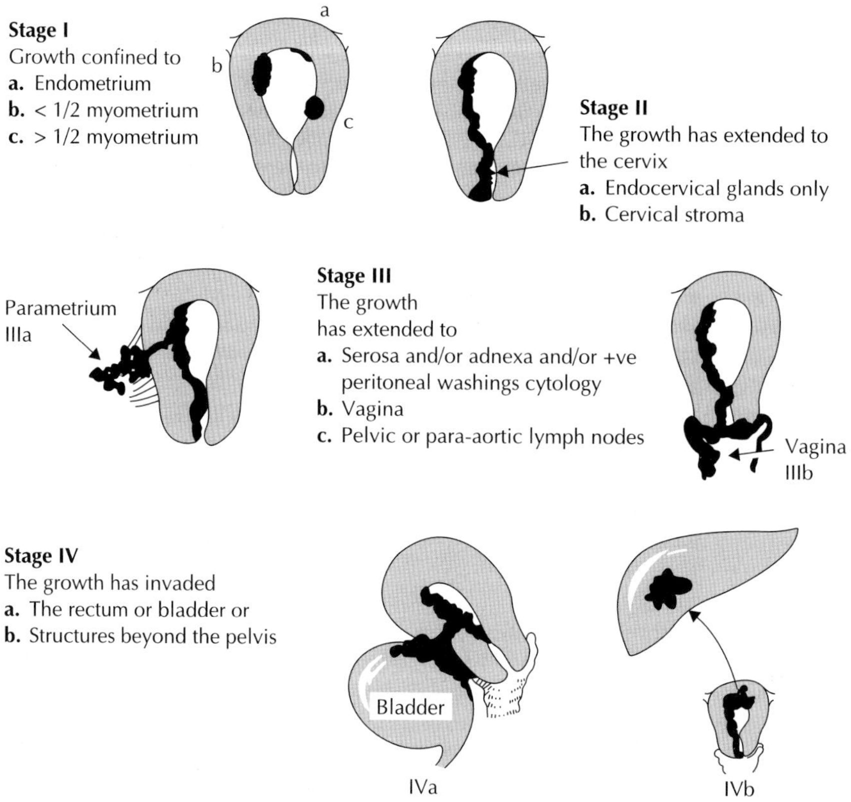

Stage I
Growth confined to
a. Endometrium
b. < 1/2 myometrium
c. > 1/2 myometrium

Stage II
The growth has extended to
the cervix
a. Endocervical glands only
b. Cervical stroma

Parametrium
IIIa

Stage III
The growth
has extended to
a. Serosa and/or adnexa and/or +ve
peritoneal washings cytology
b. Vagina
c. Pelvic or para-aortic lymph nodes

Vagina
IIIb

Stage IV
The growth has invaded
a. The rectum or bladder or
b. Structures beyond the pelvis

Bladder

IVa

IVb

Histological grading, G1, G2 or G3, is applied to stages I, II and III only.

Figure 11.7   FIGO staging for endometrial cancer.
(Reprinted from *Gynaecology Illustrated* (5th edn), McKay Hart & Norman, 'Diseases of the uterus', p. 222, ©2000, with permission from Elsevier)

and bilateral salpingo-oophorectomy and sampling of peritoneal fluid. Pelvic and para-aortic lymph nodes are either sampled or removed. In patients with stage Ia and Ib, grade 1 or 2 disease, no further treatment may be required. However those with later stage disease or poorly differentiated (grade 3) tumours will require a radical hysterectomy and possibly post-operative radiotherapy.

Post-operative considerations for patients undergoing abdominal surgery for gynaecological malignancies

The patient who has undergone abdominal surgery for a gynaecological malignancy normally returns to the ward post-operatively with an intravenous infusion or blood transfusion in progress, one or two Redivac drains, a urinary catheter, a patient-controlled analgesia pump and she will usually be receiving oxygen therapy. If the bowel has been involved she may also have a stoma and/or a nasogastric tube. The usual post-operative monitoring and care will be undertaken as discussed in Chapter 3 with the addition of observation of vaginal blood loss, a small amount of which is normal, but large amounts and the presence of large clots should be reported. Sometimes if the operation has been particularly long or difficult, or if the patient suffers from co-morbidity, she may be cared for in a critical care unit during the immediate post-operative period.

Recovery from a radical hysterectomy or laparotomy for gynaecological malignancy usually takes longer than that for a straightforward abdominal hysterectomy for a benign disorder. However, early mobilisation should be encouraged to avoid post-operative complications and the use of antiembolic prophylaxis should continue until the patient is fully mobile. During the second, third and fourth post-operative days the drains and infusions are usually removed. The urinary catheter may remain for up to five days. Oral fluids and diet are gradually introduced as tolerated; this will vary depending on the extent of bowel involvement.

Women who have undergone surgery for gynaecological cancer are likely to experience some psychosexual issues post-operatively. This will not normally be in the immediate post-operative period when they are more concerned with recovering from the surgery, but as they start to feel better and their minds turn towards the future, questions about their sexuality may arise. Box 11.16 shows the influences that cancer can have on sexuality. Sexual dysfunction following treatment for gynaecological malignancies is common and it seems that in general women do not receive adequate information or opportunities to discuss this with healthcare staff. Psychosexual aspects of surgery are discussed further in Chapter 5.

Fertility issues are closely related to sexuality as loss of function of the reproductive tract can lead to feelings of reduced self-esteem and loss of 'womanhood', particularly in younger women who may not yet have completed, or even started, their families. The induced menopause that occurs with removal of the ovaries can cause further distress in previously pre-menopausal women as menopausal symptoms occur suddenly and can commence as early as several days post-operatively. The decision as to whether hormone replacement therapy (HRT) can be prescribed sometimes depends on histological findings.

Vulval cancer

Although relatively rare, vulval cancers are seen in gynaecological wards, typically affecting the older age group. Surgical procedures for this type of cancer range from local excision of the tumour to radical vulvectomy and groin node dissection. This latter procedure creates pockets of dead space in the groins where fluid collects. The lack of adherence to underlying tissue delays healing and increases the risk of infection. Additionally, the anatomy of the vulva does not lend itself readily to the application of dressings and the proximity of urine and faeces may cause infection. For these reasons, the wounds frequently break down. The priorities for caring for patients undergoing radical vulvectomy are identified in Box 11.17.

Box 11.16   Influences of gynaecological cancer on sexuality.

- Disease process:
  - Pain, discomfort, fatigue and loss of desire
  - Bleeding, viral infection, vulval pruritus, vaginal discharge
  - Tumour growth affecting nerves can lead to loss of sensation and desire
- Psychological effects:
  - Impact of life-threatening illness causes mood disturbance – anger, fear, depression, anxiety
  - The disease can be viewed as a punishment for past sexual behaviours (e.g. promiscuity)
- Effects of treatment:
  - Surgery – nerve and vascular disruption may occur and possible scar tissue formation. In radical hysterectomy the vagina is shortened possibly leading to painful intercourse
  - Radiotherapy – pelvic radiotherapy causes thinning of vaginal tissue and loss of elasticity which can cause painful intercourse
  - Chemotherapy – can cause premature menopause, alopecia, nausea, etc., leading to decreased sexual desire

---

Box 11.17   Priorities of care for patients undergoing radical vulvectomy.

- Pain management
- Age-related co-morbidity
- Avoidance of complications associated with reduced mobility
- Wound care and drainage
  - Avoidance of wound infection
  - Monitoring of exudate
  - Body image disturbance
- Elimination
  - Avoidance of constipation and wound contamination
  - Management of urinary catheter
  - Return to normal voiding patterns
- Nutrition
  - High carbohydrate diet and proteins for wound healing
- Avoidance and management of lower limb lymphoedema

Box 11.18   Risk factors associated with breast cancer.

- Age
- Family history
- High socioeconomic class
- Early menarche and late menopause
- Nulliparity
- Older primigravida (later than 30 at first pregnancy)
- Obesity and diet

In addition, alcohol consumption, the use of hormone replacement therapy (HRT) and the combined oral contraceptive pill, and not breast-feeding are thought to be risk factors. However, there is no definite evidence to suggest that any particular one has a higher risk than another.

Table 11.2   The Nottingham Prognostic Index (NPI).

Score	Prognosis
< 3.4	Suggestive of a good outcome with a high chance of a cure
3.4–5.4	Suggestive of an intermediate level with a moderate chance of cure
> 5.4	Suggestive of a smaller chance of a cure

(Cancerbackup, 2006)
It is important to note that the NPI is a guide only and is not absolutely reliable.

Breast cancer

Patients with breast cancer may be cared for in general surgical wards or women's health or gynaecological wards. Breast cancer is the most common form of cancer amongst women, accounting for one in three female deaths. The incidence of the disease appears to be increasing, however mortality rates attributed to breast cancer are decreasing. Approximately 41 000 new cases were diagnosed in the UK in 2001 with approximately 13 000 deaths (Cancer Research UK, 2005). The disease tends to affect older women, especially those over the age of 55, and although older women have a higher risk of developing breast cancer they are less likely to die of the disease. Family history is an important risk factor for breast cancer and a significant number of these can be attributed to the BRCA1 and BRCA2 genes. Box 11.18 identifies the risk factors associated with breast cancer.

Pathophysiology

The majority of breast cancers are adenocarcinomas arising from the epithelia of the ducts and lobules of the breast. The most common type is ductal which accounts for approximately 80–90% of cases. Breast cancers are graded as well differentiated (grade I), intermediate (grade II) and poorly differentiated (grade III). Poorly differentiated tumours are associated with a poorer prognosis. Breast cancer has been staged according the tumour size, axillary lymph node involvement and evidence of metastasis to distant sites (tumour–nodes–metastases (TNM) staging). However, more recently, a formula has been developed to assess prognosis that considers the tumour size, lymph node stage and tumour grade. This is known as the Nottingham Prognostic Index (NPI) which, when applied, gives a score that falls into one of three bands (see Table 11.2).

Clinical manifestations of breast cancer

The most common symptom of breast cancer is a lump, which is usually hard, painless and irregular in shape. However, many women are asymptomatic and their cancers are found during screening via mammography or during self-examination. Box 11.19 lists some manifestations of breast cancer.

Box 11.19   Manifestations of breast cancer.

- Non-tender breast lump
- Nipple discharge or bleeding
- Nipple inversion
- Changes in the size or shape of the breast
- Dimpling of the skin of the breast
- Axillary lump
- Skin ulceration
- Lymphoedema of the arm
- Pain

Investigations and diagnosis

Diagnosis of breast cancer requires triple assessment, which typically involves clinical examination; imaging investigations such as a mammogram and ultrasound scan; and pathological examination such as fine needle aspiration cytology (FNAC) or biopsy under local anaesthetic. Specialist breast care centres enable rapid access to these investigations and results. It is important to gain histological evidence before treatment is commenced.

Pre-operative assessment and preparation

The usual pre-operative assessment and preparation is carried out as discussed in Chapter 1. The patient will normally have met the breast care specialist nurse before admission and this is an important point of contact. Pre-operative preparation should include counselling and information about treatment options and their effects and advice about post-operative exercises for rehabilitation. When the patient is admitted for surgery the relevant breast is marked and antithrombotic therapy prescribed.

Treatment

Unfortunately some breast cancers metastasise before diagnosis and for this reason it is considered a systemic rather than local disease. Whilst surgery and radiotherapy can achieve local control, systemic treatments such as chemotherapy are required to treat metastatic disease. These treatments are not necessarily given sequentially and trials are currently under way to assess the value of giving systemic treatment prior to surgery. This section discusses the surgical aspects of treatment only. The reader is directed to Moore-Higg *et al.* (2000) for further information about additional forms of treatment.

The aim of surgery is to achieve local control and prevent systemic relapse. Patients' individual cases are discussed at a multidisciplinary team meeting (MDM) where an individual treatment plan is developed. This could involve a combination of surgery, chemotherapy, radiotherapy and hormone manipulation. The patient may be offered all or a combination of these treatments.

The extent of the surgery is dependent upon the stage of the tumour. If possible, breast-conserving surgery is performed. This consists of either a wide local excision of the lump along with a 1 cm margin of normal tissue (lumpectomy) or a quadrantectomy, in which the entire quadrant of the breast is removed. If conservative surgery is not appropriate, a mastectomy may be performed. This involves removal of the complete breast and axillary tail and sampling of axillary lymph nodes or axillary node clearance. Breast reconstructive surgery can be offered either immediately or at a later date.

Post-operative considerations

When the patient returns to the ward following breast surgery she will usually have an intravenous infusion in progress, and a gentle suction drain in situ. The usual post-operative monitoring is undertaken as described in Chapter 3. When taking blood pressure, siting intravenous infusions or performing venepuncture, it is important that the unaffected side is used.

Deep breathing exercises are particularly important for these patients, as pain from the incision may reduce lung expansion. The patient is taught a range of exercises to improve shoulder and arm mobility and reduce the risk of lymphoedema. Lymphoedema occurs when the cancer or its treatment affects the lymph nodes in the axilla and the normal lymphatic drainage is impeded. Fluid collects in the tissues of the arm causing pain, swelling, reduced mobility and increased susceptibility to infection. Patients need to be aware of the potential complication and how to avoid it (see CancerHelp, 2006). Prior to discharge the patient will usually be given a soft breast prosthesis to be used until the wound has healed.

Like patients who have undergone surgery for a gynaecological malignancy, patients who have had breast surgery for cancer will experience a range of emotions including shock, denial and anxiety. Alterations in body image are common and some patients, particularly those who are younger, will suffer persistent psychological or sexual problems. These issues are discussed further in Chapter 5.

Self-test questions

Circle the correct answer(s). Some questions may have more than one correct response.

1. After the menopause, uterine fibroids have a tendency to:
   a. Get bigger
   b. Get smaller
   c. Multiply
   d. Become malignant

2. Which of the following treatments for uterine fibroids aim to conserve fertility?
   a. Laparoscopic-assisted vaginal hysterectomy
   b. Total abdominal hysterectomy
   c. Myomectomy
   d. GnRH analogues

3. Which of the following terms is used to refer to a third degree uterine prolapse?
   a. Cystocele
   b. Rectocele
   c. Urethrocele
   d. Procidentia

4. Which of the following is defined as 'the involuntary leaking of urine that occurs when intravesical pressure exceeds maximum urethral closure pressure in the absence of detrusor contraction'?
   a. Genital prolapse
   b. Detrusor instability
   c. Genuine stress incontinence
   d. Enterocele

5. Cystometry is used to investigate which of the following disorders?
   a. Genuine stress incontinence
   b. Detrusor instability
   c. Uterine fibroids
   d. Ectopic pregnancy

6. Which of the following is a common cause of ectopic pregnancy?
   a. Salpingectomy
   b. Salpingotomy
   c. Salpingitis
   d. Salpingo-oophorectomy

7. The area of the cervix where squamous metaplasia has occurred is referred to as:
   a. The transformation zone
   b. The squamo-columnar junction
   c. The endocervix
   d. The ectocervix

8. A history of infection with the sexually transmitted human papilloma virus is a risk factor for which cancer?
   a. Cervical
   b. Endometrial
   c. Ovarian
   d. Breast

9. Which type of ovarian cyst may contain hair, teeth, skin and sebaceous glands?
   a. Endometriotic cysts
   b. Dermoid cysts
   c. Follicular cysts
   d. Chocolate cysts

10. Which of the following is **not** a risk factor for endometrial cancer?
   a. Early menarche and late menopause
   b. Use of unopposed oestrogen in HRT
   c. History of multiple sexual partners
   d. History of endometrial hyperplasia

References and further reading

Anders K (2001) 'Chapter 18 – Disorders of micturition' *in*: Gangar EA (ed.) (2001) *Gynaecological Nursing – a practical guide*. London: Churchill Livingstone

Barron M (2001) 'Chapter 11 – Endometriosis' *in*: Gangar EA (ed.) (2001) *Gynaecological Nursing – a practical guide*. London: Churchill Livingstone

Baum M & Schipper H (2002) *Breast Cancer* (2nd edn). London: Fast Facts, Health Press Limited

Bullock BA & Henze RL (2000) *Focus on Pathophysiology*. Maryland: Lippincott

Cancerbackup (2006) *The Nottingham Prognostic Index for Breast Cancer* (online). www.cancerbackup.org.uk (Accessed 08.01.07)

CancerHelp (2006) *What is Lymphoedema?* (online) www.cancerhelp.org.uk (Accessed 08.01.07)

Cancer Research UK (2005) *Breast Cancer* (online) www.cancerhelp.org.uk (Accessed 08.01.07)

Clayton SG, Campbell S & Monga A (eds) (2000) *Gynaecology by Ten Teachers* (17th edn). London: Hodder Arnold

Gangar EA (ed.) (2001) *Gynaecological Nursing – a practical guide*. London: Churchill Livingstone

Gauthier SP & Carcio HA (2000) 'Normal and altered female reproductive function' *in*: Bullock BA & Henze RL (2000) *op cit*

Hollis H (2001) 'Chapter 14 – Cancer of the ovary' *in*: Gangar EA (ed.) (2001) *op cit*

Hughes C (2001) 'Chapter 13 – Cancer of the uterine cervix' *in*: Gangar EA (ed.) (2001) *op cit*

McKay Hart D & Norman J (2000) *Gynaecology Illustrated* (5th edn). London: Churchill Livingstone

Moore-Higgs GJ, Huff BC, Gossfield LM & Eriksson JH (2000) *Women and Cancer: a gynecologic oncology nursing perspective* (2nd edn). Massachusetts: Jones and Bartlett

NHS Executive (1999) *Improving outcomes in gynaecological cancers*. London: DoH

Otto JH (2000) 'Neoplasia' *in*: Bullock BA & Henze RL (2000) *op cit*

Rosevear SK (2002) *Handbook of Gynaecological Management*. Oxford: Blackwell Science

Whitton A, Mitchem L & Nicholl R (2001) 'Chapter 5 – Early pregnancy disorders' *in*: Gangar EA (ed.) (2001) *op cit*

12 Orthopaedic Surgery

Ann Newman

Introduction

Treatment and care of patients with orthopaedic conditions has changed dramatically. Advances in surgical techniques and concurrent development of the skills and knowledge of nurses and other healthcare professionals have led to a wide range of treatment options and a reduction in length of stay for patients following orthopaedic and trauma surgery.

Orthopaedic services encompass the whole age spectrum from infants and children to the elderly, providing a range of challenges to health professionals. They deal with traumatic injuries, degenerative joint disease, sports injuries, autoimmune conditions and metabolic bone disorders. Collaboration with many disciplines, including rheumatologists, neurologists, plastic surgeons and allied health professionals, ensures that patients receive optimum treatment pathways.

Generally patients tend to be classified as either orthopaedic – those admitted for elective surgery, or trauma patients – those whose episode of care was unforeseen and unplanned. These two groups of patients have a number of similar priorities in their care but also, distinct differences and individual needs to be addressed. The importance of pre-assessment and preparation for elective surgical patients and the priorities for the individual requiring emergency surgery have been discussed in

---

Box 12.1 Aims of the chapter.

- To explore a number of patient groups common to orthopaedic and trauma wards within district general hospitals
- To discuss the pathophysiology of certain disorders along with the treatment, nursing care and potential complications of the condition and treatment
- To discuss the specific needs of the orthopaedic patient, including specialist orthopaedic nursing issues such as monitoring for compartment syndrome and fat embolism, and care of an external cast

---

Chapter 1. Pain is a particular problem for many orthopaedic patients so this chapter should be read in conjunction with Chapter 4. The stress of sudden injury and admission to hospital presents a different set of issues for those caring for this diverse group of patients. Many will have multiple medical pathologies that may affect their recovery from surgery or traumatic injury. Box 12.1 identifies the aims of this chapter.

Osteoarthritis

Osteoarthritis is the leading cause of physical disability in individuals over the age of 65 (Nuki, 2002), causing more than 2 million people a year to visit their GP (Arthritis and Rheumatism Council, 2002). It is not an inflammatory disease and does not cause systemic symptoms. Some authors question whether it is one disorder or many having a single final common pathway (Felson, 2000). A number of factors increase the risk of an individual developing osteoarthritis; these include obesity, injuries to the joint or joint surfaces, congenital abnormalities of the joint and pathologies within the joint such as septic arthritis (Dickson & Hosie, 2003). There are specific differences in the development of osteoarthritis relating to age and gender, and sex hormones and other hormones appear to have a role in the development and progression of the disorder (Altizer, 1998). Age alone is not considered a cause of osteoarthritis, but it may impair tissue repair after injury and therefore be an indirect cause (Adams & Hamblen, 2001).

Pathophysiology

Osteoarthritis is often described as 'wear and tear' to the joint and many consider it an inevitable part of the ageing process. However, the disorder has a complex pathophysiology and is more than just erosion of the joint surfaces (Jester, 2004). The underlying processes remain the subject of much research.

The disorder is generally considered primarily one of the hyaline cartilage. The normal joint is able to withstand the stresses encountered during everyday activity. When osteoarthritis develops, either the stresses applied to the joint are excessive, or the structure of the cartilage changes so that it softens and fails to withstand normal amounts of stress. The cartilage surface becomes frayed, a process called fibrillation. Researchers are now exploring the role of the bone directly under the cartilage (subchondral bone) in the development of the disease, and the possibility that changes in the bone occur first, followed by changes in the cartilage (Nuki, 2002). Figure 12.1 demonstrates the development of arthritis.

With ageing, the body's ability to replace destroyed chondrocytes (the cells which produce cartilage) reduces. Gradually the articular cartilage is eroded at the points of maximal stress, exposing the bone underneath. As the cartilage wears away, the space between the ends of the bones (joint space) narrows; this narrowing can be seen in a plain X-ray.

The exposed bone becomes glossy and shiny as the protection of the cartilage is lost; this is called

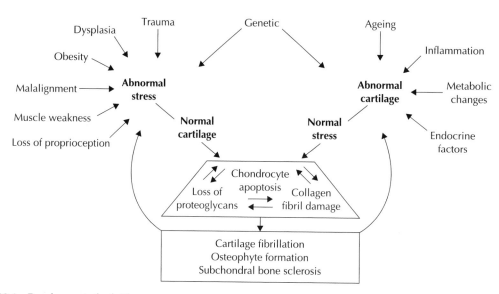

Figure 12.1   Development of arthritis.
(Reprinted from *Osteoarthritis: Risk Factors and Pathogenesis Rheumatic Disease Topical Reviews*, Nuki (2002) with permission from Professor George Nuki and the Arthritis Research Campaign)

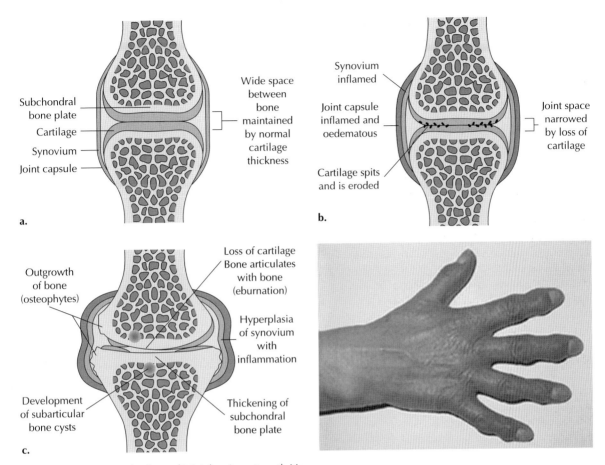

a.

Subchondral bone plate
Cartilage
Synovium
Joint capsule

Wide space between bone maintained by normal cartilage thickness

b.

Synovium inflamed
Joint capsule inflamed and oedematous
Cartilage spits and is eroded

Joint space narrowed by loss of cartilage

c.

Outgrowth of bone (osteophytes)
Development of subarticular bone cysts

Loss of cartilage
Bone articulates with bone (eburnation)
Hyperplasia of synovium with inflammation
Thickening of subchondral bone plate

Figure 12.2   Diagram of a diseased joint showing osteoarthritis.
(Reprinted from *Pathology* (2nd edn), Stevens & Lowe, Fig 24.12 (2000) with permission from Elsevier)

eburnation. The subchondral bone becomes thicker and harder. This is described as sclerosis and can be seen on X-ray as a white line along the contours of the joint. As the disease progresses, intra-articular cysts may be formed, again at the point of maximal stress. Hypertrophy of bone at the joint margins occurs and forms osteophytes (outgrowths of bone). Both cysts, if present, and osteophytes can be seen on X-ray (Figure 12.2). Eventually bone surfaces may become eroded and misshapen.

Osteoarthritis does not have any primary inflammatory features. However, secondary inflammation of the synovial membrane and joint capsule can occur as a result of the disease process, and lead to joints becoming warm and swollen. Box 12.2 lists the signs and symptoms of osteoarthritis.

Box 12.2   Signs and symptoms of osteoarthritis.

- Pain that increases on movement, worsens and eventually disturbs sleep patterns
- Stiffness and reduction in the range of movements of the joint
- Shortening of the affected leg
- Movements can be accompanied by palpable or audible crepitus
- Change in gait pattern
- Deformity is a feature in some joints in the later stages
- Osteophytes can be palpated in some joints
- Effusion of the joint can occur
- Radiographic features – osteophytes, reduced joint space, subchondral cysts, sclerosis of the bone, joint deformity

Diagnosis

A diagnosis of osteoarthritis is usually determined by the history along with physical and radiological examination. It is not easily confused with inflammatory forms of arthritis as X-rays of the joint show sclerosis of the bone rather than rarefaction; the joint is not normally warm to touch; and biochemical markers (such as erythrocyte sedimentation rate, ESR) that indicate inflammatory processes are not raised.

Treatment

Treatment of the individual with osteoarthritis should be based on a thorough assessment of the individual rather than on radiological findings. There is often a mismatch between the severity of symptoms and the radiological findings. Patients with severe destruction of bone may only report mild discomfort and those with minimal radiographic changes may report more severe symptoms (Jester, 2004). Guidelines for the care and treatment of patients with osteoarthritis are being developed by the National Institute for Health and Clinical Excellence (NICE, 2004).

There are a number of options for the treatment of osteoarthritis before the decision is taken to operate, though these are beyond the scope of this book. These options include weight loss, physiotherapy and analgesia. Oral and intra-articular chondroprotective agents are also now being used to slow down the degradation of the hyaline cartilage. Glucosamine and chondroitin are two food supplements which have been found to have chondroprotective properties – their efficacy is being investigated. A range of surgical treatments are available including osteotomy, arthrodesis, joint resurfacing and joint replacement. Caring for a patient undergoing joint replacement will be discussed later in this chapter.

Rheumatoid arthritis

Rheumatoid arthritis is rarely seen as a serious public health issue yet it is the single largest cause of disability in the UK (Bradly & Tennent, 1993, in Bath *et al.*, 1999). It is a systemic autoimmune arthritis that affects connective tissue, with the brunt of the disease process falling on the synovium (Dandy & Edwards, 2003). The condition is characterised by symmetrical poly-arthritis that initially affects the small joints of the hands and feet, though other larger joints become involved as the disease progresses. Patients can have severe deformities of their hands that, without suitable aids and adaptations, impair their ability to perform activities of living.

Along with the severe impact on joints, the systemic manifestations of rheumatoid arthritis have a significant effect on the individual's everyday life. These need to be carefully considered when organising care for the individual with rheumatoid arthritis who is undergoing surgery, or who has become acutely ill with an unrelated problem.

Pathophysiology

Normally, the immune and inflammatory responses in the body are self-limiting. However, the immune system of patients with rheumatoid arthritis has lost the ability to recognise self from non-self and the inflammatory response continues as the antigen is not destroyed (Ryan, 2002).

It is believed that an antigen initiates an auto-immune response; although the trigger for initiating this is unclear. A number of factors may be involved, for example viral infections, stress and trauma in individuals with a genetic disposition (Arthur, 1998). Hormonal factors are also implicated, as the majority of sufferers are women and the disease is more prevalent after the menarche and before the menopause (Flasher & Church, 2004).

The condition progresses within joints, bursae and tendon sheaths, which are all lined with synovial membrane. Flasher & Church (2004) identify three phases: cellular changes; inflammatory response; and destructive phase (see Box 12.3). Figure 12.3 shows the process of joint destruction in this condition. Although a disease of connective tissue, rheumatoid arthritis also has a number of systemic features that can affect the individual (see Box 12.4).

Diagnosis

The American Rheumatism Association (1987) Revised Criteria for the Classification of Rheumatoid

Box 12.3   Joint changes in rheumatoid arthritis.

Phase 1 Cellular changes
- Changes occur within the synovial membrane that becomes highly vascular, cellular proliferation occurs
- The synovial membrane thickens and becomes oedematous
- Rheumatoid factor is produced in some individuals at this point
- The inflammatory process begins and immune complexes are formed within the joint

Phase 2 Inflammatory response
- Complement is activated. This is a normal defence mechanism against antigens, which attracts neutrophils to the synovial fluid
- The neutrophils phagocytose the immune complexes and release further inflammatory chemicals, sustaining the immune response

Phase 3 Destructive phase
- This occurs due to the continuance of the inflammatory response
- High levels of lysosomes accumulate within the synovial fluid which damages the hyaline cartilage
- A further destructive element called the pannus is formed from fibrin that collects on the synovium
- The pannus invades the joint surfaces near the synovium and secretes prostaglandins and proteases
- These cause further destruction of hyaline cartilage
- Once the protection of the cartilage is removed, the bone is eroded

(Adapted from Flasher & Church, 2004)

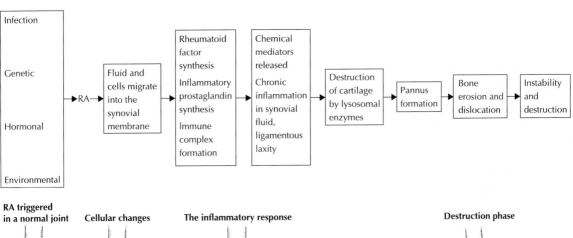

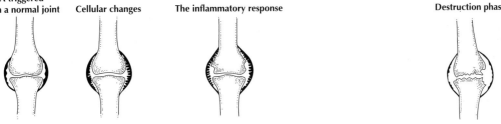

Figure 12.3   Joint destruction in rheumatoid arthritis.
(Reprinted from *Nursing the Orthopaedic and Trauma Patient*, Kneale & Davis (eds), Fig 15.2 (2004) with permission from Elsevier)

Arthritis provides the standards for diagnosis in practice (Arnett *et al.*, 1988). For a positive diagnosis of rheumatoid arthritis four or more of the criteria must be present in the patient (Box 12.5).

Patient assessment

Patients with active rheumatoid arthritis are closely monitored by their GP, a rheumatology nurse

---

Box 12.4   Systemic features of rheumatoid arthritis.

- Pain
- Early morning stiffness
- Fatigue and lethargy
- Anaemia
- Weight loss
- Nodules
- Vasculitis
- Sjögren's syndrome – dry eyes, mouth and other mucous membranes
- Neurological problems – e.g. carpal tunnel syndrome, cervical spine subluxation
- Lymphadenopathy
- GI tract problems – e.g. amyloidosis
- Cardiac problems – e.g. pericarditis
- Lung involvement – e.g. pulmonary inflammation

Box 12.5   The American Rheumatism Association 1987 Revised Criteria for the Classification of Rheumatoid Arthritis.

1. Morning stiffness in and around the joints for at least 1 hour before maximal improvement
2. Soft tissue swelling of 3 or more joint areas observed by a physician
3. Swelling of the proximal interphalangeal, metacarpophalangeal or wrist joints
4. Symmetric swelling
5. Rheumatoid nodules
6. The presence of rheumatoid factor
7. Radiographic erosions and/or periarticular osteopenia in hand and/or wrist joints

(Criteria 1–4 must have been present for more than 6 weeks)
(Reproduced with permission from Arnett *et al.*, 1988)

---

specialist or rheumatology consultant. Haematological investigations form one aspect of diagnosis, assessment and monitoring of disease activity and its response to treatment (see Table 12.1).

The effects of the condition on the patient's joints and the ability to carry out activities of living are assessed, as well as haematological investigations. Specific assessments should include the patient's level of pain, using the most appropriate tool for the individual such as a visual analogue scale, body maps, pain diary or a combination of these. Other tests and scoring systems have been developed

that assess grip strength, the number of swollen and tender joints and functional ability. Examples of these are the Disease Activity Score and the Ritchie Articular Index. When used in combination with the ESR and C-reactive protein (CRP) levels, scoring tools can help assess the efficacy of drug therapy (Sturdy, 1998a). It is not within the scope of this chapter to discuss specific assessments; further information on them can be found in any rheumatology nursing textbook.

Table 12.1   Haematological investigations and their use in patients with rheumatoid arthritis.

Investigation	Use
Rheumatoid factor	Not present in all patients. High levels typically correlate with severe disease and a poorer prognosis
Erythrocyte sedimentation rate (ESR)	Raised in RA and is used as a marker of disease activity and efficacy of drug treatment
C-reactive protein (CRP)	Raised in RA and is used as a marker of disease activity and efficacy of drug treatment
Haemoglobin levels (Hb)	Anaemia is common in patients with active RA, as the body cannot release stored iron to be used in the production of erythrocytes.
White cell count (WBC/WCC)	A raised WBC can be normal from the inflammatory process. With a sudden raise, infections should be excluded. Immunosuppression can be caused by some drug therapies and increase the risk of infection
Liver function tests (LFT)	To monitor for hepatotoxicity as a side-effect of drug therapies
Urea and electrolytes	To monitor for renal toxicity as a side-effect of drug therapies

Treatment

There are four main treatment aims for rheumatoid arthritis: relief of symptoms, preservation of function, prevention of structural damage and deformity and maintenance of the patient's normal lifestyle (Akil & Amon, 1996). Treatment primarily involves the use of drugs that reduce or modify the body's inflammatory response. Alongside drug therapy, education, information and support are needed. Advice about joint protection, to reduce the stress of everyday activities on the joints affected, is crucial to maintain longer-term function and reduce structural damage.

Some sufferers find complementary therapies helpful, although patients should be advised against stopping conventional therapies and relying on complementary therapies alone (Flasher & Church, 2004). Stopping conventional drug treatment can cause the disease to 'flare': the disease becomes more active and its impact on the individual is greater.

Surgical interventions have a role in the treatment of patients with rheumatoid arthritis. They can be used for a number of reasons including pain relief, preservation of function and maintenance of independence, and for cosmetic purposes. Surgery poses its own risks for individuals with rheumatoid arthritis and the systemic effects of the disease should be considered when planning care with the patient.

Implications of rheumatoid arthritis on pre- and post-operative care

The specific pre- and post-operative care will be affected by the site of surgery, the patient's pattern of disease and the joints affected (Sturdy, 1998b). There are, however, a number of important issues that must be considered when caring for any patient with rheumatoid arthritis.

The individual with rheumatoid arthritis has to be carefully assessed prior to surgery, whatever procedure is to be undertaken. As part of the pre-operative assessment an X-ray of the cervical spine is required (Fellows et al., 1999; Flasher & Church, 2004). There is radiological evidence of subluxation of the cervical spine in 30–40% of individuals with rheumatoid arthritis. On intubation, this may

compromise the respiratory centre of the medulla (O'Brien & Cody, 2004). Many of these patients demonstrate no clinical symptoms of nerve root compression, which is why history-taking alone is not adequate (Collins et al., 1991, cited by Cox, 1999). Some authors recommend the fitting of a soft collar prior to surgery (Sturdy, 1998b; Cox, 1999).

Other specific pre-operative assessment may include that of circulation to the limb. This may be difficult due to vasculitis, which can occur in rheumatoid arthritis and therefore Doppler studies may be needed to assess circulation (Cox, 1999). In severe cases cardiac and respiratory problems such as pericarditis, valve defects and reduced lung vital capacity may be present, so thorough assessments of the cardiovascular and respiratory systems are needed.

Where possible, continuation of the individual's usual drug regimen is maintained. Patients should miss as few of their normal doses of medication as possible to reduce the risk of a post-operative flare of the disease (Cox, 1999). This should be reviewed on an individual basis as certain drugs, such as anti-tumour necrosis factor drugs, must be stopped prior to surgery as they interfere with wound healing. Opinion varies about stopping methotrexate, given to reduce the autoimmune response, prior to surgery and individual hospital policies should be consulted. Some patients may also be at risk of delayed wound healing due to anaemia and poor nutrition, which are often associated with rheumatoid arthritis and can be compounded by surgery.

Pain has already been identified as a major symptom of rheumatoid arthritis and following surgery patients will have the added problem of acute post-operative pain. When considering strategies such as patient-controlled analgesia, the ability of the patient with rheumatoid arthritis to manipulate the handset needs to be considered. Ideally the patient should be given the opportunity to try the handset prior to going to theatre as deformity may not preclude its use.

Many patients with rheumatoid arthritis will be on long-term steroids to control their symptoms. The presence of abnormally high plasma steroid levels can suppress the body's normal mechanism of steroid secretion (Sturdy, 1998a). This means that supplementary doses of steroids may be required following trauma or surgery and local policies should be consulted on this.

Early morning stiffness can be a particular problem; the time this lasts will vary between individuals. This must be considered when planning care with the patient and time for the stiffness to wear off should be incorporated into the patient's daily routine in hospital, as they would do at home. Fatigue can also be increased by the anxiety of admission to hospital. Rehabilitation programmes that include realistic goals should be planned that take account of both early morning stiffness and times when the patient's energy levels are greatest.

Skin care is of paramount importance. Individuals with rheumatoid arthritis may have their skin integrity affected by a number of features of the disease process and its treatment (e.g. anaemia, poor nutrition and steroid therapy). Rheumatoid nodules – firm, subcutaneous, moveable lesions that can develop over bony prominences – are susceptible to trauma (Douglas & Byrne, 1998). These patients will also have reduced mobility and therefore be at risk of developing pressure ulcers if appropriate assessment and provision of suitable mattresses is not undertaken. Operating theatre staff should be contacted prior to the patient going to theatre so that appropriate equipment can be provided to give protection during the perioperative period. Regular assessment of pressure ulcer risk and evaluation of care are imperative and should be carried out throughout the patient's stay in hospital.

Joint involvement will differ between individuals, as does their ability to perform activities of living. Hand involvement may mean that special cutlery is needed; food may need to be cut up and water jugs only half filled to allow the patient to be independent with eating and drinking. Walking aids with appropriate handles will be needed: the patient may bring their own into hospital. Upper limb involvement may affect the ability to wash and dress. Time and space should be allowed to encourage independence where possible; washing and dressing aids may be provided by the occupational therapist. The impact of rheumatoid arthritis on the patient's ability to undertake activities of living and the coping strategies they have adopted should be discussed at pre-assessment clinic and then reassessed following surgery. The addition of intravenous lines and drains can further compromise independence (Sturdy, 1998b).

Joints are at risk from inappropriate positioning and lack of support when the patient is in theatre or being nursed in bed. They should be supported and carefully positioned when the patient is anaesthetised to avoid damage (Cox, 1999) and this principle should be applied to all aspects of care. Special care should also be taken during moving and handling of the patient to avoid joint damage and compromising skin integrity.

A number of patients with rheumatoid arthritis will develop dry mucous membranes, for example in the eyes and mouth. This cannot be cured but can be treated using eye drops and false saliva that should be prescribed on the patient's drug chart. During the immediate post-operative period special attention should be paid to eye care because of the risk of corneal damage from dry eyes (Cox, 1999). A dry mouth will also impair the patient's ability to talk and eat so mouthwashes and fresh drinking water should be within easy reach to ensure adequate hydration and nutrition.

Joint replacement surgery

Joint replacement surgery is carried out after all conservative treatment has been tried and has become ineffective. At this point the patient's sleep is being interrupted due to pain. The hip and knee are the most commonly replaced joints, but shoulder, elbow, ankle and finger joints can also be replaced. In 2000 more than 44 000 hip replacements and 35 000 knee replacements were performed, costing £405 million (Arthritis and Rheumatism Council, 2002). The aspects of care common to all joint replacements will be addressed. For issues regarding specific procedures specialist orthopaedic texts should be consulted.

Pre-operative assessment and preparation

All patients undergoing joint replacement surgery will normally be assessed in a pre-assessment clinic before their admission to hospital. In some trusts assessment will commence as soon as the patient is placed on the waiting list, ensuring that there is adequate time to optimise the patient's physical and psychological condition in readiness for surgery. This process also aims to reduce length of stay post-operatively. The general principles of pre-operative assessment have been discussed in Chapter 1. For patients undergoing elective orthopaedic surgery, there are certain specific issues that must be considered before the patient can proceed to surgery. Thorough physical examination of the limb and joint must be undertaken including the range of movement, presence of fixed deformities, gait pattern and use of walking aids.

A key role of pre-assessment clinics is the eradication of local and systemic infection (Fellows *et al.*, 1999). The skin condition of the limb is assessed and any skin or nail-bed infections identified. Elective surgery will usually not be undertaken if the patient has any leg ulcers, open wounds, skin, nail or other infections as this increases the risk of the joint replacement becoming infected. Should this occur it could be catastrophic for the patient and require the joint to be removed or worse, the limb to be amputated.

All patients should be screened for methicillin-resistant *Staphylococcus aureus* (MRSA). If detected on the patient's skin it does not normally prevent surgery, however the patient's GP should be contacted so that eradication treatment can commence prior to admission. On admission such patients may be nursed in a side room, and will receive prophylactic antibiotics to reduce the risk of developing MRSA in their wound. The precise treatment will depend on hospital policy.

It is important that the patient has realistic expectations of the outcome of the surgery and is motivated to undertake the post-operative exercise regimens. These issues should be discussed in advance with the patient (Jester, 2004). Discharge planning also commences at this point and the patient is given an expected discharge date. The need for aids and adaptations in the home can be identified. In many cases these can be delivered and fitted before the patient is admitted to hospital, thus avoiding delays in discharge.

Intra- and post-operative care issues in patients undergoing joint replacement surgery

The development of infection poses a serious risk to the patient undergoing orthopaedic surgery. A number of steps can be undertaken to minimise the risk at all stages of the patient's journey from good staff handwashing techniques and wound care, to surgical technique and the use of equipment in theatre. Patients receiving metal implants are given prophylactic systemic antibiotics, as this seems to reduce the number of post-operative infections (Hill & Davis, 2000). Antibiotics should be given prior to the first incision and at least 5 minutes before the tourniquet is inflated, if used, to allow adequate perfusion of the bone and tissues in the limb on which the surgery is to be performed (Bannister *et al.*, 1998, cited by Hill & Davis, 2000).

The use of ultra-clean air theatres have been recommended by the British Orthopaedic Association (BOA). Filtered air systems can significantly reduce the number of airborne bacteria and in orthopaedic theatres laminar flow systems have been shown to be effective in removing particles from around the patient (Gould & Kneale, 2004). The air passes rapidly through a series of filters and is then extracted either through the opposite wall or floor (Gould & Kneale, 2004). Ideally these theatres should be dedicated to clean elective orthopaedic surgery only. With the combination of clean air theatres and the use of prophylactic antibiotics the infection rate following hip replacement has been quoted as low as 0.3% (Lidwel, 1986, cited by BOA, 1999).

Blood loss can pose a significant risk to the orthopaedic patient and can lead to hypovolaemic shock. On return to the ward, the vital signs are closely monitored. The amount of blood lost depends on a number of factors including the anaesthetic technique; operative approach; duration of the procedure; use of bone cement; pre-operative use of aspirin and other non-steroidal anti-inflammatory drugs. Thus during the intra- and immediate post-operative period it is important that blood lost is documented within the patient's notes and, if appropriate, action taken. Advances in surgical techniques have the potential to reduce significantly the amount of blood lost during the procedure. Additionally, the use of autologous transfusions can reduce the number of post-operative homologous blood transfusions (blood from anonymous donor) required.

Autologous blood transfusions can be carried out in three ways (see Chapter 1). In orthopaedic surgery the reinfusion of blood collected in specialist drainage systems (e.g. Bellavac®) during the immediate post-operative period is some-times used. Blood collected in this way is safe and of good quality and minimises the risk to the patients of transfusion reactions and transmission of infection.

Neurovascular observations on the limb are crucial following surgery. This includes observa-tion of the colour and warmth of the limb, checking the limb has normal sensation and that the patient can move it. Pedal or radial pulses should be checked according to the site of the surgery. This must be commenced in recovery and continued on the ward as part of routine post-operative monitor-ing. Any variation from the normal for the patient should be documented and reported to medical staff immediately, though it should be remembered that some patients will have had epidural anaesthe-sia and therefore may not have normal sensation in the limb for a number of hours.

The use of wound drainage systems in ortho-paedic surgery has been under debate recently and the benefits questioned (Hill & Davis, 2000). In theory their use should limit the risk of wound infection by reducing the incidence of haematoma formation (O'Brien et al., 1997). However, some authors suggest that, while the insertion of drains does no harm, the non-use of a drain does have a number of benefits for the patient. The discomfort of drain removal and the potential problems of drain site ooze are removed (O'Brien et al., 1997). Parker & Roberts (2003) suggest that there is no conclusive proof to support or refute the use of suction drains and consider further randomised controlled trials are needed. If drains are used the level of drainage should be marked on return to the ward and subsequent drainage monitored. The amount of fluid lost into the drain should be meas-ured at midnight and documented on the patient's fluid chart.

The closed suction drains are inserted through separate stab wounds and not the surgical incision but in contrast to general surgical cases, they are not secured with sutures, so care is needed when handling such patients. Hill & Davis (2000) suggest drains should be removed no longer than 24 hours following surgery because if left any longer there is a significant risk of infection (Overgard, 1993, cited by Hill & Davis, 2000). When removing the drain, universal precautions should be followed. Follow-ing assessment of the wound drain sites should be covered with an appropriate dressing and moni-tored for signs of infection.

Post-operative deep vein thrombosis and pul-monary embolism pose a significant threat to the patient following orthopaedic surgery. Prophylaxis of thromboembolism has been discussed in Chapter 3. Individual hospital protocols should be consulted regarding the timing of administration of anticoagulation pre-operatively for patients to receive epidural analgesia, due to the potentially increased risk of bleeding into the spinal canal with anticoagulation. Intermittent pneumatic compres-sion devices may also be used with orthopaedic patients either using foot or calf pumps. The advan-tage of these is that they pose no threat of increased bleeding and do not require haematological moni-toring (Davis, 2004).

Individual orthopaedic procedures will have specific post-operative care issues and following surgery the operation notes for the patient should always be checked for special instructions or restrictions. Patients will generally be able to com-mence mobilising on the first post-operative day unless their general condition precludes this, for example if the blood pressure is low, or on specific instructions from the surgeon. Further informa-tion regarding specific orthopaedic procedures is discussed in specialist orthopaedic nursing texts. Box 12.6 outlines care issues following hip and knee arthroplasty.

Low back pain

Low back pain is a common problem and the World Health Organization (2003) estimates that 80% of persons will be affected at some point. Between 80% and 85% of back pain has no known cause. Back pain can be caused by a number of conditions (Box 12.7) and in many cases it is not possible to make a specific diagnosis and identify precise causes (Adams & Hamblen, 2001).

Those assessing individuals with back pain need to be aware of features described as 'red flags' (Box 12.8). These are specific signs and symptoms that suggest that there may be a serious underlying condition, such as malignancy, which is causing the back pain.

Spinal surgery should only be undertaken for clearly defined clinical reasons. Dandy & Edwards

Box 12.6   Specific care issues following joint replacement surgery.

Hip replacement
- To reduce the risk of dislocation the following
  - The operated leg should be nursed in abduction to reduce the risk of dislocation, patients should be educated **not** to cross their legs
  - Hip should not be flexed to more than 90 degrees – the height of the patient's chair will need to be assessed to ensure correct height; and they may need to use raised toilet seats
  - Patients should avoid twisting at the hip
  - Patients can be rolled onto either hip but care must be taken to ensure the legs remain in abduction during the procedure
  - Patients will need to get out of bed on the operated side

Knee replacement
- To avoid the knee becoming stiff the patient should be encouraged to carry out exercises as shown by the physiotherapist
- No pillows or rolled-up towels should be left under the knee, other than when needed for exercising, as this may cause the knee to become fixed in a flexed position
- When sitting out the patient should be encouraged to alternate between having the operated leg elevated on a foot stool and sitting with the knee bent to encourage both extension and flexion of the knee
- Ice packs can be used to reduce swelling

Box 12.7   Potential causes of low back pain.

- Muscle sprains or strains
- Prolapsed intervertebral disc
- Osteoarthritis of the lumbar spine (lumbar spondylosis)
- Spondylolisthesis
- Spondylolysis
- Spinal stenosis
- Rheumatoid arthritis
- Ankylosing spondylitis
- Primary cancer or metastatic tumour
- Infection, e.g. tuberculosis or infective discitis
- Osteoporosis

Box 12.8   'Red flags' in patients with back pain.

- History of cancer
- Significant trauma
- Weight loss
- Temperature > 37.8°C
- Risk factors for infection
- Neurological deficits
- Minor trauma in patients:
  - Over 50 years
  - Known to have osteoporosis
  - Taking corticosteroids
- Failure to improve over 1 month

(Reprinted from *The Musculoskeletal System Basic Science and Clinical Conditions*, 3rd edn, p. 63, Sambrook P, Schrieber L, Taylor T & Ellis A (eds) (2001) with permission from Elsevier)

(2003) limit the reasons for surgery to the following: disc excision for established disc protrusions with neurological signs; instability caused by spondylolisthesis (bony outgrowths) or unstable discs; scoliosis, kyphosis and other spinal deformities and certain tumours and infections. They also specifically state that backache is not a reason for undergoing spinal surgery.

Spinal surgery often involves major procedures, many of which will only be carried out in specialist centres. Within a district general hospital only less complex spinal decompression procedures, such as discectomies, and spinal fusions are undertaken.

Pre- and post-operative care for patients undergoing elective spinal surgery

As well as the general principles of caring for patients undergoing surgery discussed in Chapter 1 there are a number of specific issues related to those patients undergoing spinal surgery due to the risks of damage to spinal nerves and the dura mater, which covers the spinal cord and spinal nerves within the spinal canal. These are at risk due to the close proximity of all the structures (see Figure 12.4). Particular procedures may also require specific interventions and local policies should be consulted in these cases.

The risk of developing a deep vein thrombosis following orthopaedic surgery has been highlighted

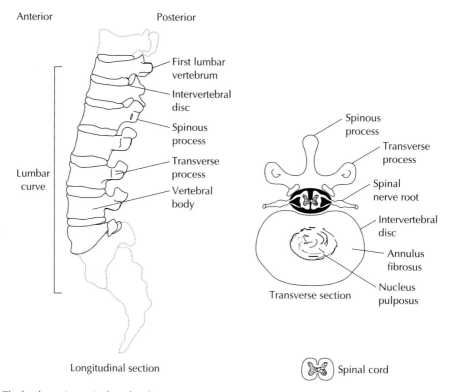

Figure 12.4   The lumbar spine, spinal cord and nerve roots.

earlier. Caution needs to be taken regarding the administration of anticoagulants prior to spinal surgery as increased bleeding at the surgical site may occur, which will reduce visualisation of the operative field. It can also increase the risk of haematoma formation at the operation site, which could cause pressure on the spinal cord with serious consequences. Local hospital protocols should therefore be consulted.

Pre-operative assessment of the patient's pain should be undertaken and the presence of any neurological deficit identified. For example, does the pain radiate down the leg; if so, how far? Is there any numbness or pins and needles and what part of the leg is affected? This information is important so that any deterioration in the patient's condition can be detected. Reassessment of pain and neurological symptoms form an important part of care following spinal surgery and should form part of the routine when carrying out post-operative observations. Any increase in numbness or pins

and needles should be documented and reported to medical staff.

The patient's ability to pass urine both pre- and post-operatively is important as difficulty in micturition and urinary retention can be a sign of compression of the spinal nerves within the vertebral canal. Should these symptoms occur they must be immediately reported to medical staff.

A rare but potentially serious complication of spinal surgery is a dural tear (damage to the dura mater that surrounds the brain and spinal cord); this may lead to cerebrospinal fluid leaking. If this has been noted during surgery it will be repaired during the operation and documented in the post-operative notes. The patient will usually be required to remain flat for 48–72 hours after surgery; this allows the dura to heal (Schoen, 2000). However, an appreciation of the signs and symptoms of a dural tear is important when caring for all patients in the recovery unit or the ward, to ensure early detection of any tears not noticed during surgery (see Box 12.9).

Fractures

McRae & Esser (2002) define a fracture as being when there is a loss of continuity of the substance of the bone, which can range from a hairline or microscopic disruption to where there are a large number of separate bone fragments. The causes of fractures are summarised in Box 12.10.

A number of descriptions, classifications and terminologies can be applied to fractures, all of which provide a different level or amount of information. Closed fractures are those where there is no break in the skin or there are superficial wounds that are unconnected to the fracture. Open fractures have a wound that provides continuity from the outside to the fracture site, allowing bacterial access and increasing the risk of infection at the fracture site. Fractures can be described in a number of ways including according to the pattern of the injury, their position (e.g. shaft of femur) and some have more in-depth classification systems (e.g. fractures involving the growth plate in children). Types of fractures are shown in Figure 12.5 and the signs and symptoms of a fracture are listed in Box 12.11.

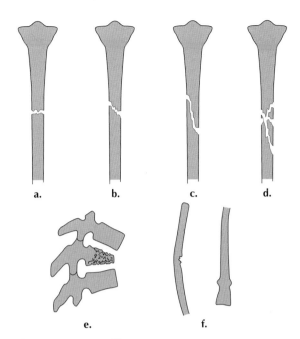

Figure 12.5   Types of fracture.
a. Transverse fracture; b. Oblique fracture; c. Spiral fracture; d. Comminuted fracture; e. Compression fracture; f. Greenstick fracture
(Reprinted from *Outline of Fractures* (11th edn), Crawford Adams & Hamblen, Fig 1.2, p. 5 (1999), with permission from Elsevier)

Complications of fractures

Bone is a living tissue and each bone has its own blood supply and therefore will bleed when fractured. In general terms the larger the bone the greater the blood loss will be. Added to this is the potential for bone ends to damage blood vessels that may run alongside the bone. Patients admitted to the ward with fractures must therefore be closely monitored for signs of shock. Patients with femoral,

Box 12.12   Complications of a fracture.

- Compartment syndrome
- Fat embolism
- Neurovascular damage
- Fracture blisters
- Shock and haemorrhage
- Osteomyelitis

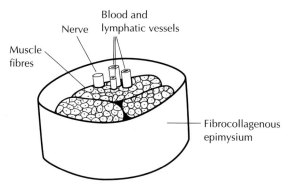

Figure 12.6   Compartment syndrome.
The muscle fibres, their nerves, blood and lymphatic vessels within the epimysium form a non-distensible **compartment**. Compression of this compartment will raise local pressure and may cause muscle and nerve ischaemia, oedema and, ultimately, cell necrosis.

pelvic or multiple fractures are at greatest risk of significant blood loss.

Complications following a fracture can occur in the first few hours or days following the injury or may develop over a number of weeks or months. They can be directly related to the fracture or be general complications that may arise following any surgery, hospitalisation and associated immobility (for example, pain, venous thromboembolism and shock). Major complications of fractures are shown in Box 12.12.

Compartment syndrome

This is an orthopaedic emergency and all patients admitted with fractures or soft tissue injury must be monitored for this condition. A compartment is a group of muscles that work synergistically, contained within a layer of fascia (Love, 1998) (see Figure 12.6). Fascia is a tough, relatively inelastic connective tissue. Acute compartment syndrome can be caused either by conditions that cause external compression of the compartment such as tight bandaging and casts, positioning following injury or during surgery; or by conditions that cause an increase in the compartment content such as bleeding and oedema. Capillary blood flow is reduced within the muscle compartment and this leads to tissue death. This is irreversible; healthy muscle tissue is replaced by fibrous scar tissue that can lead to contractures or paralysis of the limb (Dandy & Edwards, 2003). Myoglobin molecules released when muscle tissue dies can damage the renal tubules and cause acute renal failure, in severe cases leading to the patient's death. Hence, monitoring urine output and colour is important to ensure early identification of renal failure.

Compartment syndrome can develop within a few hours of an injury and therefore observation for this complication should commence in the emergency department and be continued on the ward throughout the patient's stay, and will form part of patient education for those discharged in casts. Love (1998) cites McQueen (1996) suggesting that the first 12–24 hours post-injury or surgery is the most critical time for developing compartment syndrome. The signs and symptoms of compartment syndrome are shown in Box 12.13.

Pain, often greater than that of the initial injury and unrelieved by analgesia, is frequently the first sign of developing compartment syndrome. Therefore regular assessment of pain and neurovascular status of the limb should be undertaken on all patients admitted with limb injuries, including soft tissue damage without bony injury, and following limb surgery. Any complaints of increased pain should lead to further assessment of the neurovascular status of the limb, its colour, warmth, sensation and movement. All of these symptoms are only easily identifiable in the conscious patient and nurses must be extra vigilant in cases where the patient has cognitive impairment or a reduced level of consciousness. Accurate documentation of findings following assessment of the limb is vital.

Initial treatment of a fracture includes elevation of the limb to reduce swelling and therefore reduce the risk of compartment syndrome developing. However, where compartment syndrome is suspected, the limb should be nursed at heart level. Limb elevation decreases arterial pressure within

---

Box 12.13   Signs and symptoms of compartment syndrome.

Pain – worse than the initial injury and unrelieved by analgesia, caused by muscle ischaemia and necrosis
Pain on passive stretching – passive movement of the patient's fingers, toes, foot can elicit pain in the muscle group
Paraesthesia – abnormal sensations, pins and needles, tingling, burning, numbness due to compression of the nerves within the compartment
Paralysis – inability to undertake active movements, usually a late sign
Pressure – compartment feels swollen and tense on palpation, area is taut and firm to touch
Pallor – the area of skin over the compartment may have altered coloration due to compression of arterial blood supply, skin tense and shiny
Pulses – pulses may be present in compartment syndrome. Absence of pulses is a late and serious complication

(Love, 1998; Tucker, 1998; Lucas & Davis, 2004)

---

the compartment and therefore further reduces tissue perfusion and oxygenation. Ice therapy must also be removed, as again this will reduce local blood flow and therefore diminish oxygen supply to the area (Love, 1998). Adequate hydration of the patient is important to maintain mean arterial pressure, so if the patient requires surgery, intravenous fluids should be commenced as required. Patients and their relatives will be anxious and upset. It is important to provide reassurance and keep the patient informed and involved in their care.

If compartment syndrome is suspected, the medical staff must be informed immediately. Early treatment is important to avoid permanent muscle damage and involves relieving the source of the pressure. In its simplest form this may be cutting tight bandages to restore circulation. Where the cause of the pressure is due to an increase in the content of the compartment, this will include surgery to cut through the fascia that encloses the compartment. This is called a fasciotomy and it will relieve tissue pressure and re-establish tissue perfusion. Following fasciotomy the incisions are left open and dressed prior to return to the ward. The patient will then need to return to theatre in three to five days, depending on position, in order for the wounds to be evaluated and closed or skin

grafts applied. During this time, risk of infection is a major issue for the patient.

Fat embolism

Fat embolism syndrome is a major cause of morbidity and mortality following trauma and long bone fracture, most frequently following femoral shaft and pelvic fractures. Some authors also consider fat embolism as a potential complication of hip replacement surgery (Temple, 2004). The pathophysiology of fat embolism is not fully understood and is contentious. One theory is that fat droplets are released following disruption of bone marrow and adipose tissue following injury and they enter the circulatory system through damaged vessels at the site of the injury. Others suggest that circulating blood triglycerides split into glycerol and fat, thus generating a large number of circulating fat particles (Dandy & Edwards, 2003). Signs and symptoms develop following both mechanical obstruction and chemical changes within the lungs and other tissues due to the presence of the fat particles. The timescale for the development of fat embolism syndrome is uncertain. Santy (2004) suggests observing for its signs for 72 hours following a fracture of the femoral shaft. The clinical features of fat embolism syndrome are listed in Box 12.14.

Treatment of long bone fractures

Initial treatment following a fracture will be stabilisation of the patient, ensuring accurate assessment

---

Box 12.14   Clinical features of fat embolism.

- Hypoxia
- Tachypnoea
- Tachycardia
- Confusion
- Change of mood
- Drowsiness
- Reduced level of consciousness
- Petechial rash (caused by small cutaneous haemorrhages) on the anterior portion of the body including chest, neck, upper arms, axilla, shoulder, oral mucous membranes and conjunctiva

(Dandy & Edwards, 2003)

(see Chapter 13), with fluid replacement resuscitation as necessary and adequate pain relief. This will be followed by reduction of the fracture to give correct alignment of the bone ends, if required, and immobilisation of the fracture if necessary (Crawford Adams & Hamblen, 1999). Fractures can be immobilised using a variety of techniques: external splintage, internal fixation using metal implants, external fixation and traction.

External splintage

External splintage often takes the form of a rigid cast using plaster of Paris or a range of synthetic materials that are resin-based (Royal College of Nursing Society of Orthopaedic and Trauma Nursing (RCN/SOTN), 2000). Care of the cast starts prior to its application, which should be undertaken by a skilled and competent practitioner. Once the cast has been applied it takes time to dry. For plaster of Paris this may be from 24 to 48 hours, during which time it must be left uncovered (Prior & Miles, 1999). The smell and colour of a plaster of Paris cast will also change as it dries, from grey and musty smelling to white and odourless (Lucas & Davis, 2004). Synthetic casts dry much more quickly, taking only 30–60 minutes (Prior & Miles, 1999). Table 12.2 summarises the principles of caring for a drying plaster cast.

As discussed earlier, compartment syndrome can be caused by casts that are too tight and good care of the plaster should minimise the risk of neurovascular complications occurring. Therefore following application of a cast the limb should be elevated to reduce swelling and aid venous return (Lucas & Davis, 2004). Assessment of the circulation to the limb should form an integral part of care at all times and, where able, the patient should be educated to report any signs of neurovascular impairment to a member of the healthcare team.

Skin integrity can be compromised through the application of a cast and correct handling of a wet cast is important. Areas of skin at risk include those over bony prominences under the cast and at the edges of the cast. Only exposed skin can be examined visually, therefore the nurse needs to listen to the patient and act on complaints of wetness, burning pain beneath the cast, local areas of heat on the plaster, appearance of discharge though the cast or an offensive smell from the cast, as all are signs of underlying pressure ulcers (Powell, 1986, cited by Lucas & Davis, 2004). Patients should be educated not to use pointed objects to relieve itching under the cast as this can also lead to the development of sores. Casts are often applied immediately following surgery; any bleeding through the plaster should be marked, timed and dated to allow further bleeding to be monitored.

On a practical level for the patient, casts can be heavy and make undertaking activities of living difficult. Individual assessment of the impact on each patient will be needed. Special consideration of the cast and its impact on moving and handling the patient is also important.

Internal fixation

Internal fixation of the fracture is used when adequate stabilisation of the fracture cannot be achieved by other means, where a patient has fractures of more than one bone; where there is a fracture in which the blood supply to the limb is

Table 12.2   Principles of caring for a drying plaster cast.

Care	Rationale
Rest limb on pillows	Avoids causing undue pressure or deformities in the cast that may cause pressure on the underlying skin
Cover pillows with absorbent materials and change regularly	Aids drying
Leave the cast exposed	Drying occurs as the water in the cast evaporates
Use the palms of the hand rather than the finger tips to handle a drying cast	Avoids making dents in the cast, which can cause pressure on underlying skin
Do not use external heat to aid drying	Heat will be transmitted through to the skin and could cause burns

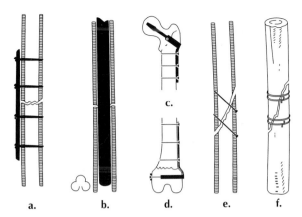

Figure 12.7   Example of internal fixator devices.
a. Plate and screws; b. Intramedullary nail; c. Screw plate
and screws; d. Nail-plate; e. Oblique transfixion (for spiral
or oblique fractures).
(Reprinted from *Outline of Fractures* (11th edn), Crawford
Adams & Hamblen, p. 44 (1999), with permission from
Elsevier)

jeopardised and blood vessels need to be protected;
or where the fracture involves joint surfaces or the
fracture ends are displaced (Dandy & Edwards,
2003). Internal fixation of fractures can be achieved
by using a wide range of devices including screws,
nails, plates and wires; the choice of device used is
dependent on the site and pattern of the fracture
(Crawford Adams & Hamblen, 1999). Figure 12.7
shows some examples of internal fixation devices.

The care of patients following any internal fixation of a fracture follow the same general principles
of pre- and post-operative care as discussed in
Chapters 1 and 3. Many of the issues discussed
within this chapter related to care of patients following joint replacement surgery are also relevant
to patients having internal fixation of fractures and
readers should refer to that section. When caring
for these patients both pre- and post-operatively,
the risks of developing compartment syndrome
and fat embolism must be considered. It is important to observe for the signs and symptoms of these
and other complications of fractures and, if appropriate, measures should be taken to reduce the risk
of them, such as elevation of the limb and the use of
ice therapy to reduce swelling. Reducing the risk
of infection, screening for MRSA and the administration of prophylactic antibiotics and appropriate
wound care are also of particular importance to this
group of patients.

External fixation

With this method of fracture treatment bone
ends are held together with pins and wires that
are inserted through the skin (McRae & Esser,
2002). External fixation is used particularly in the
management of open fractures where, due to the
increased risk of infection, internal fixation is
deemed inappropriate or where the fracture is too
complex to be immobilised by internal fixation or
external splintage (Santy, 2000). Figure 12.8 is an
example of external fixation.

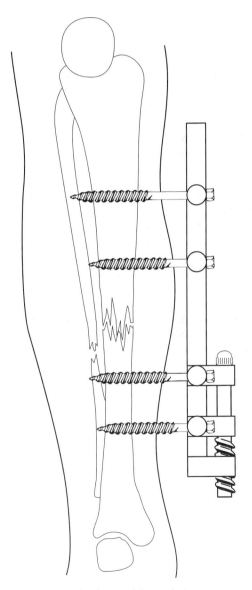

Figure 12.8   Example of external fixator device.

Table 12.3   RCN/SOTN Consensus Guidelines for pin site care.

Guideline	
Summary guidelines	Rationale
Apply absorbent low adherent, sterile immediate post-operative dressings	To absorb blood and exudate
Inspect the wound within 24 hours of surgery	For patient comfort and the early assessment of potential problems
Re-dress all pin sites after 24 hours	There is likely to be exudate and bleeding
No solution should be used on the immediate post-op dressing	There is no reliable evidence to support any of the solutions currently used to clean/dress pin sites
Use only sterile normal saline or water to clean any exudates or dried blood away from the area around the pins	There is no reliable evidence to support any of the solutions currently used to clean/dress pin sites
Use a dressing that applies a small amount of pressure and keep it continuously in place	To prevent tenting of the skin along the pin
Only remove dressings infrequently as required. Aseptic technique must be rigorously maintained at all times during pin site care and observation	To prevent cross-infection
Observe the pin site dressings regularly, at least daily in the immediate post-operative period. Observe for increased tenderness or pain at the pin site, increased level of exudates, presence of pus, an odour from the site and any increased inflammatory process	To identify problems at an early stage
Take seriously any complaints from the patient	Patients often identify problems earliest
Clean pin sites daily with non-shedding material (e.g. gauze) and normal saline or water only to clean away exudates or dried blood. Otherwise do not clean	There is no evidence to support the use of anything else, and other solutions may cause damage
Leave the wound dry after cleaning	Moisture encourages colonisation
Meet general hygiene needs with showering	There seems little support for sterile cleansing after this effective washing. Bathing in personal bath water is to be discouraged
Gently remove scabs and crusts around the pin site. Clean or rub dry with gauze. Do not massage	Allows visualisation of the wound and encourages free drainage of exudates which may harbour infection
Keep metal work socially clean	To remove social contamination and wound exudates
Teach patient to shower at home and dry the fixator with a clean towel used only for this purpose. Actively clean pin sites only if exudates present	Tampering pin sites excessively can lead to infection
Educate patient family and community staff to look for signs of infection	To identify problems early
Provide as much written and verbal information to patients and carers as possible	To reduce anxiety, increase compliance and provide support
Provide opportunities to contact other patients and support groups	To provide psychological support and information
Keep patient regimes simple and provide instruction and evaluation. Expect non- or poor compliance	To increase compliance
Provide psychosocial support	Percutaneous pins amount to a major insult to self-image

(Reprinted from *Journal of Orthopaedic Nursing 5*, Lee-Smith, Santy, Davis, Jester & Kneale, 'Pin Site management, Towards a consensus: part 1', p. 41 (2001) with permission from Elsevier)

The main nursing issue for a patient with an external fixator is minimising the risk of infection through appropriate pin site management. Where the pin or wire enters the patient's skin, each pin site offers a potential access for infection and appropriate wound care is of paramount importance as the pin tract offers direct contact with bone. Santy & Temple (2003) found no randomised controlled trials to support any particular method of pin site care and highlighted the need for significant work in this area. The Royal College of Nursing Society of Orthopaedic and Trauma Nursing have produced consensus guidelines based on the best available evidence and these currently stand as best practice in pin site care. These are shown in Table 12.3.

Pain assessment must be carried out regularly and adequate analgesia provided. Once the fixator is applied and the fracture stabilised, the limb may feel less painful (Bryant, 1998). Alongside this, regular assessment of the neurovascular status of the limb and observation for signs of compartment syndrome must be undertaken as with other forms of fracture immobilisation.

Care needs to be taken to avoid damage to the skin on the other limb or other parts of the body by the fixator and adaptations to clothing may be required. Staff should also take care to avoid damage to themselves when caring for patients with external fixators, especially when undertaking moving and handling techniques.

External fixation can also have a psychological impact as the frame can be viewed as a major disfigurement to the individual (Santy, 2000). Sensitivity is required when caring for the patient and their family and addressing their feelings towards the frame, throughout the acute and re-habilitation phases of the patient's treatment. Sims *et al.* (1999) highlight the role that the patient's family and friends play in helping the patient avoid feeling isolated and depressed.

Traction

Traction may be applied to the patient prior to surgery and the insertion of internal fixation devices or application of external fixation. In some patients whose injury is not suitable for other methods of immobilisation or whose medical condition is too poor to undergo anaesthesia, traction will be used

---

> **Box 12.15**   Uses of traction.
>
> - To relieve muscle spasm and pain
> - To restore and maintain alignment of bone following fractures and or dislocations
> - To help re-establish blood flow and nerve function
> - To facilitate easier treatment and dressing of soft tissue injuries
> - For resting injured or inflamed joints whilst keeping them in a functional position
> - To permit movement of joints while fractures heal
> - Slow correction of deformities that have been caused by contraction of soft tissues from disease or injury
> - To facilitate easier movement of the patient in the bed
>
> (Adapted from RCN SOTN, 2002)

as the main method of treatment. Traction simply means pulling and has a number of uses in relation to the treatment of orthopaedic patients (see Box 12.15).

Traction is either fixed, where the pull is between two points, or sliding or balanced traction, where the pull is balanced between weights and the patient's body weight (RCN SOTN, 2002). It can be applied either as skin traction or skeletal traction. Care must be used in the application and continued management of a patient in traction as badly applied traction can cause a number of problems and discomfort for the patient and even impede their recovery and rehabilitation.

Skin traction

Skin traction can be applied to the arm or leg using non-adhesive or adhesive traction kits. The benefit of the non-adhesive kit is that patients are at less risk of skin reactions. Adhesive skin traction should not be used on patients with frail or friable skin. Padding should be applied over bony prominences; the traction extensions are then placed over the limb and bandaged in position using either a spiral or figure of eight bandage (RCN SOTN, 2002). Care must be taken not to apply the bandage too tightly as this may lead to compartment syndrome. Joints should be left free of bandaging to avoid constriction of blood vessels and nerves in these areas and allow some movement of the joint (RCN SOTN, 2002). A small piece of tape should be used to secure the bandage, not tape that encircles the whole circumference of the limb, which may constrict the circulation.

Skeletal traction

In skeletal traction the pulling force is applied directly through the bone via pins. This method of traction has the advantage that greater amounts of weight can be applied and is the preferred method of application if the traction is required for a long time (Lucas & Davis, 2004). Patients with skeletal traction will require appropriate management of the pin sites.

Care of the patient in traction

Many of the principles of patient care have been discussed above and will relate to the reason why the patient is in traction. Patients are at risk of compartment syndrome; therefore regular neurovascular assessment of the limb should be undertaken. As the patients are immobile, they are at risk of associated complications such as deep vein thrombosis, pulmonary embolism, chest infection, constipation and urinary retention. Problems with skin integrity are a particular risk, not just on pressure points but also under the bandages of skin traction. Leg troughs can be used to relieve pressure from the heel. Bandages should be removed at least daily and the skin inspected (RCN SOTN, 2002). Adequate pain relief must be given prior to this. Box 12.16 lists the principles of management of the traction system.

It should also be appreciated that the patient on traction may have a number of anxieties associated with their admission to hospital and the psychological care of the patient and their family is as important as the management of the traction system itself.

Hip fractures

This section relates to the care of patients with a fracture of the proximal femur (commonly called hip fractures), particularly those over 65, as in this age group the injury can be as devastating and have as serious consequences as multiple trauma in the younger population. Santy (2004) highlights the

---

Box 12.16   Management of the traction system.

- The amount of weight used in the traction system must be recorded clearly in the medical and nursing notes.
- The traction system should be checked by a trained healthcare professional at least once every 8 hours and always after any procedure, e.g. moving the patient, physiotherapy or X-ray, to ensure that the system has not been altered and that the pull of the traction is in collect alignment.
- All hinged clamps in the structure should be tight and checked regularly.
- Only traction cord should be used for traction as it does not stretch and should be appropriate diameter for the pulleys used within the system. It should sit within the pulleys at all times and run freely within them.
- Only one length of cord should be used. Short lengths of cord should not be knotted together as this would prevent the cord running freely over the pulleys and there is the potential for the knots to separate, thus putting the patient at risk.
- The cords must be attached to equipment (e.g. weights) securely by non-slip knots.
- Adhesive tape should be applied to the ends of traction cord to stop it fraying as this may lead to possible disruption of the traction. Knots should not be covered.
- The weights must hang freely at all times and not rest on the floor. If the weights rest on the floor, the pulling forces of the traction system are lost or reduced.
- When skeletal traction is used, the pointed ends of pins or wires must be covered as they are a potential source of injury to the patient and staff.
- Weights should only be hung over the patient when another safety cord is used. This must be checked regularly.
- If required, counter-traction must be maintained at all times.

(Adapted from RCN SOTN, 2002; Lucas & Davis, 2004)

---

challenges of caring for this frail and vulnerable group. Hip fractures take up 20% of orthopaedic beds (Parrott, 2000), and can mean that these patients are often seen as routine and not as individuals who are acutely ill or may become so. However, multiple medical pathologies are often seen in this group and individuals may be at increased risk of renal failure and cardiovascular complications and therefore should be closely monitored during the acute phase of their treatment. Within the last ten years the treatment of patients with hip fractures has come under increasing scrutiny and drives formulated to improve the care for patients (Audit Commission, 2000).

The hip joint is a synovial ball and socket joint. It has a joint capsule and is supported by accessory ligaments. Fractures can occur within the capsule (intracapsular) or outside the capsule (extracapsular). The exact position of the fracture is significant for the surgeon, as it determines the type of surgical treatment and allows the nurse to discuss treatment and post-operative care with the patient and their family. Intracapsular fractures can cut off the blood supply to the head of the femur leading to avascular necrosis (death) of the femoral head. It is for this reason that this type of fracture in the individual over 65 is generally treated using a hemiarthroplasty (Santy, 2004). The position of the fracture also makes accurate reduction of the fracture difficult (Dandy & Edwards, 2003). Extracapsular fractures are treated with internal fixation devices such as a dynamic hip screw. Figure 12.9 shows an Austin Moore prosthesis.

Some patients may be considered too frail or sick to undergo anaesthetic and these patients may be treated conservatively. This can take 12 weeks or more in the older person and is not without risk. Bed rest for this long has a number of potential complications, particularly in the older frail person, and for this reason spinal anaesthesia is increasingly being used so that the surgery can take place. Guidelines suggest that regional anaesthesia should be the anaesthetic of choice for patients having

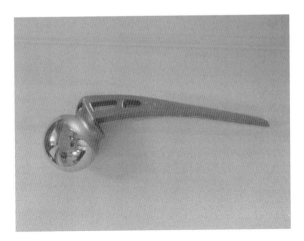

Figure 12.9 Austin Moore prosthesis.

surgery for hip fracture (SIGN, 2002). A review of the evidence failed to demonstrate clear conclusions regarding the benefit of this in the reduction of mortality or outcomes other than a reduction in the incidence of post-operative confusion (Parker *et al.*, 2004).

Pain management needs to be given careful consideration as unrelieved acute pain can increase the risk of life-threatening complications in older people with co-existing medical pathologies (Briggs, 2003). Pain management can be complicated by a number of cultural and psychological issues and in the older person confusion and cognitive impairment can also make effective pain assessment and management difficult. Murdoch & Larsen (2004) consider that those with cognitive impairment are less likely to have their pain identified than are cognitively intact individuals. They go on to suggest that behavioural tools should be used as a method of pain assessment along with acting on verbal reports of pain, though highlight the need for further research to validate their effectiveness.

Skin traction was historically used as one method of pre-operative pain management for this injury, but evidence now suggests that the benefits of this are limited and that supporting the leg on a pillow or other soft appliance is equally effective; however, further research into this area is required (Parker & Handoll, 2003).

Opiate analgesia can be used effectively both pre-operatively and in the immediate and early post-operative period. The route of their administration needs to be considered as the reduction of muscle tone found in older patients can cause the fluid in intramuscular injections to pool at the injection site and thus delay the drug's action (Gould, 1999). Small intravenous doses of opiate analgesia allow accurate titration against pain scores and patient condition and they are also advantageous in the shocked patient who is peripherally shut down, where absorption of intramuscular doses of analgesia is unpredictable. The older person may be more susceptible to the side-effects of opiate analgesia such as respiratory depression, suppression of coughing and changes in levels of consciousness in the normal doses prescribed. However, opiates can be used safely in this group with appropriate monitoring (Seers, 1999), therefore smaller, more frequent doses with close monitoring of vital signs are needed in these patients

(American Geriatric Society, 2002, cited by Briggs, 2003).

Recently attention has been given to the use of femoral nerve blocks as a method of pain relief with some success in this group of patients. In a small study Candal-Couto *et al.* (2005) demonstrated benefits in the use of a modified nerve block with improved pain scores using a visual analogue scale. Fletcher *et al.* (2003), in a randomised controlled trial of 50 patients, demonstrated that pain relief was achieved more rapidly and less opiate analgesia was required in patients who received 3-in-1 femoral nerve blocks and intravenous morphine when compared with those who received intravenous morphine alone. However, a systematic review of randomised controlled trials failed to demonstrate any clear benefits of this method of pain relief in this group of patients (Parker *et al.*, 2005). Further evaluative work in this area is needed, as the use of this method of pain management is not without risks and requires adequate training in the administration technique.

Regular simple oral analgesia such as paracetamol should be included in the patient's treatment regimen as this can be effective. However Santy (2004) reminds us to exercise caution in overestimating such drugs' efficacy when the pain is severe. Non-steroidal anti-inflammatory drugs can have a role to play but should be used with caution in the older person as they are associated with increased side-effects such as renal impairment and drug interactions (Briggs, 2003).

Best practice advocates that patients who are fit for surgery should be operated on by an experienced surgeon within 24 hours of admission to hospital or within 24 hours once fit for surgery (SIGN, 2002). In an ideal patient pathway, this would occur and the patient would only be fasted once and for the minimum amount of time. In reality this does not always occur. Adequate hydration must be maintained to avoid further complications for the patient; therefore intravenous fluid replacement is essential. This should be commenced in the emergency department and continued into the post-operative period. Care should be taken to avoid fluid overload and the use of infusion devices should be used where available. The National Confidential Enquiry into Perioperative Deaths (NCEPOD) reports in 1999 and 2002 have identified continued deficits in this area of care.

Hypoxaemia will slow the patient's recovery from the anaesthetic and subsequent rehabilitation process. It is also a common cause of acute confusion in the older person. Not only is acute confusion distressing for the family, it also makes other aspects of the patient's care, such as pain assessment and management, more difficult. Oxygen saturation should be monitored routinely in the pre-operative period and oxygen prescribed if indicated by the results. The evidence suggests that oxygen should be prescribed for at least 6 hours post-anaesthetic (general or regional) and should be continued at night for 48 hours post-operatively, or longer as determined by pulse oximetry (SIGN, 2002).

A large percentage of patients are admitted to hospital in less than optimal nutritional status (McWhirter & Pennington, 1994). The effect of the injury and subsequent surgery will increase the individual's nutritional requirements further. A review of the evidence into the benefits of nutritional supplements in patients with hip fractures found that the strongest evidence existed for the use of protein and energy feeds (Avenell & Handoll, 2005). However, these should not be given to the patients immediately before or at mealtimes, as they will reduce the amount the patient eats and therefore their daily calorie intake.

The psychological needs of the patient and their family must also be addressed at this very stressful time. They will have major concerns surrounding the impending surgery, the long-term outcome and potential for rehabilitation. These need to be dealt with to facilitate the patient's recovery and rehabilitation. Delirium (acute confusion) may also occur due to a number of precipitating factors. Nurses caring for patients with hip fractures need to be aware of these and be able to assess for the potential cause in individual cases. As Norman (1999) highlights, the successful management of the delirious patient relies on the prompt diagnosis and treatment of the underlying cause. Box 12.17 lists the causes of acute confusion.

Prevention of pressure ulcer formation should be commenced as soon as the patient is admitted to hospital. Many of them will have been lying on the floor for a number of hours before being discovered and an ambulance called, thus meaning that a sore, though not apparent, may have already formed. The length of time that the individual was lying on the floor must be documented in the nursing notes

---

Box 12.17   Examples of causes of delirium in older people.

- Cardiovascular disease
- Infection – especially urinary tract and chest
- Carcinomatosis
- Transient ischaemia
- Drugs
- Drug interactions
- Drug withdrawal
- Hypoglycaemia
- Dehydration
- Electrolyte imbalance
- Anoxia from any cause

(Adapted from Byrne (1994) in Norman (1999))

---

and skin integrity assessed as soon as possible with the appearance of skin accurately documented. Risk assessment scoring must be carried out on admission and appropriate interventions implemented. This should be repeated as the patient's condition alters.

Early mobilisation acts as one method of reducing the risk of pressure ulcer formation. It also has the added benefits of improved circulation and can reduce the risk of venous thromboembolism. The evidence to support the use of graduated compression stockings can seem confusing and the choice of best anticoagulant is inconclusive. However, in the review of the evidence by SIGN (2002), aspirin 150 mg for 35 days for all patients, intermittent pneumatic compression and early mobilisation were suggested as best practice in reducing the risk of developing venous thromboembolism in this patient group, with heparin being reserved for those who were at high risk of venous thromboembolism. Most noticeable in this advice is the absence of the use of graduated compression stockings; however, as patients admitted with hip fracture often have leg ulcers or have frail skin, this may also make the use of graduated compression stockings inappropriate.

Other considerations

Patients within an orthopaedic and trauma ward may have a wide range of conditions and have undergone a wider range of different procedures. Some patients will have sustained multiple trauma, with fractures to more than one bone and damage to other organs, and the information in Chapter 13 has specific relevance to this group of patients. Trauma patients may also have suffered head injury and/or spinal injury at the time of the accident and this can further complicate the care they require. Care of the patient with head injuries or a spinal fracture with or without spinal cord injury are specialist areas in themselves. Patients will be admitted to orthopaedic wards with a range of spinal fractures, and may have halo traction applied in a district general hospital. The complex nature of the care required by both these patient groups is outside the remit of this chapter and readers should consult specialist texts on the subjects.

Self-test questions

1. Identify the main differences between osteoarthritis and rheumatoid arthritis.
2. List five systemic effects of rheumatoid arthritis.
3. Prior to undergoing elective orthopaedic surgery the patient will be assessed for the presence of systemic and local infections. Why?
4. What does neurovascular observation following limb surgery include?
5. **True** or **false**? Wound drainage systems are generally not secured using sutures when used in orthopaedic surgery.
6. List five specific features of the symptoms that you need to identify when admitting a patient with back pain prior to surgery.
7. What are the signs and symptoms of compartment syndrome?
8. Other than compartment syndrome what is another potentially serious complication that may follow a fracture of the shaft of a long bone?
9. What principles should be adhered to whilst casts used to treat fractures are drying?
10. What do SIGN (2002) recommend as prophylaxis of deep vein thrombosis in patients with hip fractures?

References and further reading

Adams JC & Hamblen DL (2001) *Outline of Orthopaedics* (13th edn). Edinburgh: Churchill Livingstone

Akil M & Amon R (1996) *in*: Snaith M (ed.) (1996) *ABC of Rheumatology*. London: BMJ Publishing Group

Altizer L (1998) 'Chapter 15 – Degenerative disorders' *in*: Maher A, Salmond S & Pellino T (eds) (1998) *Orthopaedic Nursing* (2nd edn). Philadelphia: WB Saunders

Arnett F, Edworthy S, Bloch D *et al.* (1988) 'The American Rheumatism Association 1987 Revised criteria for the classification of rheumatoid arthritis' *Arthritis and Rheumatism* 31(3): 315–324

Arthritis and Rheumatism Council (2002) *Factfile – arthritis at a glance* (online). www.arc.org.uk/about_arth/FactFile.pdf (Accessed 10.01.07)

Arthur (1998) 'Chapter 2 – The rheumatic conditions – an overview' *in*: Hill J (ed.) (1998) *Rheumatology Nursing*. Edinburgh: Churchill Livingstone

Audit Commission (2000) *United They Stand: Co-ordinating Care for Elderly Patients with Hip Fracture* (online). www.audit-commission.gov.uk/Products/NATIONAL-REPORT/251D3429-93AE-4F4A-B912-8D89E87F749F/hipvfmi.pdf (Accessed 10.01.07)

Avenell A & Handoll HHG (2005) 'Nutritional supplementation for hip fracture aftercare in older people' *The Cochrane Database of Systematic Reviews* 2005, Issue 2. Chichester: John Wiley & Sons, Ltd

Bath J, Hooper J, Giles M, Steel D, Reed E & Woodland J (1999) 'Patients' perceptions of rheumatoid arthritis' *Nursing Standard* 14(3): 35–38

Briggs E (2003) 'The nursing management of pain in older people' *Nursing Standard* 17(18): 47–53

British Orthopaedic Association (1999) *BOA Recommendation on Sterile Procedures in Operating Theatres* (online) www.boa.ac.uk/site/showpublications.aspx?ID=59 (Accessed 10.01.07)

British Orthopaedic Association (no date) *Knee Replacements: A Guide to Good Practice* (online). www.boa.ac.uk/site/showpublications.aspx?ID=59 (Accessed 10.01.07)

Bryant (1998) 'Chapter 11 – Modalities for immobilisation' *in*: Maher A, Salmond S & Pellino T (eds) (1998) *Orthopaedic Nursing* (2nd edn). Philadelphia: WB Saunders

Candal-Couto J, McVie J, Haslam N, Innes A & Rushmer J (2005) 'Pre-operative analgesia for patients with femoral neck fractures using a modified facia iliaca block technique' *Injury: International Journal of the Care of the Injured* 36: 505–510

Cox M (1999) 'Rheumatology Part 3: the role of surgery' *Professional Nurse* 14(6): 427–430

Crawford Adams J & Hamblen DL (1999) *Outline of Fractures* (11th edn). Edinburgh: Churchill Livingstone

Dandy D & Edwards D (2003) *Essential Orthopaedics and Trauma*. Edinburgh: Churchill Livingstone

Davis P (2004) 'Chapter 5 – Why move?' *in*: Kneale J & Davis P (eds) (2004) *Nursing the Orthopaedic and Trauma Patient*. Edinburgh: Churchill Livingstone

Department of Health (2001) *National Service Framework for Older People*. London: Department of Health

Dickson DJ & Hosie G (2003) *Your Questions Answered: Osteoarthritis*. Edinburgh: Churchill Livingstone

Douglas J & Byrne J (1998) 'Chapter 10 – Skin and nutrition' *in*: Hill J (ed.) (1998) *Rheumatology Nursing*. Edinburgh: Churchill Livingstone

Fellows H, Abbott D, Barton K, Burgess L, Clare A & Lucas B (1999) *Orthopaedic Pre-Admission Clinics*. London: Royal College of Nursing

Felson (2000) 'Osteoarthritis: New Insights Part 1: the disease and its risk factors' *Annals of Internal Medicine* 133(8): 635–646

Flasher N & Church S (2004) 'Chapter 15 – Care of patients with rheumatoid arthritis' *in*: Kneale J & Davis P (eds) (2004) *Nursing the Orthopaedic and Trauma Patient*. Edinburgh: Churchill Livingstone

Fletcher A, Rigby A & Heyes F (2003) 'Three in one femoral nerve block as analgesia for fractured neck of femur in the emergency department' *Annals of Emergency Medicine* 41: 227–233

Gould D (1999) 'Chapter 14 – Drugs and older people' *in*: Redfern S & Ross F (eds) (1999) *Nursing Older People*. Edinburgh: Churchill Livingstone

Gould D & Kneale J (2004) 'Chapter 10 – Process and prevention of infection' *in*: Kneale J & Davis P (eds) (2004) *Nursing the Orthopaedic and Trauma Patient*. Edinburgh: Churchill Livingstone

Hill J (ed.) (1998) *Rheumatology Nursing*. Edinburgh: Churchill Livingstone

Hill N & Davis P (2000) 'Nursing care of total joint replacement' *Journal of Orthopaedic Nursing* 4(1): 41–45

Jester R (2004) 'Chapter 17 – Osteoarthritis and total joint replacement' *in*: Kneale J & Davis P (eds) (2004) *Nursing the Orthopaedic and Trauma Patient*. Edinburgh: Churchill Livingstone

Kneale J & Davis P (eds) (2004) *Nursing the Orthopaedic and Trauma Patient*. Edinburgh: Churchill Livingstone

Lee-Smith J, Santy J, Davis P, Jester R & Kneale J (2001) 'Pin site management. Towards a consensus: part 1' *Journal of Orthopaedic Nursing* 5(1): 37–42

Love C (1998) 'A discussion and analysis of nurse-led pain assessment for the early detection of compartment syndrome' *Journal of Orthopaedic Nursing* 2(3): 160–167

Lucas B & Davis P (2004) 'Chapter 6 – Why restricting movement is important' *in*: Kneale J & Davis P (eds) *op.cit.*

Maher A, Salmond S & Pellino T (eds) (1998) *Orthopaedic Nursing* (2nd edn). Philadelphia: WB Saunders

McRae R & Esser M (2002) *Practical Fracture Treatment* (4th edn). Edinburgh: Churchill Livingstone

McWhirter JP & Pennington CR (1994) 'Incidence and recognition of malnutrition in hospital' *British Medical Journal* 308: 495–498

Murdoch J & Larsen D (2004) 'Assessing pain in cognitively impaired older adults' *Nursing Standard* 18(38): 33–39

National Confidential Enquiry into Perioperative Deaths (1999) *Extremes of Age* (online). www.ncepod.org.uk/1999.htm (Accessed 10.01.07)

National Confidential Enquiry into Perioperative Deaths (2002) *Functioning as a team?* (online). www.ncepod.org.uk/pdf/2002/02full.pdf (Accessed 10.01.07)

National Institute for Health and Clinical Excellence (2004) *Osteoarthritis* (online). www.nice.org.uk/pdf/Osteoarthritis_Remit.pdf (Accessed 10.01.07)

Norman I (1999) 'Chapter 30 – Acute confusional states (delirium) in later life' *in:* Redfern S & Ross F (1999) (eds) *op.cit.*

Nuki G (2002) *Osteoarthritis: Risk Factors and Pathogenesis Rheumatic Disease Topical Reviews* (online). www.arc.org.uk/about_arth/med_reports/series4/tr/6609/6609.htm (Accessed 10.01.07)

O'Brien S & Cody J (2004) 'Chapter 12 – Patient admission: planned and emergency' *in:* Kneale J & Davis P (eds) *op.cit.*

O'Brien S, Gallagher P, Engela D, James P, Kernohan G, Connolly D, Milligan K, Kettle P & Beverland D (1997) 'The use of wound drains in total hip replacement surgery' *Journal of Orthopaedic Nursing* 1(2): 77–83

Parker MJ, Griffiths R & Appadu B (2005) 'Nerve blocks (subcostal, lateral cutaneous, femoral, triple, psoas) for hip fractures' *The Cochrane Database of Systematic Reviews*, Issue 4. Chichester: John Wiley & Sons, Ltd

Parker MJ & Handoll HHG (2003) 'Pre-operative traction for fractures of the proximal femur in adults' *The Cochrane Database of Systematic Reviews* Issue 4. Chichester: John Wiley & Sons, Ltd

Parker MJ, Handoll HHG & Griffiths R (2004) 'Anaesthesia for hip fracture surgery in adults' *The Cochrane Database of Systematic Reviews*, Issue 4. Chichester: John Wiley & Sons, Ltd

Parker MJ & Roberts C (2003) 'Closed suction surgical wound drainage after orthopaedic surgery' *The Cochrane Database of Systematic Reviews* Issue 4. Chichester: John Wiley & Sons, Ltd

Parrott S (2000) *The Economic Cost of Hip Fracture in the UK* (online). www.dti.gov.uk/files/file21463.pdf (Accessed 10.01.07)

Prior M & Miles S (1999) 'Principles of casting' *Journal of Orthopaedic Nursing* 3(3): 162–170

RCN SOTN (2000) *A Framework for Casting Standards*. London: Royal College of Nursing

RCN SOTN (2002) *A Traction Manual*. London: Royal College of Nursing

Redfern S & Ross F (eds) (1999) *Nursing Older People*. Edinburgh: Churchill Livingstone

Ryan S (2002) 'Rheumatoid arthritis' *Nursing Standard* 16(20): 45–52, 54–55

Sambrook P, Schrieber L, Taylor T & Ellis A (eds) (2001) *The Musculoskeletal System: Basic Science and Clinical Conditions*. London: Churchill Livingstone

Santy J (2000) 'Nursing the patient with an external fixator' *Nursing Standard* 14(31): 47–52

Santy J (2004) 'Chapter 24 – Care of patients with lower limb injuries and conditions' *in:* Kneale J & Davis P (eds) *op.cit.*

Santy J & Temple J(2003) 'Pin site care for preventing infections associated with external bone fixators and pins' *The Cochrane Database of Systematic Reviews* Issue 4. Chichester: John Wiley & Sons, Ltd

Schoen D (2000) *Adult Orthopaedic Nursing*. Philadelphia: Lippincott

Seers K (1999) 'Chapter 29 – Pain and older people' *in:* Redfern S & Ross F (eds) *op.cit.*

SIGN (2002) *Guideline 56 Prevention and management of hip fracture in older people* (online). www.sign.ac.uk/guidelines/fulltext/56/index.html (Accessed 10.01.07)

Sims M *et al.* (1999) *External Fixators*. London: Royal College of Nursing

Smeltzer SC & Bare BG (2000) *Brunner & Suddarth's Textbook of Medical-Surgical Nursing* (9th edn). Philadelphia: Lippincott

Stevens A & Lowe J (2000) *Pathology* (2nd edn). London: Mosby

Sturdy C (1998a) 'Chapter 4 – Assessing rheumatic patients' *in:* Hill J (ed.) *op.cit.*

Sturdy C (1998b) 'Chapter 14 – Surgical interventions' *in* Hill J (ed.) *op.cit.*

Temple J (2004) 'Total hip replacement' *Nursing Standard* 19(3): 44–51

Tucker K (1998) 'Compartment syndrome: the nurse's vital role' *Journal of Orthopaedic Nursing* 2(1): 33–36

World Heath Organization (2003) *The Burden of Musculoskeletal Conditions at the Start of the New Millennium*. Report of a WHO Scientific Group WHO Technical Report Series Number 919 (online). www.ota.org/downloads/bjdExecSum.pdf (Accessed 22.01.07)

13 Identifying and Managing Life-threatening Situations

Tim Collins and Catherine I Plowright

Introduction

Evidence suggests that acutely ill patients receive sub-optimal care before admission to intensive care (ITU) (McQuillan *et al.*, 1998; Goldhill *et al.*, 1999; NCEPOD, 2005). Before admission to ITU or cardiac arrest, patients frequently show signs and symptoms of physiological deterioration. McQuillan *et al.* (1998) and Goldhill (2000) found that health professionals lacked essential knowledge in identifying, assessing and managing acutely unwell patients in hospital wards. McArthur-Rouse (2001) and Department of Health (2001) recommend that all ward staff learn to identify patients at risk of developing critical illness. The evidence suggests that early identification and appropriate management of unstable patients improves prognosis and reduces admission to ITU and the incidence of cardiac arrest (McQuillan *et al.*, 1998; Goldhill, 2000).

The Department of Health (2000, 2001) recommends that all nurses undertake high-dependency training. This chapter explores critical care issues relevant to practitioners working within the surgical ward environment. The physiological early warning signs and symptoms of critical illness will be discussed with reference to the role of critical care outreach teams and their impact on managing the unwell surgical patient. The causes, management and role of the nurse in cardiorespiratory arrest will also be considered.

The physiology of shock and its surgical causes will be discussed. Clinical shock can occur in any surgical patient and healthcare professionals must identify this early and respond appropriately, otherwise the patient outcome is reduced. The most common type of surgical shock is hypovolaemic; however, septic, cardiogenic, anaphylactic and neurogenic causes may also occur. These five types of shock are treated differently and nurses need to know the differences in order to correct them appropriately.

The chapter will discuss the management of four critical conditions that can occur in surgical patients and require urgent attention. These are the management of hypoxia, acute hypotension, reduced conscious levels and oliguria. The altered physiology of these serious conditions and the corrective interventions will be discussed. This chapter aims to provide an overview of how to identify, assess and manage patients who are at risk of becoming or are critically ill (Box 13.1).

Early warning signs and symptoms of critical illness

It has been evident for a number of years that patients in hospital show signs of deterioration that are observed by medical and nursing staff but not acted upon prior to cardiac arrest (Franklin &

Mathew, 1994; Rich, 1999). Comparable findings are also evident in patients who have been admitted to a critical care area of a hospital (Goldhill, 1997; McQuillan *et al.*, 1998; Goldhill *et al.*, 1999; NCE-POD, 2005). Therefore, it is suggested that if there is early identification and management of the deteriorating patient in a ward then the outcomes will be improved.

To identify a deteriorating patient, a number of tools have been developed such as the Early Warning Score System (EWSS) by Morgan *et al.* (1997), the Modified Early Warning System (MEWS) developed for surgical patients by Stenhouse *et al.* (2000) and validated by Subbe *et al.* (2001) for medical patients. Whichever tool is used (it may not be one of the above) it will be based on predefined physiological parameters, to assist in prompt identification and management of deteriorating patients. The tools use physiological parameters such as pulse/heart rate, systolic blood pressure, respiratory rate, temperature, urine output and conscious level of the patient. Scores are allocated to each of the physiological parameters and a total score obtained which indicates whether further assistance is required.

Critical care outreach

Further assistance is often provided by outreach teams. These originated in the United Kingdom following the Audit Commission Report (1999) and the Department of Health Report (2000), which both investigated critical care services. Outreach services have three key roles, which are outlined in Box 13.2.

Outreach teams vary throughout the country according to locally available resources. Examples range from nurse-led teams providing a service 24 hours a day, 7 days a week, to single nurses providing a service 5 days a week. Some teams include doctors and/or physiotherapists and some hospitals have no such service (Department of Health, 2003). However the service is organised, the core function of the outreach team is as described in Box 13.2.

Systematic assessment of the acutely unwell patient

When a patient is identified as being at risk of deterioration, a regular, comprehensive systematic assessment is needed. Many professionals use an ABCDE method of assessment as taught in life support courses such as ALS (Advanced Life Support) provider course, ALERT™ (Acute Life Threatening Events Recognition and Treatment) (Smith, 2003) and CCrISP (Care of the Critically Ill Surgical Patient) (Anderson, 2003). The use of a systematic approach to assessment is valuable when the healthcare professional is under pressure (Anderson, 2003), as often occurs when faced with a deteriorating acutely unwell patient. The ABCDE system aims to make the patient safe, rather than making a diagnosis (Smith, 2003). It is important to remember that if the patient is unwell he or she should be monitored with all the aids available, for example a pulse oximeter, heart monitor and non-invasive blood pressure monitor.

Airway

The airway can be assessed using the look, listen and feel method. If the patient is awake and talking easily, generally the airway is being maintained. If there are indications of airway difficulties such as noisy breathing, simple airway adjuncts such as an oropharyngeal airway, or head tilt chin lift/jaw thrust manoeuvre may be needed along with oxygen therapy. Further information on airway management can be found later in this chapter.

Breathing

Breathing also can be assessed using the look, listen and feel method. The respiratory rate should be taken. Further information is provided in the section discussing hypoxia.

Circulation

Hypovolaemia is a major common cause of circulatory collapse (Anderson, 2003; Smith, 2003) and the main treatment is to administer intravenous fluids rapidly. Again the look, listen and feel method is useful to assess the circulation. This includes feeling the temperature of the skin and peripheries, feeling the pulse rate and checking on capillary refill times. Further information is available in the section discussing management of hypotension.

Disability

There are three areas to be assessed in this section (Anderson, 2003; Smith, 2003). The first is the rapid assessment of the patient's neurological status using the AVPU method (see Box 13.3), then the pupils can be checked to see if they are equal and reacting to light. Lastly the patient's blood sugar is checked as hypoglycaemia is common and affects consciousness. Further information is provided in

---

> **Box 13.3**   AVPU scale for assessing conscious levels.
>
> **A**   Alert
> **V**   Responds to Voice
> **P**   Responds to Pain
> **U**   Unresponsive

---

the section on the management of the patient with altered levels of consciousness.

Exposure

The patient needs to be fully exposed to enable a full examination. It is the healthcare professional's role to ensure that dignity and privacy are maintained and that the patient does not become cold.

Clinical shock

Clinical shock is a life-threatening condition requiring immediate attention. It is an acute state in which tissue perfusion fails to maintain the supply of oxygen and nutrients for normal cell homeostasis (Collins, 2000). Shock involves many body organs and must be reversed or death may occur. To maintain normal cell function the heart circulates oxygen and nutrients for the cells to produce adenosine triphosphate (ATP) for production of cell energy. This process is termed 'aerobic respiration'. In shock this is impaired and cells become deprived of oxygen and glucose. In order to survive energy is produced by 'anaerobic respiration'. This is less effective, produces less energy than aerobic respiration and results in accumulation of lactic acid, which ultimately impairs cellular homeostasis and exacerbates systemic metabolic acidosis and organ hypoxia (Collins, 2000). There are three reasons why tissue perfusion might become inadequate and clinical shock develops:

- A decreased circulating blood volume
- A failure of the heart to pump effectively
- A massive increase in peripheral vasodilation

There are four stages of shock (see Table 13.1) and the earlier the shock is treated, the better the outcome for the patient. Therefore, healthcare professionals should constantly observe for shock and

Table 13.1 The four stages of shock.

Stage of shock	Physiology	Signs and symptoms
Initial stage The shock is in the initial stages	Cells initially become hypoxic and ATP production reduces. Cells then start to convert ATP into energy by anaerobic respiration. Lactic acid is produced as a by-product and begins to accumulate	There may be few signs and symptoms at the initial stage; however, if the shock continues and is not reversed the patient will develop abnormal signs and symptoms
Compensatory stage The body tries to intervene and overcome the progressing shock	Metabolic acidosis occurs due to build-up of lactic acid. Initial hypotension is detected by the baroreceptors and corrected by the release of adrenaline and noradrenaline. This causes vasoconstriction at the skin, GI tract and kidneys, which concentrates blood supply to the heart and brain as the brain is particularly susceptible to hypoxia and cell damage	<ul><li>Hyperventilation to compensate for metabolic acidosis and hypoxia</li><li>Tachycardia due to increased catecholamine release (adrenaline) and attempt to increase cardiac output</li><li>Delayed capillary refill time > 2 seconds due to vasoconstriction</li><li>Decreased urine output</li><li>Confusion, agitation due to cerebral hypoxia</li></ul> NB. Blood pressure will be maintained due to compensatory mechanisms
Progressive stage The compensatory mechanisms that the body initially implemented are failing	If the originating problem of the shock, e.g. blood loss, has not been corrected, organ perfusion will reduce, resulting in widespread hypoxia and multi-organ failure	<ul><li>All the above</li><li>Hypotension</li><li>Severe metabolic acidosis</li><li>Severe hypoxia</li></ul>
Refractory or irreversible stage	The vital organs have failed and the shock can no longer be reversed. Death is imminent	Gross abnormal observations and metabolic disturbances

commence treatment early (Collins, 2000; Smeltzer & Bare, 2000). Shock can be classified as either hypovolaemic, cardiogenic or distributive (Hand, 2001).

Hypovolaemic shock

Hypovolaemic shock is the most common type of shock that is found in the surgical patient. Hypovolaemic shock occurs when circulating fluid volume is reduced. This causes a reduction in cardiac output and results in a low perfusion state (Collins, 2000). Hypovolaemia often results from haemorrhage, which can be either internal or external; or fluid loss from extracellular compartments (see Box 13.4).

Treatment

The standard ABCDE approach should be utilised in assessing a patient suspected of hypovolaemic

---

Box 13.4 Causes of hypovolaemic shock.

- External haemorrhage (e.g. arterial bleed)
- Internal haemorrhage (e.g. ruptured spleen, ruptured internal blood vessel)
- Trauma
- Fractures
- Severe vomiting and diarrhoea
- Bowel obstruction
- Pancreatitis
- Peritonitis
- Burns
- Third space fluid shift movements
- Inappropriate diuretic therapy

---

shock. Treatment involves optimising ventilation and oxygenation by administering oxygen therapy, correcting the cause of hypovolaemia and fluid resuscitation. This may involve the patient requiring urgent surgery to treat the cause of the hypovolaemia. Patients require frequent monitoring

Table 13.2   Signs, symptoms and management of hypovolaemic shock.

Signs and symptoms	Treatment	Regularly record and observe the following
• Hyperventilation • Rapid weak and thready pulse • Delayed capillary refill (> 2 seconds) • Cold and pale peripheral digits (vasoconstriction) • Oliguria (reduced below 0.5 mL/kg/hour and concentrated) • Confusion and agitation • Reduced level of consciousness • Bleeding may be obvious • Excessive blood loss from wound drains • Abdomen may be hard, distended and painful • Blood results will show falling haemoglobin • Arterial blood gases (ABG) will show metabolic acidosis • Elevated lactate level (normal < 1.5) • CVP (if inserted) will be low (normal = 0–8 mmHg (Woodrow, 2000)) • Hypotension (late sign)	• Assess and manage as per ABCDE method • Call expert help from surgeon, anaesthetist and critical care outreach team • Treat the direct cause of hypovolaemic shock • Obtain blood for FBC, clotting screen, cross-match, urea and electrolytes (U&E) and ABGs • IV cannulae (two) • CVP line insertion • Fluid resuscitation (blood products) • High-flow oxygen therapy • Transfer to operating theatre for surgery	• Respiratory rate, depth and pattern • The patient's pulse (weak and thready due to low stroke volume) • Blood pressure (note mean arterial BP and pulse pressure) • Oxygen saturation (may be inaccurate if vasoconstricted) • Core and peripheral temperature • Capillary refill (delayed > 2 seconds) • Hourly urine measurements • Fluid balance • Drain loss or blood loss from obvious bleeding sites or orifices • Glasgow Coma Score • Pain scoring • CVP recordings (if inserted)

of all vital signs including Glasgow Coma Score, blood results and arterial blood gases. (Table 13.2 summarises the signs, symptoms and management of hypovolaemic shock.) Immediate referral should be made to senior surgeons, anaesthetists and critical care outreach teams, as the prognosis diminishes the longer untreated hypovolaemic shock persists. There are four classifications of hypovolaemic shock that are dependent upon the patient's blood loss: the more severe the blood loss, the more critical the patient (see Table 13.3). Refer to the rest of this chapter for the management of disordered vital signs.

Cardiogenic shock

This is characterised by left ventricular pump failure which causes reduced tissue perfusion. This may occur following myocardial infarction and is associated with a mortality rate of 80% (Moore & Woodrow, 2004). Treatment involves supporting the failing heart; increasing blood pressure using inotropic support and improving oxygen delivery to the cells (see Table 13.4).

Table 13.3   Four classes of hypovolaemic shock.

Blood loss	Observations
Class 1 Up to 15% blood loss	Usually few clinical signs. The body's compensatory mechanisms are activated to cope with the blood loss (patients who are young and fit can tolerate significant blood loss before vital signs become abnormal)
Class 2 15–30% blood loss	• Tachycardia (weak and thready pulse) • Hyperventilation • Vasoconstriction (delayed capillary refill >2 seconds) • Cool skin • Oliguria (below 0.5 mL/kg/hr) • Concentrated urine • Confusion and agitation NB Changes in all observations except for blood pressure
Class 3 30–40% blood loss	• Dramatic deterioration in all vital signs • Severe tachycardia and hypotension develops
Class 4 Above 40% blood loss	• Immediate threat to life • Cardiorespiratory arrest impending • Drastic surgery and treatment required

Table 13.4   Causes, signs, symptoms and treatment of cardiogenic shock.

Causes	Signs and symptoms	Treatment
• Myocardial infarction • Cardiomyopathy • Trauma • Cardiac tamponade • Valve disease • Pericardial infection • Pulmonary embolism • Arrhythmias	• Fast, weak and thready pulse • Systolic BP < 90 mmHg • Cold and clammy • Hypoxic • Oliguria • Confused/agitated • Pulmonary oedema • Dysrhythmias	• Oxygen therapy • Non-invasive ventilation (NIV) • Invasive ventilation • Inotropic support • Organ support

Distributive shock

This comprises three types, septic shock, anaphylactic shock and neurogenic shock. Distributive shock is characterised by loss of blood vessel tone and enlargement of the vascular compartment that diverts the intravascular fluid volume away from the heart (Hand, 2001). Although blood volume remains normal, the subsequent vasodilation reduces venous return, cardiac output and tissue perfusion.

Septic shock

Septic shock is the most common type of distributive shock and can arise from a variety of overwhelming toxins. It can be caused by Gram-negative and Gram-positive bacteria. Box 13.5 identifies the risk factors for developing septic shock. When infective organisms invade body tissues an immune response occurs. This involves various chemical mediators (interleukins, tumour necrosis factor, platelet activating factor and myocardial depressant factor) being released (Hand, 2001). Initially these mediators produce an early hyperdynamic state comprising fever, vasodilation and increased cardiac output. Septic shock characteristically presents with severe vasodilation and leakage of fluid into the interstitial spaces. This results in hypovolaemia and poor tissue perfusion (see Box 13.6).

The chemical mediators also cause micro-thrombus formation, which obstructs blood flow to the organs and cells (Hand, 2001). This further exacerbates the condition. If untreated the patient will develop a hypodynamic state in which cardiac

Box 13.5   Risk factors for developing septic shock.

- Older people
- The very young
- Intravenous drug users
- Those with existing infection
- Loss of skin integrity due to wounds, burns, pressure sores, ulcers
- Major surgical operations particularly colorectal surgery
- Faecal peritonitis
- Any indwelling medical devices (as below):
  - CVP lines
  - IV cannulae
  - Urinary catheters
  - Abdominal drains
  - Chest drains
  - Pacemakers
  - Endotracheal tubes
- Genetic predisposition
- Immunosuppression (as below):
  - Malignancy
  - HIV/AIDS
  - Diabetes
  - Alcoholism
  - Immunosuppressant drugs
  - Malnutrition
  - Neutropenia

output falls and the prognosis decreases. Treatment involves increasing circulatory volume and perfusion, and giving antibiotics and cardio-respiratory support. The management of sepsis is continuously being researched and developed. The Surviving Sepsis Campaign (2005) website provides current sepsis information aimed specifically at healthcare professionals.

Box 13.6   Signs and symptoms of septic shock.

- Fever (core > 38.3°C)
- Hypothermia (< 36°C)
- Patient may have warm peripheral circulation (not always)
- Altered mental status
- Tachycardia
- Hypotension (systolic < 90 mmHg)
- Tachypnoea
- Hypoxaemia
- Oliguria
- Leukocytosis (WBC count > 12 000/μL)
- Leukopenia (WBC count < 4000/μL)
- Thrombocytopenia
- Coagulation abnormalities
- Hyperglycaemia
- High-risk category for developing sepsis

NB Patients may not present with all these signs and symptoms

Box 13.7   Causes of neurogenic shock.

- Injury or stroke to the brain stem
- Spinal cord injury
- Emotional trauma
- Depressive drugs (usually anaesthetic agents)

Table 13.5   Causes, signs and symptoms of anaphylactic shock.

Causes	Signs and symptoms
<ul><li>Antibiotics</li><li>Vaccinations</li><li>Transfusion of incorrectly cross-matched blood</li><li>Drugs</li><li>Nuts</li><li>Eggs</li><li>Fruit</li><li>Latex</li><li>Insect bites</li></ul>	<ul><li>Respiratory distress</li><li>Cardiovascular collapse</li><li>Hypotension</li><li>Tachycardia</li><li>Anxiety</li><li>Urticaria (skin rash)</li><li>Sensations of burning or itching of the skin</li><li>Gastrointestinal cramps</li><li>Bronchospasm</li><li>Oedema</li><li>Airway compromise</li><li>Recent history of administration of potential anaphylactic antigen</li></ul>

Neurogenic shock

This type of shock occurs due to loss of sympathetic nerve activity from the brain's vasomotor centre due to disease, drugs or traumatic injury (Collins, 2000) (Box 13.7). The loss of sympathetic impulses causes massive vasodilation, resulting in a significant decrease in peripheral vascular resistance, which reduces venous return and cardiac output. Treatment involves fluid resuscitation to increase circulatory volume, oxygen therapy and vasoconstrictors to counteract the vasodilation.

Anaphylactic shock

This results from a severe allergic reaction in which an antigen–antibody reaction occurs. There are numerous antigens that can cause anaphylaxis (Table 13.5). Once the antigen is inside the body, the allergen provokes an extensive defence reaction, including vasodilation and increased vascular permeability, which allow fluid to leak out of vessels into the interstitial spaces (Hand, 2001). This is a medical emergency and death can occur within minutes unless treatment is commenced. The airway is at risk of swelling and occluding in severe anaphylactic shock. Immediate airway maintenance should be achieved by a senior anaesthetist. Treatment involves administering high flow oxygen; adrenaline (for its vasoconstriction action and for relaxing smooth muscle); intravenous antihistamine; intravenous steroids; and fluid resuscitation. Readers are recommended to review the current anaphylactic shock algorithm from the Resuscitation Council.

The hypoxic patient

Respiratory assessment

Deterioration in respiratory function may occur when patients become critically ill and if alterations are identified early and managed, then outcomes will be improved (McQuillan *et al.*, 1998). Respiratory assessment is used to determine the oxygen transportation abilities and, if possible, the same nurse should be involved in the monitoring of respiratory function throughout a shift (Moore, 2004).

Table 13.6   Assessment of efficiency of breathing.

Look	• Count the respiratory rate for a full minute (the normal range varies between textbooks but as a general rule should be between 12 to 18 breaths per minute) • Is the rhythm normal? (inspiration should be slightly longer than expiration) • Undertake oximetry reading • Are chest movements symmetrical? • Is the patient using any accessory muscles? • Is the patient cyanosed? • Are there any chest wall deformities or is there clubbing of fingers? • Is the patient producing any sputum? If so what colour? How much? And is this normal for the patient?
Listen	• What is the patient's mental status? An alteration may indicate hypoxaemia • What does the breathing sound like? • Can the patient talk in full sentences without getting breathless?
Feel	• Can you feel vibrations when you place your palm on the patient's chest? • Is there any tenderness?

(Adapted from Sheppard & Wright, 2000; Jevon & Ewens, 2002; Bickley, 2004; Moore, 2004)

Table 13.7   How to differentiate between peripheral and central cyanosis.

Peripheral cyanosis	Central cyanosis
• There is adequate oxygenation of the blood • Poor local circulation • Common causes include hypovolaemia, cardiogenic shock, the cold • The extremities are blue • The tongue and lips are pink	• Poor oxygenation of the blood with oxygen saturations 85–90% • Common causes include pneumonia, acute asthma, pulmonary oedema • The lips, nail-beds and tongue are blue-tinged

(Adapted from Lumb, 2000; Smith, 2003)

Assessment of respiratory function involves more than counting the respiratory rate or undertaking pulse oximetry. It is known that a change in respiratory rate is an early indicator of deterioration, which may precede collapse or cardiac arrest (Fieselmann et al., 1993; Goldhill et al., 1999). However, in everyday practice respiratory rate monitoring does not occur for every patient. Chellel et al. (2002) found that 55% of all patients they surveyed had no respiratory rates recorded in the previous eight hours and 36% had no oxygen saturation recorded.

Table 13.6 explains how to assess the efficiency of breathing by looking, listening and feeling. There are differences between peripheral and central cyanosis, which are summarised in Table 13.7. See Chapter 3 for normal range of arterial blood gases.

Hypoxia

The main function of the respiratory system is to deliver oxygen to and remove carbon dioxide from the body cells via the blood. Failure to do so will result in respiratory failure. Hypoxia occurs when the patient's cells have inadequate oxygen (Jevon & Ewens, 2002). Respiratory failure is a syndrome where one or other of the gas exchange functions is inadequate (Sharma, 2005).

Respiratory failure

There are two types of respiratory failure, which are summarised in Table 13.8.

Table 13.8   Type 1 and type 2 respiratory failure.

Type 1	Type 2
<ul><li>The patient has hypoxia without hypercapnia</li><li>It often occurs acutely and with diseases that affect the lung tissue, e.g. pneumonia, pulmonary oedema, infective conditions (Dougherty & Lister, 2004)</li><li>Defined as the patient having a PaO_2 of less than 8 kPa and a $PaCO_2$ of less than 6 kPa (The British Thoracic Society, 2002)</li></ul>	<ul><li>The patient has hypoxia *and* hypercapnia</li><li>Caused by reduced lung compliance and an increase in airway resistance</li><li>Causes include chronic obstructive pulmonary disease (COPD), chest wall deformities, neuromuscular disorders affecting the respiratory muscles and drug overdoses (Dougherty & Lister, 2004)</li><li>Defined as the patient having a PaO_2 of less than 8 kPa and a $PaCO_2$ of greater than 6 kPa (The British Thoracic Society, 2002)</li><li>Type 2 failure occurs in 10–15% of patients who have COPD (Bateman & Leach, 1998)</li></ul>

Recognition of hypoxia

Healthcare professionals should recognise hypoxia as early as possible in order to manage the situation before the patient becomes too unwell. Early signs of hypoxia include irritability, altered conscious levels, confusion, tiredness, restlessness, anxiety or headaches (Moore, 2004). If the situation is not recognised at this stage the next stage is confusion and aggression, lethargy, increased respiratory rate, hypotension, and cardiac rhythm problems. If not managed correctly the patient will become cyanosed, oxygen saturations will deteriorate, and coma and respiratory arrest will follow (Moore, 2004).

The earlier the hypoxia is identified, the earlier treatment can commence. It is useful to consider all patients who develop new confusion or agitation as being potentially hypoxic.

Causes of hypoxia

There are a number of reasons why patients become hypoxic, including:

- Airway problems
- Acute respiratory failure
- Neuromuscular disorders
- Acute lung injury
- Trauma
- Altered levels of consciousness
- Post-operatively

The treatment of patients who are hypoxic will depend on the underlying reason but the first-line treatment is oxygen therapy (Smith, 2003).

Oxygen therapy

If hypoxia is not urgently treated with oxygen, then the effects may be brain damage and/or cardiac problems leading to cardiac arrest. Oxygen is a prescription-only medicine so it must be prescribed before administration. The prescription should include not only the percentage to be administered but also the type of oxygen delivery system (Bateman & Leach, 1998; Sheppard & Wright, 2000; Smith, 2003).

Information regarding oxygen therapy can at times be confusing, especially for patients who have type 2 respiratory failure, but the following needs to be remembered:

'Patients do not die from a raised carbon dioxide level alone: they die from hypoxaemia'.

(Smith, 2003, p. 35)

This re-emphasises the need for all patients who are hypoxic to receive oxygen. Patients who have type 1 respiratory failure (no chronic obstructive pulmonary disease – COPD) should be administered 100% oxygen via a mask with an oxygen reservoir (see Figure 13.1). The purpose of this is to achieve oxygen saturations of 100% or at least 90% (Smith, 2003).

Patients who have known COPD (type 2 respiratory failure) also require oxygen therapy. However, a very small number of them are at risk of respiratory depression if they are given high concentrations of oxygen, because their main respiratory stimulus is a hypoxic drive (Marieb, 2001). Even when well these patients normally have high carbon dioxide levels. If they are given too high a

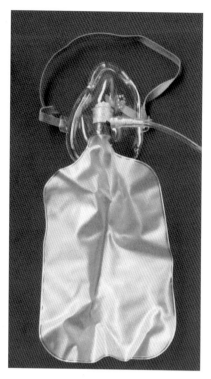

Figure 13.1   Mask with an oxygen reservoir.
(Reprinted with kind permission of Respironics (UK) Ltd)

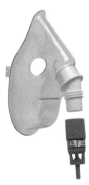

Figure 13.2   Venturi systems.
(Reprinted with kind permission of Respironics (UK) Ltd)

percentage of oxygen it will lead to respiratory depression (MacKenzie, 2004).

The goal of oxygen therapy for these patients is to achieve an oxygen saturation of 90% (Smith, 2003). The recommendation is to administer initially 35% oxygen using a venturi-type delivery system (see Figure 13.2) and to adjust the percentage incrementally in order to achieve the desired oxygen saturation (Smith, 2003).

All patients who require oxygen when they are acutely unwell require close monitoring of their respiratory rate, respiratory pattern, conscious level (using the AVPU scale), and oxygen saturations using a pulse oximeter; as well as all other vital observations, including their colour. Additionally arterial blood gases should be monitored. It is important that oxygen therapy is not removed from the patient whilst taking blood gases (Smith, 2003). If the arterial carbon dioxide ($PaCO_2$) starts to rise in a patient with a type 1 respiratory failure then it is a good indication that the patient is beginning to tire and may need further respiratory support. However, if the arterial carbon dioxide ($PaCO_2$) starts to rise in a patient with a type 2 respiratory failure the nurse should consider having the oxygen percentage reduced.

The hypotensive patient

Physiological factors responsible for blood pressure

Blood pressure is produced by a person's cardiac output and vascular resistance:

$$BP = cardiac\ output \times vascular\ resistance$$

Three factors affect cardiac output – preload, myocardial contractility and afterload (Smith, 2003) (see Figure 13.3).

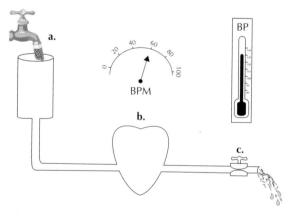

Figure 13.3   Factors influencing cardiac output.
a. Preload; b. Cardiac contractility; and c. Afterload (vascular resistance)
(Reprinted with kind permission of Professor GB Smith and Learning Media Development, University of Portsmouth)

Preload is the amount of blood returning to the heart from the tissues: if there is hypovolaemia there will be unsatisfactory filling of the heart and the cardiac output will fall. Myocardial contractility is concerned with how well the heart contracts and pumps blood into the arteries: if contractility diminishes, the cardiac output will be reduced. The afterload is a measure of the resistance that the blood encounters on ejection from the left ventricle. If the vascular resistance is raised then the cardiac output falls, as there is a greater resistance against which the heart has to empty (Smith, 2003).

Recognising the signs of reduced organ perfusion

Signs of reduced perfusion should be recognised early so that they can be managed. The signs to observe for include a reduction in urine output to less than 1 mL/kg/hour, an altered neurological status, and decreased skin perfusion resulting in cool or cold hands and feet (Smith, 2003).

The cerebral blood pressure is autoregulated between 60 and 140 mmHg and if it falls below this there will be alterations in conscious level. This can result in a reduction in AVPU score or a fall in Glasgow Coma Score of 2 or more points. The renal blood pressure is autoregulated between 70 and 170 mmHg and any reduction will result in a reduction in urine production. If the urine output falls below 1 mL/kg/hour, it may be that blood pressure and renal perfusion are inadequate (Smith, 2003).

Management of hypotension

Hypotension (low blood pressure) is defined in adults as a systolic blood pressure of less than 100 mmHg (Marieb, 2001). Organ perfusion is dependent on an adequate blood pressure, and for the majority of organs, the mean blood pressure needs to be above 70 mmHg for normal perfusion and function.

When a patient is hypotensive it is important to assess whether it is as a result of a reduction in preload, contractility or afterload (Smith, 2003). If not identified and treated appropriately then organ perfusion will be reduced and the patient will become more unwell. The patient's history is important as well as evidence from the notes and charts to identify the cause of the hypotension. This may or may not be obvious, and may include, for example, observable signs of haemorrhage (reduced preload) or myocardial infarction (contractility problems).

The commonest cause of hypotension is hypovolaemia (Smith, 2003) and this is also the easiest to treat. The management of this is to administer 500 mL of crystalloid fluid as quickly as possible and within 5 to 10 minutes: if the patient has a myocardial cause for the hypotension, the amount of fluid should be reduced to 250 mL (Smith, 2003). If there is a reduction in heart rate, a quicker capillary refill time, an improved urine output and an improvement in conscious level, then it can be considered that there is a good response to the fluid. If, however, the response is not so good, then the fluid administration has to be repeated. If cardiac function gives cause for concern, then it is important to closely monitor and observe for an increase in heart rate and listen to the lungs for crepitations, both of which are indicators of fluid overload (Smith, 2003). The aim of the fluid replacement should be to achieve a systolic blood pressure of at least 100 mmHg and, if the hypotension continues, further advice is required as the patient may require inotropic drugs to assist the improvement in blood pressure (Smith, 2003).

The oliguric patient

The functions of the kidneys are described in any text book on anatomy and physiology but in summary they are:

- Excretion of water soluble waste products of metabolism and drugs
- Fluid, electrolyte and hydrogen ion homeostasis
- A number of endocrine functions

In health we produce 1.5 to 2 litres per day of urine (this equates to >1 mL/kg/hour) (Anderson, 2003; Smith, 2003). For people to produce urine the following have to be present:

- No impediment to urine flow
- Normal kidney function
- An adequate blood supply to the kidneys

Urine is produced by a process of filtration followed by selective reabsorption and then the secretion of the urine. The renal system regulates electrolyte and fluid balance by increasing or restricting the filtrate produced, and by the ability of the renal tubules to absorb or excrete electrolyte and waste products of metabolism.

Normal urine is straw-coloured and clear and has little odour. Abnormalities include changes such as pale, dark, cloudy or frothy appearance and changes in odour, and each has its own significance (Jevon & Ewens, 2002; Dougherty & Lister, 2004). A valuable tool is to undertake a 'dipstick' urinalysis, which will show the presence or absence of a number of things such as ketones, blood, glucose, pH, and specific gravity. The procedure to do this is explained in *The Royal Marsden Manual* (Dougherty & Lister, 2004). There are also a number of electronic devices on the market today that will undertake a urinalysis. The 'dipstick' urinalysis is valuable because it measures the specific gravity: this is an indication of the ability of the renal system to concentrate or dilute the urine. A raised specific gravity above 1.025 may indicate dehydration, whereas a low specific gravity below 1.010 may be a sign of overhydration (Cook, 1996).

Significance of poor renal perfusion and blood pressure

The efficiency of the renal system is determined by the renal blood supply and in a healthy adult is about 1000–1200 mL of blood per minute. The renal blood supply is kept constant at mean arterial pressures (MAP) of between 70 and 170 mmHg by the process known as autoregulation (Smith, 2003). If a patient's mean arterial pressure falls below the lower limit of 70 mmHg, this results in a reduction in renal blood supply, which will result in a reduced urine output. The body will start to compensate by increasing retention of water and electrolytes in an attempt to maintain the circulatory volume. The result will be a reduced urine volume with a higher specific gravity.

Oliguria

Most patients admitted to critical care areas from general wards are dehydrated (Kishen, 2002) and

Table 13.9 Examples of fluid input and output.

Input	Output
● Oral fluids	● Urine
● Intravenous fluids and drugs	● Nasogastric tube drainage
	● Vomit
● Blood	● Diarrhoea
● Enteral/parenteral feed	● Colostomy/ileostomy
	● Wound drainage

as oliguria is an early sign of a patient's potential worsening condition, it should be acted upon early. Oliguria is defined as a urine production of between 100 and 400 mL of urine a day. If patients produce less than 100 mL of urine per day, this is defined as anuria and absolute anuria is where there is no urine production.

When monitoring fluid balance, all fluid gains and losses must be recorded in order to provide an accurate record of fluid balance (Carroll, 2000). Examples of types of fluid input and output can be found in Table 13.9. Fluid balance charts are sometimes very poorly completed: Reid *et al.* (2004) found that none of the fluid balance charts they examined were correctly completed, and Chellel *et al.* (2002) found that just over 40% of fluid balance charts were correctly completed. Reid *et al.* (2004) found:

'. . . one patient's chart had no fluid records on the first day, while for the other two days, total input was recorded to be 5500 mL more than the total volume of output. Inappropriate comments were common on the charts, such as "wet pad", "toilet?" "I forgot to measure", "estimated", "sips" and even ??????? . . .' (p. 38)

This is inappropriate when caring for patients who have the potential to deteriorate as there is no mechanism to record urine output or fluid balance accurately.

Management of oliguria

The purpose of monitoring urine output and fluid balance via fluid charts is to ensure that patients have a urine output of at least 0.5 mL/kg/hour (Smith, 2003). Appropriate action must be taken if a patient shows signs of oliguria, anuria or absolute anuria. In the first instance, the patency of the urinary catheter should be checked following the local hospital protocol or that described in *The Royal Marsden Manual* (Dougherty & Lister, 2004). For patients who do not have urinary catheters in situ and who are showing signs and symptoms of becoming acutely unwell, it is important to gain their consent and insert a urinary catheter because monitoring of fluid balance is essential. It is also important to examine the abdomen to assess whether a distended bladder can be palpated or not.

If after the patency of the urinary catheter has been checked and there is no obstruction to the urine flow and still there is little or no urine production, the nurse must refer the patient to the doctor. Patients should not be allowed to have a low hourly urine output (0.5 mL/kg/hour) for more than two hours consecutively, without it being referred for further investigation and treatment. It is also necessary to undertake a urinalysis to determine the specific gravity as this will give a good indication as to whether the patient is dehydrated or not.

Reducing urine volumes is one of the most common reasons for a doctor to be called to review a patient (Anderson, 2003). The first thing that should be considered is whether the patient is adequately perfused. If the oliguria is due to a reduction in either cardiac output or renal blood flow or a fall in mean arterial pressure (less than 70 mmHg) then it can potentially be corrected as long as the treatment is given immediately. The treatment is the rapid infusion of intravenous fluids as described earlier.

Diuretics should not be administered to patients just to promote urine flow, even if prescribed, as these will make the dehydrated patient more dehydrated. The only exception to this would be if there were definite signs of fluid overload, for example, dyspnoea, evidence of pulmonary oedema, neck vein distension or increased respiratory rate. It may not always be appropriate to rely upon the fluid balance chart when assessing whether the patient is overloaded because, as mentioned previously, these are not always accurate.

If the administration of fluids does not maintain a systolic blood pressure above 100 mmHg, then further advice must be sought from a more senior member of the medical team or the outreach critical care team as the patient may require administration of inotropic drugs (these increase myocardial contractility). The administration of additional intravenous fluids should be considered before commencing inotropes.

Box 13.8   Common causes of a decreased conscious level.

- Cerebral infarction
- Cerebral neoplasm
- Drugs (e.g. opiates)
- Head injury
- Hypoxaemia
- Hypotension
- Hypercapnia
- Hypoglycaemia
- Hyponatraemia
- Hypothermia
- Hyperthermia
- Hypothyroidism
- Hepatic encephalopathy
- Intracranial haemorrhage
- Intracranial infection
- Seizures

(Smith, 2003)

Management of a patient with reduced consciousness

A reduction in the level of consciousness is common in critical illness and may be caused by a variety of conditions (see Box 13.8). When managing a patient with decreased levels of consciousness it is imperative that the airway is maintained, as this may be obstructed by the tongue. The airway may also be at risk from inhalation of secretions or vomit. Therefore, when assessing patients with altered consciousness, airway manoeuvres and adjuncts may be used to establish a patent airway. Smith (2003) recommends the use of the AVPU scale (Box 13.3) as this provides an initial rapid assessment that is easy to use and can be easily remembered. AVPU is used in conjunction with the ABCDE assessment process and the pupils should also be examined for size, equality and reaction to light. The Glasgow Coma Scale (GCS) (Teasdale & Jennet, 1974) (Box 13.9) can also be used to assess the patient's eye opening, motor and verbal response. It is recommended that patients with a GCS of 8 or below should be intubated, as the airway may be compromised. This should be done using the rapid sequence intubation technique involving full anaesthetic and neuromuscular blockade drugs (Price *et al.*, 2003). (Rapid sequence intubation is discussed in Chapter 2.)

Box 13.9   Glasgow Coma Score

Eye opening	Spontaneous	4
	To speech	3
	To pain	2
	No response	1
Best motor response	Obeys commands	6
	Localises to pain	5
	Withdraws to pain	4
	Abnormal flexion to pain	3
	Extensor response to pain	2
	No response	1
Best verbal response	Orientated	5
	Confused conversation	4
	Uses inappropriate words	3
	Incomprehensible sounds	2
	No response	1

If GCS is 8 or below OR falls by 2 points – seek expert help.
   When using the GCS, it is beneficial to quantify the patient's response to stimulation in descriptive terms rather than a numerical number. Try to describe conscious levels by breaking down the GCS to each stimulus, e.g. E-2, M-3, V-3 rather than GCS = 8, as this gives more precise information to which response is compromised.

(Reprinted from *The Lancet, 2*, Teasdale G & Jennett B, Assessment of coma and impaired consciousness: a practical scale, 81–84, ©1974 with permission from Elsevier)

Box 13.10   Management of altered consciousness.

- Assess using ABCDE approach
- Ensure airway is patient (use airway manoeuvres and adjuncts if necessary)
- High flow oxygen
- AVPU, GCS and pupil response
- Refer to critical care outreach and seek expert help
- Give IV fluids to maintain systolic BP above 100 mmHg
- Reverse any possible drug-induced CNS depression (e.g. naloxone for opiate overdose)
- Maintain blood glucose above 3 mmol/L and administer IV glucose if necessary
- Place patient horizontally in the recovery position

(Adapted from Smith, 2003)

Pupil assessment is vital as changes in size, equality and reactivity to light may give an indication of raised intracranial pressure (Price *et al.*, 2003). They should be regularly observed and documented. Patients who have pupils that are dilated and unreactive on one side need immediate medical intervention. The blood glucose needs to be measured in all patients with decreased levels of consciousness and if this is below 3 mmol/L, intravenous glucose solution should be administered (Smith, 2003). Although hypoxaemia, hypotension and hypercapnia are all causes of altered consciousness, they will also exacerbate secondary brain damage and should be corrected (Smith, 2003) (see Box 13.10).

Cardiorespiratory arrest

There is a high mortality following cardiorespiratory arrest and it is important to identify those at risk and try to prevent cardiac arrest from occurring. The evidence suggests that 80% of hospital cardiac arrests are not sudden events and that patients show signs of deterioration in vital signs before the cardiac arrest occurs (Resuscitation Council, 2001). Health professionals must recognise patients at risk of cardiac arrest and instigate preventive care. Generally, the causes of cardiopulmonary arrest can be classified under three headings: airway obstruction, breathing inadequacy and cardiac abnormalities (see Table 13.10).

The UK Resuscitation Council produces evidence-based guidelines that all healthcare professionals should follow when performing cardiopulmonary resuscitation (CPR). To ensure that these CPR guidelines are based upon latest research, the guidelines are updated at appropriate intervals and the reader should review the current guidelines from the UK Resuscitation Council via their website.

The foundations of resuscitation practice are based upon the ABC approach: airway, breathing and circulation:

- *Airway* – It is essential that an airway is patent in the unconscious patient; this can be achieved by positioning (e.g. head tilt chin lift manoeuvre, jaw thrust or airway adjuncts such as oropharyngeal, nasopharyngeal, laryngeal mask airways and endotracheal intubation). Nurses can insert oropharyngeal airways (Figure 13.4) and some hospitals train nurses in advanced airway management such as laryngeal mask insertion.

Table 13.10   Potential causes of cardiac arrest.

Airway obstruction	Breathing inadequacy	Cardiac abnormalities
• Central nervous system depression • Foreign body, e.g. vomit • Trauma • Inflammation • Laryngospasm • Bronchospasm • Airway occlusion	• Decreased respiratory drive, e.g. opiates/drugs • Hypoxaemia • Neurological lesions (e.g. brain tumours) • Respiratory muscle weakness (Guillain–Barré syndrome) • Restrictive chest defect (e.g. chest burns) • Pulmonary embolism • Pneumothorax • Severe asthma • Severe COPD • Lung pathology • Hypothermia	• Myocardial infarction • Ischaemia • Drugs • Electrolyte imbalance • Hypertensive heart disease • Valve disease • Cardiac tamponade • Asphyxia • Hypovolaemia • Clinical shock

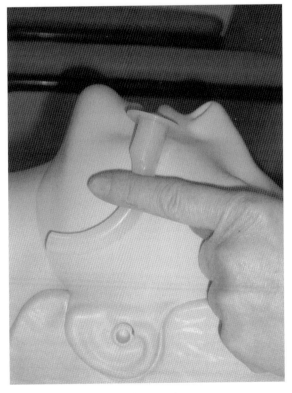

Figure 13.4   Sizing an oropharyngeal airway. Estimate the size by measuring the vertical distance of airway between the patient's incisors to the angle of the jaw. Insert the airway into the oral cavity initially in the 'upside down' position as far as the junction between the hard and soft palate and then rotate it through 180 degrees and then insert airway fully into the oropharynx. (Resuscitation Council, 2001).

- *Breathing* – It is important to 'look, listen and feel' for breathing for a maximum of 10 seconds. If breathing is absent or ineffective, ventilation with high flow oxygen will need to be commenced via either a pocket mask or bag-valve mask using the two-person technique (see Figure 13.5). When using this equipment the practitioner should ensure that the patient's chest is rising and falling on ventilation.

- *Circulation* – If there are no clear signs of circulation upon checking the carotid pulse for a maximum of 10 seconds, chest compressions should be commenced. The correct location for chest compressions must be found: using the fingers the nearest lower rib edge is identified; the fingers are then slid up to the bottom of the sternum. With the middle finger on this point, the index finger is placed on the sternum. Then the heel of the hand is put above the index finger and the hands are interlocked keeping the arms straight, and the sternum is pressed down 4–5 cm (Resuscitation Council, 2001), (see Figure 13.6).

Equipment and drugs used in cardiac arrest

The UK Resuscitation Council (2001) states that there are four key interventions that contribute to a successful outcome following cardiac arrest. This is called the 'chain of survival' and comprises four key interventions:

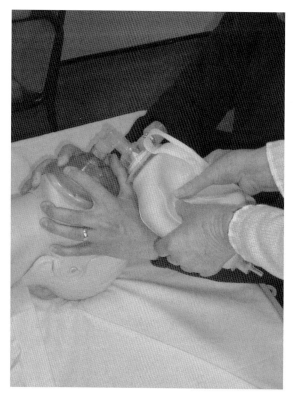

Figure 13.5   Bag valve mask ventilation using the two-person technique.

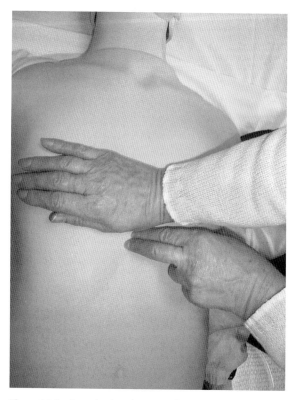

Figure 13.6   Locating hand position for chest compressions.

- Early access to the emergency services or cardiac arrest team
- Early basic life support (BLS) to buy time
- Early defibrillation to restart the heart
- Early advanced life support (ALS) to stabilise

The cardiac arrest team should be summoned immediately when a patient is found in peri-arrest or cardiac arrest. Staff must also ensure that the cardiac arrest trolley and defibrillator are brought to the bedside. The cardiac arrest team consists of a minimum of two doctors; however, the composition of the team will vary between hospitals and may also consist of specialist nurses and operating department practitioners (ODPs) who have undertaken advanced training in resuscitation (see Table 13.11).

The management of the cardiac arrest depends upon which cardiac arrest rhythm the patient is in. This is why the patient is immediately attached to a defibrillator, which will show the cardiac rhythm (Table 13.12). See the Resuscitation Council UK website for cardiac arrest treatment algorithms.

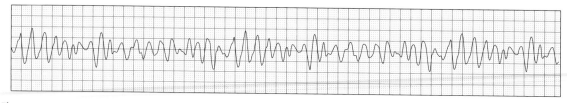

Figure 13.7   Coarse ventricular fibrillation (VF).

Table 13.11   Role and composition of cardiac arrest team.

Resuscitation team leader	The team leader is normally a senior doctor who is at minimum an Advanced Life Support Provider. The team leader is responsible for directing and co-ordinating the resuscitation attempt and ensures safety during the resuscitation. They are also responsible for ending the attempt, documentation and communicating with relatives.
Medical practitioner	To undertake IV cannulation and drug administration (however some nurses are trained to undertake this procedure).
Medical practitioner	Defibrillation (some nurses are trained to undertake this procedure).
Anaesthetist	Undertakes advanced airway interventions including endotracheal intubation.
Anaesthetist assistant	This may be either a specialist ITU, anaesthetic nurse or an ODP who assists the anaesthetist in airway and ventilatory management.
Hospital nurse practitioner	The hospital nurse practitioner would be trained at advanced resuscitation and would support the medical and ward staff. They may also be required to obtain specialist equipment from other parts of the hospital.
Resuscitation officer	Specialist practitioners who are responsible for teaching and ensuring best practice in resuscitation. They have extensive critical care experience and have advanced training in resuscitation. They will provide advice and support at the resuscitation and will also audit the CPR attempt.
Ward nurses	They will provide valuable assistance to the cardiac arrest team by initiating hospital life support with possible defibrillation. They will brief the team leader on the patient's condition as the resuscitation team may have not been previously involved in the patient's care. Ward staff assist the team with chest compressions, assisting with medical procedures, acting as runners for additional equipment and taking samples to the laboratory for urgent analysis.

Table 13.12   Cardiac arrest rhythms.

Figure 13.7 Coarse ventricular fibrillation (VF)	VF is where the ventricles are in a flutter and subsequently fibrillating. This produces a bizarre and chaotic ECG that reflects disorganised electrical activity in the myocardium. All patients in true VF will have no pulse. The priority for VF is immediate defibrillation as the chances of successful defibrillation drop by 7–10% every minute that treatment is delayed (Jevon, 2002). Left untreated, coarse VF will go into fine VF and then to asystole. VF is present in approximately 30% of in-hospital cardiac arrests and is presenting rhythm in 90% of patients who have acute MI and then suffer a cardiac arrest (Jevon, 2002).
Fig.13.8 Ventricular tachycardia (VT) Can be either pulseless or non-pulseless.	This is where the QRS complex is broad (> 0.12 seconds) and tachycardic. VT causes profound loss of cardiac output particularly at higher rates. Patients in VT can either present with a pulse or be pulseless. Pulseless VT cardiac arrest is treated the same as VF and requires immediate defibrillation. Patients who are in VT but have a pulse are generally critically ill and require either prompt cardioversion or anti-arrhythmic medication.
Figure 13.9 Asystole	Ventricular standstill is present due to the suppression of the heart's natural pacemakers. No palpable pulse will be present. Occurs in 25% of in-hospital cardiac arrest and is associated with a poor outcome (Gwinnutt et al., 2000). Asystole is unresponsive to defibrillation, and treatment focuses upon effective CPR, adrenaline and drug administration and trying to reverse the potential cause of the cardiac arrest.
Figure 13.10 Pulseless electrical activity (PEA) Formerly known as electromechanical dissociation or EMD.	PEA is where the heart is still producing electrical activity seen on an ECG but is not producing a pulse. The ECG may look like sinus rhythm but no pulse is present. There are many causes of PEA, related to electrolyte imbalance, pulmonary embolism, cardiac tamponade, tension pneumothorax and hypovolaemia. PEA is the presenting rhythm in around 35% of in-hospital cardiac arrests (Gwinnutt et al., 2000). Like asystole it, too, is associated with a poor outcome. Treatment focuses upon effective CPR, adrenaline and drug administration and trying to reverse the potential causes of the cardiac arrest.

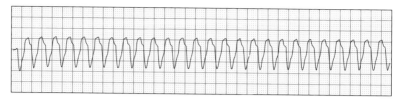

Figure 13.8   Ventricular tachycardia (VT).

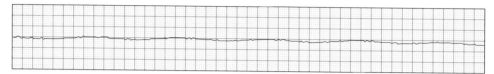

Figure 13.9   Asystole.

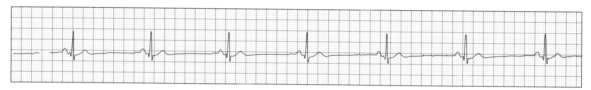

Figure 13.10   Pulseless electrical activity (PEA).

Defibrillation

It is recommended within hospitals that healthcare staff should be attempting defibrillation within three minutes of collapse; this is being facilitated by the increased availability of automated external defibrillators (AED). Staff should only use defibrillators if they have been trained to do so according to their local policy. Manual defibrillators require more expertise than AEDs; however, they are still regularly used within hospitals and specially trained nurses with knowledge of rhythm recognition can undertake this skill. Defibrillation is defined as the termination of ventricular fibrillation (VF) or ventricular tachycardia (VT) at five seconds after shock delivery (Resuscitation Council, 2001). An electrical current is passed across the myocardium to depolarise the cardiac muscle, to allow the heart's pacemaker to resume control of the cardiac cycle (Jevon, 2002). When using either a manual or AED defibrillator, safety is paramount.

There should be no direct or indirect contact with the patient, for example touching drip stands that are connected to the bed, otherwise electrocution may occur.

Drugs used in cardiac arrest

Drugs may be considered after defibrillation (if indicated) and when chest compressions and ventilation have been started. However, there is limited scientific evidence supporting their use (Resuscitation Council, 2001). The three drugs that are generally indicated for the immediate management of cardiac arrest are adrenaline (epinephrine), atropine and amiodarone (see Box 13.11). Emergency drugs are usually prepared in pre-filled syringes that save time in drawing up. There are different manufacturers for pre-filled syringes and staff must be familiar with the type used in their hospital.

Box 13.11   Drugs used in cardiac arrest.

Adrenaline (epinephrine) – Adrenaline causes an increase in peripheral vasoconstriction, which results in an increase in cerebral and coronary perfusion. This makes chest compressions more effective at perfusing blood to the essential organs.

Atropine – Atropine blocks the effect of the vagus nerve on both the sinoatrial (SA) and atrioventricular (AV) nodes, this increases sinus automaticity and improves AV node conduction. This drug is mainly effective in severe bradycardia, as it will increase the patient's heart rate.

Amiodarone – Amiodarone increases the duration of the action potential in atrial and ventricular myocardium. This drug helps to suppress cardiac arrhythmias such as ventricular tachycardia, atrial fibrillation, etc.

As with any drug it is essential that the healthcare professional is aware of the dosage and side-effects. It is recommended that the nurse looks these drugs up in the *British National Formulary* (BNF) and refers to the current ALS Resuscitation Council guidelines on emergency drug administration.

Self-test questions

1. Identify the six main physiological signs and symptoms that a deteriorating patient will show.
2. When assessing acutely unwell patients the ABCDE method of assessment should be used. What does ABCDE stand for?
3. Circle the correct statement relating to hypovolaemic shock:
   a. Hypovolaemic shock is rarely found in surgical patients
   b. Hypovolaemia is only caused by trauma and subsequent blood loss
   c. Hypovolaemia occurs when circulating fluid volume is reduced which causes reduced cardiac output and results in a low perfusion state
   d. Hypotension occurs early in hypovolaemic shock
4. Circle the correct statement relating to cardiogenic shock:
   a. Cardiogenic shock results in a drug allergy which causes heart failure
   b. Cardiogenic shock has a good survival rate with only a 20% mortality rate
   c. Patients with cardiogenic shock often show signs of tachycardia, and hypertension
   d. Cardiogenic shock may occur following myocardial infarction, cardiomyopathy, trauma, cardiac tamponade and valve disease
5. Circle the correct statement relating to septic shock:
   a. Patients with septic shock always have an elevated temperature above 38.3°C
   b. Septic shock involves organisms invading the body and an immune response where chemical mediators are released causing initial vasodilation and a hyperdynamic state
   c. Vasodilators are prescribed to counteract the vasoconstriction
   d. Only post-operative patients can develop septic shock
6. Circle the correct response to the following statement:
   a. High flow oxygen therapy should never be given to a patient who has signs of hypoxia but has chronic obstructive pulmonary disease (COPD). **True** or **false?**
7. Complete the following statement:
   The management of hypotension and oliguria should be to give a __ mL fluid challenge and then monitor its response. If the patient has a history of underlying cardiac problems then __ mL of intravenous fluid is given instead, and then the response is assessed.
8. AVPU is used to assess conscious levels. What does AVPU stand for?
9. List four reasons why patients may become hypoxic.
10. Circle the correct statement relating to cardiac arrest management:
    a. Ventricular fibrillation and ventricular tachycardia cardiac arrests are treated with defibrillation
    b. Ventricular fibrillation has a poor outcome
    c. Asystole is always defibrillated
    d. Ventricular tachycardia is treated with atropine 3 mg

References and further reading

Adam SK & Osborne S (2005) *Critical Care Nursing* (2nd edn). Gosport: Oxford University Press

Anderson ID (ed.) (2003) *Care of the Critically Ill Surgical Patient* (2nd edn). London: Arnold

Audit Commission (1999) *Critical to Success: The place of efficient and effective critical care services within the acute hospital.* London: Audit Commission

Bateman NT & Leach RM (1998) 'ABC of Oxygen: Acute Oxygen Therapy' *British Medical Journal* 317(7161): 798–801

Bickley LS (2004) *Bates' Pocket Guide to Physical Examination and History Taking* (4th edn). Philadelphia: Williams and Wilkins

British Thoracic Society (2002) 'Non-invasive ventilation in acute respiratory failure' *Thorax* 57(3): 192–211

Carroll H (2000) 'Fluid and electrolytes' *in*: Sheppard M & Wright M (eds) (2000) *Principles and Practice of High Dependency Nursing.* London: Baillière Tindall

Chellel A, Fraser J, Fender V, Higgs D, Buras-Rees S, Hook L, Mummery L, Cook C, Parsons C & Thomas C (2002) 'Nursing observations on ward patients at risk of critical illness' *Nursing Times* 98 (46): 36–38

Collins T (2000) 'Understanding Shock' *Nursing Standard* 14(49): 35–41

Cook R (1996) 'Urinalysis: ensuring accurate urine testing' *Nursing Standard* 10(46): 220–225

Department of Health (2000) *Comprehensive Critical Care: A Review of Adult Critical Care Services.* London: Department of Health

Department of Health (2001) *The Nursing Contribution to the Provision of Comprehensive Critical Care for Adults.* London: Department of Health

Department of Health (2003) *Critical Care Outreach: Progress in Developing Services.* London: Department of Health

Dougherty L & Lister S (eds) (2004) *The Royal Marsden Hospital Manual of Clinical Nursing Procedures* (6th edn). Oxford: Blackwell

Fieselmann J, Hendryx MS, Helms CM & Wakefield DS (1993) 'Respiratory rate predicts cardiopulmonary arrest for internal medicine patients' *Journal of Internal Medicine* 8(7): 354–360

Franklin C & Mathew J (1994) 'Developing strategies to prevent in hospital cardiac arrest: analysing responses of physicians and nurses in the hours before the event' *Critical Care Medicine* 22(2): 244–247

Goldhill DR (1997) 'Introducing the post-operative care team: Additional support, expertise and equipment for general post-operative patient' *British Medical Journal* 314(7078): 389

Goldhill D, White S & Sumner A (1999) 'Physiological values and procedures in the 24 hours before ICU admission from the ward' *Anaesthesia* 54: 529–534

Goldhill D (2000) 'Medical Emergency Teams' *Care of the Critically Ill* 16(6): 209–212

Gwinnutt C, Columb M & Harris R (2000) 'Outcome after cardiac arrest in adults in UK hospitals: effect of the 1997 guidelines' *Resuscitation* 47: 125–135

Hand H (2001) 'Shock' *Nursing Standard* 15(48): 45–55

Jevon P & Ewens B (2002) *Monitoring the Critically Ill Patient.* Oxford: Blackwell

Kishen R (2002) 'Managing acute renal failure in the critically ill: Where are we today?' *Care of the Critically Ill* 18(6): 170–172

Lumb A (2000) *Nunn's Applied Respiratory Physiology* (5th edn). Oxford: Butterworth-Heinmann

MacKenzie E (2004) 'Respiratory Therapy' *in*: Dougherty L, Lister S (eds) (2004) *The Royal Marsden Hospital Manual of Clinical Nursing Procedures* (6th edn). Oxford: Blackwell

Marieb EN (2001) *Human Anatomy and Physiology* (5th edn). New York: Benjamin Cummings

McArthur-Rouse FJ (2001). 'Critical care outreach services and early warning scoring systems: a review of the literature' *Journal of Advanced Nursing* 36(5): 696–704

McQuillan P, Pilkington S, Allan A, Taylor B, Short A, Morgan G, Nielson M, Barrett D & Smith G (1998) 'Confidential inquiry into quality of care before admission to intensive care' *British Medical Journal* 316: 1853–1858

Moore T & Woodrow P (2004) *High dependency nursing care, observation, intervention and support.* London: Routledge

Moore T 'Respiratory Assessment' *in*: Moore T & Woodrow P (eds) (2004) *High dependency nursing care, observation, intervention and support.* London: Routledge

Morgan RJM, Williams F & Wright MM (1997) 'An early warning scoring system for detecting developing critical illness' *Clinical Intensive Care* 8: 100

National Confidential Enquiry into Perioperative Outcome and Death (NCEPOD) (2005) *An Acute Problem 2005* (online). www.ncepod.org.uk/2005.htm (Accessed 11.01.07)

Price A, Collins T & Gallagher A (2003) 'Nursing the acute head injury, a review of the evidence' *Nursing in Critical Care* 8(3): 126–133

Reid J, Robb E, Stone D, Bowden P, Baker R, Irving S & Waller M (2004) 'Improving the monitoring and assessment of fluid balance' *Nursing Times* 100(20): 36–39

Resuscitation Council UK (2001) *Advanced Life Support Course provider manual* (4th edn). Rochester: Resuscitation Council

Resuscitation Council UK (2004) *Cardiopulmonary Resuscitation Standards for Clinical Practice and Training.* Rochester: Resuscitation Council

Resuscitation Council UK (2005) (online). www.resus.org.uk (Accessed 11.01.07)

Rich K (1999) 'In hospital cardiac arrest: pre-event variables and nursing response' *Clinical Nurse Specialist* 13(3): 147–153

Sharma S (2005) *Respiratory Failure*. EMedicine (online). www.emedicine.com/med/topic2011.htm (Accessed 11.01.07)

Sheppard M & Wright M (eds) (2000) *Principles and Practice of High Dependency Nursing*. London: Baillière Tindall

Smeltzer S & Bare B (2000) *Brunner & Suddarth's Textbook of Medical-Surgical Nursing* (9th edn). Philadelphia: Lippincott

Smith G (2003) ALERT™ *A Multiprofessional Course in Care of the Acutely Ill Patient*. University of Portsmouth Learning Media Development

Stenhouse C, Coates S, Tivey M, Allsop P & Parker T (2000) 'Prospective evaluation of a modified early warning score to aid earlier detection of patients developing critical illness on a surgical ward' *British Journal of Anaesthesia* 84(5): 663

Subbe CP, Kruger M, Rutherford P & Gemmel L (2001) 'Validation of a modified Early Warning Score in medical admissions' *Quarterly Journal of Medicine* 94(10): 521–526

Surviving Sepsis Campaign (2005) (online). www.survivingsepsis.com (Accessed 11.01.07)

Teasdale G & Jennett B (1974) 'Assessment of coma and impaired consciousness: a practical scale' *Lancet* 2: 81–84

Woodrow P (2000) *Intensive Care Nursing: a framework for practice*. London: Routledge

Self-test Answers

Chapter 1

1. Match each statement with the correct ASA grade:
   a. ASA = 4
   b. ASA = 1
   c. ASA = 5
   d. ASA = 2
2. **True** or **False**?
   a. False – some medications need to be discontinued, such as anticoagulants.
   b. True – this may be due to the nature of the surgery and any pre-existing disease and factors such as prolonged fasting pre-operatively and restriction of oral intake post-operatively.
   c. True – informed consent should be obtained unless the patient lacks the capacity to give it.
   d. False – there is evidence both for and against the removal of body hair from the surgical site.
3. Which of the following tests should be carried out on all surgical patients (answer **Yes** or **No**)?
   a. Blood pressure – Yes
   b. ECG – No, not necessary for asymptomatic males under 40 or females over 50 but useful if they have a cardiac history
   c. Liver blood tests – No, but use discretion dependent on patient
   d. Waterlow risk assessment – Yes

4. (c) is correct. Cardiac complications are 2–5 times more likely in patients following an emergency procedure.
5. (b) is correct. The minimum recommended fasting period before surgery is 6 hours for solid food/milk and 2 hours for clear fluid.
6. (b) is correct. The Waterlow Risk Assessment Scale is used to assess the patient's pressure sore risk.
7. Three types of autologous blood transfusion are: pre-operative donation, isovolaemic haemodilution, cell salvage.
8. Nutritional *screening* involves taking a dietary and clinical history from the patient in order to identify those at risk. Nutritional *assessment* includes more intense measurements such as anthropometric indices and biochemical indicators.
9. The aim of pre-operative skin cleansing is to reduce the bacterial skin flora, which are a common cause of wound infection and to remove dirt and microbes from the skin.
10. See Box 1.8, which lists the checks undertaken and recorded before the patient is transferred to the operating department.

Chapter 2

1. (b) is correct. The ventilation system changes the air within the operating theatre at a rate

of 20–30 changes per hour. (Air changes occur in ancillary areas at reduced rates.)

2. (b) is correct. A humid atmosphere can lead to sterile packs becoming damp and therefore contaminated.

3. (a) is correct. Narcosis (sleep), analgesia (pain relief), relaxation (muscle relaxation).

4. (c) is correct. NSAIDs work by blocking the enzyme cyclo-oxygenase (COX), which is involved in the production of prostaglandins.

5. (d) is correct. The cuff on an endotracheal tube produces an airtight seal in the trachea, preventing entry of any gastric contents.

6. (c) is correct. The brachial plexus nerve supplies the shoulders and upper limbs and runs through the axilla. This can become damaged through hyperextension of the arm by over-abduction on an arm board.

7. (c) is correct. Peri-operative hypothermia is classified as a core temperature of less than 36°C. Three categories of hypothermia have been defined; mild (32–35°C), moderate (30–32°C), and severe (below 30°C).

8. (c) is correct. Anaesthesia inhibits the autonomic nervous system and depresses the ability of the hypothalamus to regulate body temperature. Natural responses to cold, such as vasoconstriction and shivering, are also inhibited by anaesthetic agents.

9. (d) is correct. Although the scrub practitioner and surgeon often accompany the patient and contribute to the handover of care, it is the responsibility of the anaesthetist to hand over care of the patient to a qualified recovery practitioner.

10. (d) is correct. Upper airway obstruction is a common post-operative complication largely due to a loss of muscle tone resulting in the tongue falling back and obstructing the pharynx. This can often be resolved simply by lifting the patient's chin into a 'sniffing the morning air' position.

Chapter 3

1. See Table 3.2, which lists the advantages and disadvantages of oxygen therapy for the post-operative patient.

2. A narrowing pulse pressure is often indicative of falling cardiac output and/or hypovolaemia.

3. See Box 3.3, which lists the signs or symptoms of DVT.

4. The proportion of body water and electrolytes are monitored by **osmoreceptor** cells present in the **hypothalamus** and **kidneys**.

5. Three causes of reduced urine output in the post-operative patient may include increased ADH release in response to stress, bleeding, excessive pre-operative fasting, inadequate fluid replacement, impaired renal function.

6. See Box 3.2, which lists the advantages and disadvantages of surgical drains.

7. Growth hormone is needed by adults for tissue growth and repair and is released during sleep.

8. See Table 3.7, which lists the factors that increase the risk of suffering from PONV.

9. The management of pyrexia is controversial because the high temperature has a beneficial protective effect in infective states and lowering it may deprive the patient of an important host defence mechanism (Edwards, 1998). However, detrimental effects of high temperature include an increased basal metabolic rate, increased heart and respiratory rates, vasodilation. If these symptoms are present, the use of antipyretics may help to relieve them and make the patient more comfortable.

10. Prerequisites for wound healing include a diet containing protein, oxygen, a good blood supply and a clean, warm and moist environment.

Chapter 4

1. Three classifications of pain are: acute, chronic non-malignant and chronic malignant.

2. **Somatic** pain is experienced in superficial structures, muscle and fascia, and is usually described as dull or achy, well-localised and consonant with the underlying lesions; for example, post-operative pain. **Visceral** pain arises in hollow organs and is usually poorly localised, deep, squeezing and cramp-like.

3. (a) is correct. Prostaglandins, histamine, bradykinin, substance P and 5-hydroxytryptamine are released following tissue damage.

4. (b) is correct. A-beta fibres carry sensations of warmth and touch.
5. (c) is correct. A-delta fibres transmit fast pain.
6. (c) is correct. The A-delta fibres and the C-fibres synapse in the substantia gelatinosa of the dorsal horn.
7. (d) is correct. The Gate Control Theory provides an important explanation of aspects of the nature of pain, and reflects physiological, cognitive and emotional facets of the pain experience.
8. The four stages of nociception in the processes of perception and response to pain are (b): transduction, transmission, modulation and perception.
9. See Box 4.7, which lists the adverse effects of non-steroidal anti-inflammatory drugs.

Chapter 5

1. (d) is correct. The link between pre-operative stress and post-operative recovery is uncertain.
2. 'Worry' is thought to be an active process by which the patient thinks about the forthcoming surgery in such a way that the threat associated with it is reduced (Salmon, 2000).
3. (b) is correct. Giving detailed information pre-operatively is thought to benefit 'vigilant copers'.
4. (c) is correct. Information that describes how the patient will feel pre- and post-operatively is referred to as sensory.
5. (d) is correct. Altered body image can cause a range of reactions in individual patients.
6. See Box 5.8, which lists a number of reasons why sexuality is not addressed. However, you may have additional reasons.
7. See Table 5.3, which identifies a number of reasons why it is important to address sexuality issues with surgical patients.
8. See Box 5.10, which lists a number of challenges associated with caring for dying patients in an acute surgical ward. However, you may be able to add some more of your own.
9. Tissues that can be donated following death include: corneas, skin, bone, heart valves, tendon.

10. (d) is correct. Contraindications for tissue donation include recent tattoos, dementia and Alzheimer's disease.

Chapter 6

1. (a), (c) and (d) are true. Tracheostomy is undertaken to decrease, not increase, the dead space.
2. (b), (c) and (d) are true. Silver tubes are not used in the early post-operative stages.
3. All are hazards.
4. (a), (b) and (c) are true. Opinions differ about the need to use aseptic technique, although cleaning of the stoma site as appropriate is important.
5. (b), (c) and (d) are correct.
6. All are true.
7. All are serious complications.
8. (c) and (d) are caused by thyroid over-activity. (a) occurs as a result of thyroid under-activity, and (b) because of haemorrhage from the vascular wound site.
9. All are true.
10. (a) and (d) are true.

Chapter 7

1. A build-up of fatty deposits in the vessels that leads to occlusion of the arteries. The occlusion leads to poor blood flow and ischaemia to affected areas.
2. Diabetics build up fat deposits more quickly due to elevated blood sugars and older people are more at risk because of their prolonged exposure to risk factors.
3. When considering vascular problems the following should be assessed: vital signs, peripheral signs, undiagnosed/poorly controlled diabetes, abdominal signs, neurological signs, type and position of pain.
4. **Fusiform** is a weakness surrounding the vessel, **saccular** is a weakness bulging in one area and **dissecting** is where the vessel has split.
5. An **arterioplasty** is where the wall of the vessel is stretched to allow blood flow and an **endarterectomy** is where plaques are removed to improve blood flow.

6. In **carotid** arterial stenosis the patient would have transient ischaemic attacks and possibly a history of CVA; in **femoral** artery stenosis the patient would have a history of limb pain usually worsening when exercising.

7. The major complications you should be observing for following vascular surgery are: bleeding, loss of blood flow to limb(s), hypertension and hypotension, signs of neurological deterioration, wound infection.

8. You would advise a patient who wanted to reduce their risk for peripheral vascular disease to stop smoking, eat a low-fat diet, take regular exercise, take prescribed medications (e.g. anti-hypertensive medication and anti-coagulants).

9. A diabetic patient can reduce the complications of peripheral vascular disease if they take care of their feet, wear well-fitting shoes, don't ignore injuries, avoid walking barefoot; control diabetes and take medication.

10. Psychological issues that may need considering with vascular surgery include: body image, lack of motivation, depression, immobility, feelings of isolation, long-term pain.

Chapter 8

1. Oesophageal varices: obstruction of the blood flow through the portal venous system results in portal hypertension. This causes collateral veins to open between the portal and systemic veins and if the high pressure is maintained for a long period of time the collateral veins dilate leading to varices. Treatment options include intravariceal sclerotherapy, banding via endoscopy and the use of a compression balloon.

2. Three factors that may lead to development of oesophageal carcinoma are: ulceration from gastric reflux, smoking and alcohol (irritants).

3. Two investigations that patients with dysphagia should have are chest X-ray and barium swallow.

4. Investigations undertaken to fully stage an oesophageal carcinoma include: barium swallow, endoscopy, CT scan, bronchoscopy, endoscopic ultrasound and staging laparoscopy.

5. A thoracotomy is a surgical opening of the chest cavity.

6. Risk factors for carcinoma of the stomach include: predisposing conditions – chronic peptic ulceration, pernicious anaemia; environmental factors – *Helicobacter pylori* infection; genetic factors – blood group A.

7. Common routes of spread of gastric carcinoma include: portal venous to the liver, lymphatic to local nodes, transcoelomic to the pelvis.

8. Important factors in T-tube management are: record drainage accurately, empty the drainage bag regularly, check the entry site for evidence of bile leakage.

9. Physiological consequences of pancreatic auto-digestion include oedema, haemorrhage, necrosis, abscess or cyst formation.

10. Key areas of management of patients with acute pancreatitis include: pain control, suppression of pancreatic function, correction of shock, monitoring of blood glucose levels, infection management.

Chapter 9

1. Parts of the large bowel in order: ileo-caecal junction, caecum, ascending colon, hepatic flexure, transverse colon, splenic flexure, descending colon, sigmoid colon, rectum and anus.

2. Causes of gastrointestinal obstruction include: **mechanical** – adhesions, hernia, volvulus, tumour, diverticulitis, impaction, intussusception, stenosis; **non-mechanical** – paralytic ileus, electrolyte imbalance, rib, spine or pelvic trauma, drugs.

3. Inflammation of the diverticulum – small pouches or pockets in the lining of the intestine. The inflammation causes bacteria to collect in the pouches resulting in varying degrees of infection, inflammation, fever and formation of abscesses, which could eventually obstruct the lumen.

4. Risk factors for colorectal cancer include high-fat, low-fibre diet, genetic predisposition (hereditary non-polyposis colorectal cancer, familial adenomatous polyposis), smoking, inflammatory bowel disease, lack of exercise.

5. Signs and symptoms of barium contrast leak include abdominal pain, nausea and vomiting, pyrexia, signs of shock.

6. Patients receiving bowel preparation lose a large amount of fluid and therefore fluid balance needs to be maintained either through encouraging oral fluids or intravenous therapy.

7. When siting a stoma, it is important to avoid old scars, bony prominences, the umbilicus, groin creases, pubic areas, the waistline, fatty bulges or creases, underneath large breasts, areas affected by skin disorders, the site of the proposed surgical incision, a site that cannot be seen by the patient. Also consider the patient's eyesight, manual dexterity, mental state and cultural needs.

8. Patients suffering from perforated diverticulum are likely to undergo a Hartmann's procedure.

9. Principles of post-operative stoma management include: using only transparent appliances to allow for visualisation, observe stoma colour, size, output and for signs of oedema or necrosis; leaving the initial appliance in situ for at least 48 hours, emptying the bag regularly, and accurately recording output.

10. Signs of a post-operative anastomotic leak include bowel contents in the wound drain, high fever, generalised peritonitis and sepsis, elevated white blood cell count, prolonged ileus.

Chapter 10

1. Structures within the urinary system and male reproductive organs: kidneys, ureters, bladder, urethra, prostate gland, penis and testes.

2. Four aspects of urodynamic procedures: pressure, flow, electrical activity, radiographic imaging.

3. KUB = Kidneys-Ureters-Bladder. IVU = Intravenous Urography.

4. The three main focuses of renal calculi management are pain relief, confirmation of diagnosis and recognition of complications.

5. Three aspects of nephrostomy tube care are keeping the tube dry, cleaning the skin around the insertion site and changing the dressing frequently.

6. The irritative and obstructive symptoms of benign prostatic hypertrophy are: **Irritative** – urgency, frequency, nocturia, haematuria (carcinoma), UTI; **Obstructive** – slow flow, incomplete emptying, hesitancy, postmicturition dribble, dysuria.

7. Glycine is used for bladder irrigation during urological surgery because it is an isotonic and non-electrolyte solution that prevents translocation of diathermy electrical current to other parts of the body.

8. Signs and symptoms of transurethral syndrome include: **Cardiovascular effects** – chest pain, hyper- and hypotension, bradycardia, ECG changes; **CNS effects** – generalised seizures, restlessness, confusion, nausea, headache, visual disturbances.

9. Potential complications of prostate and bladder surgery include: anxiety, pain, perforation of bladder wall, UTI, urethral stricture, urinary retention, urinary incontinence, impotence, retrograde ejaculation.

10. Hormonal control of the prostate gland and its relation to benign prostatic hyperplasia: testosterone is primarily produced by the testes and converted in the prostate by the enzyme 5-alpha-reductase to dihydrotestosterone (DHT). DHT is the most active androgen in the prostate and is necessary for normal prostate growth. One form of therapy to reduce the size of the prostate in benign prostatic hyperplasia is the use of anti-androgens that reduce the level of testosterone and therefore DHT. This ultimately reduces the growth of the prostate.

Chapter 11

1. (b) is correct. Because the fibroid is oestrogen-dependent, growth ceases after the menopause and the fibroid atrophies.

2. (c) and (d) are both correct. (a) and (b) both involve hysterectomy, which renders the woman infertile.

3. (d) is correct. Procidentia is the term used to describe third-degree uterine descent in which the uterus comes to lie outside of the vulva.

4. (c) is correct. Genuine stress incontinence is differentiated from detrusor instability by

the fact that leakage of urine occurs without contraction of the detrusor muscle.

5. (a) and (b) are both correct. Cystometry is a urodynamic investigation that helps to differentiate between genuine stress incontinence and detrusor instability.

6. (c) is correct. Salpingitis is inflammation of the fallopian tubes that causes damage to the ciliated epithelium. It is usually attributed to sexually transmitted disease such as *Chlamydia trachomatis.*

7. (a) is correct. The area of metaplastic cells is called the transformation zone. In post-menopausal women, the size of the cervix is reduced and the squamo-columnar junction and part of the transformation zone come to lie in the endocervix.

8. (a) is correct. Cervical cancer is associated with previous infection with the human papillomavirus.

9. (b) is correct. Dermoid cysts or teratomas arise from the germ cells of the ovary. This type of cyst contains a variety of tissues derived from the primary germ layers.

10. (c) is correct. History of multiple sexual partners is associated with cancer of the cervix, not endometrial cancer.

Chapter 12

1. **Osteoarthritis** is a disease of articular cartilage, specific to joint, may affect one joint only, joint inflammation secondary to local irritation rather than part of the primary disease process; **rheumatoid arthritis** is a systemic autoimmune disorder, inflammatory disorder of connective tissue, synovial membrane primary focus, usually presents symmetrically i.e. both hands.

2. Systemic effects of rheumatoid arthritis include: pain, early morning stiffness, fatigue and lethargy, anaemia, weight loss, nodules, vasculitis, Sjögren's syndrome, dry eyes, mouth and other mucous membranes, neurological problems – e.g. carpal tunnel syndrome – cervical spine subluxation, lymphadenopathy, GI tract problems – e.g. amyloidosis, cardiac problems – e.g. pericarditis, lung involvement – e.g. pulmonary inflammation.

3. Infection present at the time of the surgery increases the risk of developing infection around the new joint after insertion.

4. Neurovascular observations include observing limb colour, warmth, checking for normal limb sensation and movement, and feeling for radial or pedal pulses.

5. **True.** Wound drainage systems are generally not secured in orthopaedic surgery.

6. Specific features of the symptoms to identify when admitting a patient with back pain include: Does the pain radiate down the leg, if so how far? Is there any numbness or pins and needles and what part of the leg is affected? The patient's ability to pass urine both pre- and post-operatively should be noted. This information is important so that any deterioration in the patient's condition can be detected.

7. Signs and symptoms of compartment syndrome include: pain on passive stretching of muscle group, paraesthesia (abnormal sensations, pins and needles etc), paralysis, compartment feels swollen and tense on palpation, the area of skin over the compartment may have altered colouration.

8. Other potentially serious complications that may follow a fracture of the shaft of a long bone include: fat embolism, osteomyelitis, damage to surrounding nerves and blood vessels, pulmonary embolism, deep vein thrombosis, hypovolaemic shock.

9. While casts are drying, the limb should be rested on pillows to avoid causing dents that put pressure on the underlying skin. To aid drying, the pillows should be covered with absorbent materials that are changed regularly. When handling a drying cast the palms of the hand should be used, rather than the finger tips to avoid making dents in the cast. No external heat should be used to aid drying. The limb should be elevated to reduce swelling and aid venous return. Assessment of the circulation to the limb should be undertaken regularly.

10. Aspirin 150 mg for 35 days for all patients, intermittent pneumatic compression and early mobilisation was suggested as best practice in reducing the risk of developing venous thromboembolism in this patient group, with heparin being reserved for those who were at high risk of venous thromboembolism.

Chapter 13

1. Six main physiological signs and symptoms that a deteriorating patient will show:
   i   Tachycardia due to the heart trying to compensate for reduced venous return and maintain cardiac output and circulation.
   ii Hyperventilation in an attempt to increase oxygen supply as the body is becoming hypoxic. Also, the body is attempting to correct systemic acidosis or carbon dioxide retention by increasing the respiratory rate.
   iii Hypotension due to reduced cardiac output. Hypotension is often a late sign in hypovolaemia occurring when over 30% of the circulatory fluid volume is depleted. Hypotension causes underperfusion of the vital organs such as the brain and the kidneys, eventually causing organ failure.
   iv Urine output is reduced below 0.5 mL/kg/hour. This is due to vasoconstriction of blood vessels supplying the kidneys to divert circulatory fluid volume to the core of the body, i.e. the brain and the heart. Also, if the patient is hypotensive, the nephrons will not have a driving pressure to allow filtration to occur. A poor end organ perfusion pressure will reduce urine output.
   v   Reduced level of consciousness or confusion occurs due to reduction in oxygen delivery to the brain causing cerebral depression reflected in a reduced Glasgow Coma Score. The priority is to increase oxygen perfusion to the brain.
   vi Raised temperature is not always evident in critically ill patients; however, an elevated temperature may mean that an inflammatory response is occurring in the body which is most likely to be caused by an infection. However, patients can still be critically ill and display the above signs and symptoms but have a normal temperature.

2. ABCDE stands for: Airway, Breathing, Circulation, Disability, Exposure.

3. (c) is correct. Hypovolaemia occurs when circulating fluid volume is reduced which causes reduced cardiac output and results in a low perfusion state.

4. (d) is correct. Cardiogenic shock may occur following myocardial infarction, cardiomyopathy, trauma, cardiac tamponade and valve disease.

5. (b) is correct. Septic shock involves organisms invading the body and an immune response where chemical mediators are released causing initial vasodilation and a hyperdynamic state.

6. False – Oxygen should always be given for hypoxic patients. Patients who have COPD should initially be commenced on 35% oxygen, which is increased as required to achieve oxygen saturations of 90%.

7. The management of hypotension and oliguria should be to give a **500** mL fluid challenge and then monitor the response. If the patient has a history of underlying cardiac problems, **250** mL of intravenous fluid is given instead and the response is assessed.

8. AVPU stands for Alert, Responds to Voice, Responds to Pain, Unresponsive.

9. Reasons why patients may become hypoxic include: airway problems, acute respiratory failure, neuromuscular disorders, acute lung injury, trauma, altered levels of consciousness, post-operatively.

10. (a) is correct. Ventricular fibrillation and ventricular tachycardia cardiac arrests are treated with defibrillation.

Index